Clinical Consultant

Joanne Kirk, RN, MSN
Retired Nursing Instructor
Whitehouse, Texas

Preface

The *Laboratory Manual for Nursing Health Assessment: A Best Practice Approach* has been designed for use as both a clinical tool and a study guide to accompany *Nursing Health Assessment* by Sharon Jensen. Each chapter has a corresponding textbook chapter and contains an **objectives summary, reading assignment, vocabulary list (key terms and abbreviations), study guide, alternative case study scenarios, sample documentation form/checklist, and physical assessment checklist**. The manual helps you to understand and apply the content explained in the corresponding textbook. It serves as a guide for clinical work in performing skills related to health assessment, as well as better preparing you for tests and examinations.

The following information outlines the purpose of each section of the laboratory manual:

- **Objectives Summary**. This brief paragraph explains the main points of the corresponding textbook chapter. It is useful to review both before and after reading the actual assignment.

- **Reading Assignment**. This paragraph identifies the corresponding textbook chapter from *Nursing Health Assessment*.

- **Vocabulary/Terminology**. This section identifies and defines the key terms from the corresponding textbook chapter. Some chapters also include a list of common abbreviations/acronyms associated with the chapter.

- **Study Guide**. The Study Guide portion of each chapter includes combinations of Fill in the Blank, Labeling, Matching, Sequencing,

Short Answers, and Multiple Choice questions. All these exercises allow students to reinforce knowledge, synthesize concepts, prepare for tests, and ensure their understanding of health assessment and the role of the nurse in caring for patients. An answer key to the Study Guide portion of each chapter is provided at the end of the manual.

- **Alternative Case Study Scenarios**. These scenarios, tied to the case studies in the textbook, focus on critical thinking. They ask students to consider how responses to patients would change with different assessment data, patient background, medical diagnoses, and other key variables.

- **Documentation.** Two key components of every chapter help guide students through their clinical experiences. The *Form for Use in Practice* serves as a quick checklist by which students can ensure that they are covering all key areas of the health history and physical assessment. The *Guide for Use in Practice* serves as a quick summary of all the techniques of the physical assessment, with normal findings and unexpected findings identified. In this way, students have a handy reference to ensure they are covering all key components of the assessment and also compare results against established benchmarks.

The authors and publisher sincerely hope that this product achieves the goals of assisting with learning and optimizing comprehension and application to facilitate quality health assessments and competent nursing care.

Contents

The Nurse's Role in Health Assessment

OBJECTIVE SUMMARY

Nursing is a rewarding and challenging profession that requires extensive knowledge and skills. Nurses assess health on many levels, including psychosocial, physical, emotional, spiritual, and cultural. They develop and use skills in communication to provide therapeutic responses to the concerns of patients. Wellness and health are concepts that influence the health beliefs and health behaviors of patients. Nurses explore factors related to such beliefs and behaviors to understand better how to promote health for patients and their families. They use the nursing process to care for patients by assessing completely, making nursing diagnoses, developing outcomes, planning for care, performing interventions, evaluating effectiveness, and revising interventions as needed. The foundation of this collaborative process depends on having accurate and complete assessment data.

READING ASSIGNMENT

Read Chapter 1 in Jensen's *Nursing Health Assessment: A Best-Practice Approach*.

VOCABULARY/TERMINOLOGY

Key Terms

- **Advocate:** Nursing role that encompasses keeping patients safe, communicating their needs, identifying side effects of treatment and finding better options, and helping them to

understand their diseases and treatments so they can optimize self-care.

- **Altruism:** True concern for the welfare of others.

- **Assessment:** Gathering information about the health status of the patient, analyzing and synthesizing those data, making judgments about nursing interventions based on the findings, and evaluating patient care outcomes.

- **Autonomy:** The right of patients to make decisions about their own health care.

- **Body systems assessment:** Assessment method in which a nurse examines the patient focused on a single system or clusters data related to that system together to identify issues.

- **Collaborative problems:** Problems that nurses monitor but require the expertise of other health care providers for intervention.

- **Comprehensive assessment:** An assessment that includes a complete health history and physical assessment; it is done annually on an outpatient basis, following admission to a hospital or long-term care facility, or every 8 hours for patients in intensive care.

- **Critical thinking:** Thinking that requires specific knowledge, skills, and experience and is purposeful and outcome-directed (results-oriented); driven by patient, family, and community needs; based on the nursing process, evidence-based thinking, and the scientific method; guided by professional standards and codes of ethics; and constantly re-evaluating, self-correcting, and striving to improve.

- **Cultural competence:** The complex combination of knowledge, attitudes, and skills that a health care provider uses to deliver care that considers the total context of the patient's situation across cultural boundaries.

- **Diagnosis:** Clustering of data that makes a judgment or statement about the patient's problem or condition.

- **Diagnostic reasoning:** Gathering and clustering data to draw inferences and propose diagnoses.

- **Emergency assessment:** An assessment that involves a life-threatening or unstable situation and that focuses on A—Airway (with cervical spine protection if injury suspected); B—Breathing (rate and depth, use of accessory muscles); C—Circulation (pulse rate and rhythm, skin color); and D—Disability (level of consciousness, pupils, movement).

- **Evaluation:** Judgment of the effectiveness of nursing care in meeting the patient's goals and outcomes based upon the patient's responses to the interventions.

- **Evidence-based nursing:** Approach to patient care that minimizes intuition and personal experience and instead relies upon research findings and high-grade scientific support.

- **Focused assessment:** An assessment based on the patient's issues that can occur in all health care settings; it usually involves one or two body systems and is smaller in scope than the comprehensive assessment but more in depth on the specific issue(s).

- **Functional assessment:** An assessment that focuses on the functional patterns all humans share: health perception and health management, activity and exercise, nutrition and metabolism, elimination, sleep and rest, cognition and perception, self-perception and self-concept, roles and relationships, coping and stress tolerance, sexuality and reproduction, and values and beliefs.

- **Head-to-toe assessment:** An assessment that organizes the collection of comprehensive physical data by proceeding through the entire body from head to toe.

- **Health-belief model:** Model focused on the relationship between beliefs and actions, with the host (patient), agent (disease), and environment interacting.

- **Health-promotion model:** Model that views individuals as multidimensional and in interaction with interpersonal and physical environments as they pursue health, combining individual characteristics and experiences with behavior-specific cognitions and affect, as well as with behavioral outcomes.

- **Human dignity:** Respect for patients, such as by ensuring privacy and confidentiality.

- **Illness:** State in which patients experience objective signs and subjective symptoms of sickness, with subsequent disability.

- **Integrity:** Providing honest information to patients, documenting care accurately, and reporting errors.

- **Intervention:** Any treatment, based upon clinical judgment and knowledge, that a nurse performs to enhance patient outcomes.

- **Nursing diagnosis:** Clinical judgment about individual, family, or community responses to actual or potential health problems/life processes.

- **Objective data:** Measurable findings from the health assessment, usually gathered in the physical examination.

- **Outcomes:** More specific than goals, these are the realistic and measurable desired consequences of nursing interventions.

- **Planning:** Determining resources, targeting nursing interventions, and writing the plan of care.

- **Priority setting:** An important professional nursing skill by which nurses organize activities and issues by focusing on the most important and immediate concerns first. Priorities depend upon the acuity of the situation.

- **Social justice:** Working to ensure for patients equal treatment and access to quality health care.

- **Subjective data:** Findings from the health assessment that are based on patient experiences and perceptions. They are usually revealed during the interview and health history taking.

- **Wellness:** Process by which people maintain balance and direction in the most favorable environment.

Common Abbreviations

Review the following abbreviations that you may encounter in the clinical setting. Think about how you may incorporate these abbreviations into your documentation as you progress through the course.

A-P: anterior-posterior

BP: blood pressure

CC: chief complaint

c/o: complains of

DOE: dyspnea on exertion

DTR: deep tendon reflexes

GI: gastrointestinal tract

HEENT: head, eyes, ears, nose, throat

HOH: hard of hearing

ICS: intercostal space

LLQ: left lower quadrant

LMP: last menstrual period

LUQ: left upper quadrant

NSR: normal sinus rhythm

P: pulse

PERRLA: pupils equal, round, reactive to light and accommodation

PMH: past medical history

PMI: point of maximal impulse (apical heart)

PND: paroxysmal nocturnal dyspnea

PPD: packs per day

R: respiration and right

R/O: rule out

ROM: range of motion

RLQ: right lower quadrant

RUQ: right upper quadrant

S&S: signs and symptoms

S, M, W, D: single, married, widowed, divorced

SOB: shortness of breath

T: temperature

TPR: temperature, pulse, respiration

VS: vital signs

WNL: within normal limits

STUDY GUIDE

Answer the following questions, which assist you in identifying the most important information from Chapter 1 of Jensen's *Nursing Health Assessment*.

Activity A FILL IN THE BLANK

1. Identify the roles of nursing
   A. Being members of a profession

   _____

   B. Providing care based on current evidence

   _____

   C. Managing patient care

   _____

   D. Typically performing more advanced assessments, such as examining the eyes with an ophthalmoscope or performing a gynecologic assessment

   _____

2. List the purposes of a health assessment.
   A. _____
   B. _____
   C. _____
   D. _____

Activity B MATCHING

1. *Match the type of prevention with its definition*

Answer	Type of Prevention	Definition
	1. Primary prevention	A. Focuses on preventing complications of an existing disease and promoting health to the highest level.
	2. Secondary prevention	B. Involves strategies aimed at preventing problems. Immunizations, health teaching, safety precautions, and nutrition counseling are examples.
	3. Tertiary prevention	C. Includes the early diagnosis of health problems and prompt treatment to prevent complications.

2. *Match advocacy roles with definition of role*

Answer	Advocacy Role	Definition
	1. Showing respect for patients	**A.** Social justice
	2. Providing honest information to patients, documenting care accurately, and reporting errors	**B.** Human dignity
		C. Autonomy
		D. Integrity
		E. Altruism
	3. Being truly concerned for the welfare of others	
	4. Understanding that patients have the right to make decisions about their health care	
	5. Working to ensure equal treatment and access to quality health care	

3. *Match nursing action with definition of action*

Answer	Nursing Action	Definition
	1. Collecting data	**A.** Outcomes
	2. Clustering data to make a judgment or statement about the patient's problem or condition	**B.** Goals
		C. Intervention
		D. Diagnosis
		E. Assessment
	3. Establish these as realistic and measurable	
	4. Establish these as measurable, realistic, and patient-centered	
	5. Any treatment, based upon clinical judgment and knowledge	

Activity C **SHORT ANSWER**

1. List and discuss the four broad goals within nursing.

_____

_____

_____

_____

2. Nurses work in hospice, rehabilitation centers, and homes to help patients and their families cope with disability and, when unavoidable, to facilitate the most comfortable death for patients. What are these nurses providing?

_____

_____

_____

_____

3. Explain evaluation of care.

_____

_____

_____

_____

4. List the components of critical thinking.

_____

_____

_____

_____

5. Explain cultural competence.

_____

_____

_____

_____

6. Explain what a comprehensive assessment includes for a child.

_____

_____

_____

_____

7. High-level wellness is a process by which people maintain balance and direction in the most favorable environment. What is the role of the nurse in facilitating this process?

_____

_____

_____

_____

Activity D MULTIPLE CHOICE

1. The nurse is conducting a physical assessment of a new patient. What data does the nurse collect that are measurable?
   A. Subjective
   B. Objective
   C. Primary
   D. Secondary

2. A student nurse is learning to document an initial assessment. What would the instructor tell the student that accurate documentation best provides?
   A. Data on the patient
   B. Information on which to base the care plan
   C. A baseline
   D. Information on which to base outcomes

3. An assessment that concentrates on patterns that all humans share is called what?
   A. Head-to-toe
   B. Body systems
   C. Focused
   D. Functional

4. The preceptor of the student nurse is explaining the assessment that is considered the most organized for gathering comprehensive physical data. What assessment is the preceptor talking about?
   A. Functional
   B. Focused
   C. Head-to-toe
   D. Body system

5. A patient has just been diagnosed with diabetes. What would be the most appropriate nursing diagnosis for this patient?
   A. Knowledge deficit
   B. Patient coping
   C. Nutrition: Inadequate
   D. Fear

6. Student nurses are learning about evidence-based thinking. What would they learn is a step in this process?
   A. Searching the literature for research
   B. Evaluating research evidence using their own criteria
   C. Identifying the issue or problem based on an inaccurate analysis of current nursing knowledge and practice
   D. Justifying the selection of interventions

7. A patient is brought to the emergency department by ambulance after a motor vehicle accident. What would be given the highest priority by the staff triaging the patient?
   A. Breathing
   B. Airway
   C. Circulation
   D. Disability

ALTERNATIVE CASE STUDY SCENARIOS

In Chapter 1 of *Nursing Health Assessment*, you learned about Maria Ortiz, a 52-year-old Mexican American, who has a follow-up appointment related to type 2 diabetes mellitus, which was diagnosed 2 weeks ago during an annual physical assessment. Her primary language is Spanish; while her English skills are good, she has difficulty understanding complex medical terminology. Ms. Ortiz has been married for 30 years, and her three grown children live nearby.

Ms. Ortiz is 160 cm tall, weighs 75 kg (body mass index [BMI] 29), and eats a diet high in fats and starches. Her blood glucose levels at home have been elevated. She has a history of obesity and peripheral vascular disorder. Current vital signs are temperature 36.5°C tympanic, pulse 82 beats/min, respirations 16 breaths/min, and blood pressure 138/78. Medications include an oral hypoglycemic, plavix, and a daily vitamin.

Alternative A

Mrs. Ortiz tells the clinic nurse that she is going to have a holiday dinner at her sister's house and the whole family will be there. She conveys concern about being able to follow her diet plan while eating with the whole family.

- What could the nurse do to help this patient?

- How might Mrs. Ortiz plan for family dinners in her diet plan?

Alternative B

Mrs. Ortiz tells the nurse that she is very confused about what it means to have type 2 diabetes.

- What would be the most beneficial interventions the nurse could do for Mrs. Ortiz?

- What modifications of information might be helpful for Mrs. Ortiz?

CHAPTER 2

The Interview and Therapeutic Dialogue

OBJECTIVE SUMMARY

This chapter assists you to identify the importance of the nurse–patient relationship, which is built on verbal and nonverbal communication within a specific defined setting. After completion, you should understand how you will establish the nurse–patient relationship in the clinical setting and approach patient interviews.

READING ASSIGNMENT

Read Chapter 2 in Jensen's *Nursing Health Assessment: A Best-Practice Approach*.

VOCABULARY/TERMINOLOGY

- **Active listening:** The ability to focus on patients and their perspectives.
- **Clarification:** A therapeutic communication technique that nurses use when a patient's word choice or ideas are unclear to better understand the meaning. For example, the nurse states, "Tell me what you mean by...." Clarification prompts patients to identify other facts or give more information so that the nurse better understands.
- **Closed-ended (direct) questions:** Questions that yield "yes" or "no" responses and are focused on obtaining facts. An example would be, "Do you have a family history of heart disease?"
- **Communication etiquette:** The code of conduct and good manners by which those engaged in communication show respect for others.
- **Empathy:** The ability to perceive, reason, and communicate understanding of another person's feelings without criticism. It is being able to see and feel the situation from the patient's perspective, not the nurse's.
- **Encouraging elaboration:** A technique that assists patients to more completely describe problems. These responses encourage patients to say more and continue the conversation. They show patients that the nurse is interested. The nurse may nod the head or say "Um hum," "Yes," or "Go on" to cue patients to keep talking. Another technique is to let patients know that their thoughts and feelings are common and give them permission to discuss them.
- **Focusing:** A therapeutic communication technique used when patients are straying from a topic and need redirection. An example is, "We were talking about the reaction that you had to the penicillin. Tell me more about that reaction."
- **Intercultural communication:** The sender of an intended message belongs to one culture, while the receiver is from another. Cultural differences may exist related to group or ethnicity, region, age, degree of acculturation into Western society, or a combination of these factors.
- **Open-ended questions:** Questions that require patients to give more than "yes" or "no" answers. They are broad and provide responses in the patient's own words.

- **Reflection:** Similar to restatement; however, instead of simply restating comments, the nurse summarizes the main themes of communication. The conversation may be longer, in which a patient discusses several elements related to a topic. The nurse listens carefully to the different thoughts expressed and attempts to identify their relationship. With this technique, patients gain a better understanding of the issues that underlie their thoughts, which helps to identify their feelings.

- **Restatement:** A therapeutic communication technique by which the nurse makes a simple statement, usually using the words of the patient, to prompt the patient to elaborate. Restatement provides an opportunity for patients to further understand their communication.

- **Sexual boundary violation:** The clearest example of unprofessional involvement. Sexual contact is never acceptable within the therapeutic nurse–patient relationship.

- **Silence:** Purposefully not speaking during an interview to allow patients time to gather their thoughts and provide accurate answers or to communicate nonverbal concern. Silence also gives patients a chance to decide how much information to disvclose.

- **Summarizing:** Used at the end of the interview, during the closure phase, when the nurse reviews and condenses important information into two or three of the most important findings. Doing so helps ensure that the nurse has identified important information and lets the patient know that he or she has been heard accurately.

- **Therapeutic communication:** A basic tool that the nurse uses in the caring relationship with patients. In therapeutic communication, the interaction focuses on the patient and the patient's concerns. The nurse assists patients to work through feelings and explore options related to the situation, outcomes, and treatments.

STUDY GUIDE

Answer the following questions, which assist you in identifying the most important information from Chapter 2 of Jensen's *Nursing Health Assessment*.

Activity A   FILL IN THE BLANK

1. Identify the following techniques of **therapeutic** communication.

A. A technique used to get the patient to elaborate

_____

B. A technique that assists patients to more completely describe problems

_____

C. The ability to focus on patients and their perspectives

_____

2. Identify the following types of **nontherapeutic** communication.

A. "I know this is frightening for you, but it really will be alright. You'll see."

_____

B. "I see the doctor has recommended an L5–S1 discectomy for you."

_____

C. "I know just how you feel. I care for many patients who have just been diagnosed with cancer."

_____

D. "I have some papers for you to sign. (cell phone rings) Just a minute, I need to take this call from my daughter."

_____

Activity B   MATCHING

1. *Match type of communication with the statement.*

Answer	Type of Communication	Statement
	1. Restatement	A. "So, you feel like there is a knot in your chest."
	2. Encouraging elaboration	B. "We were talking about how you felt when you were diagnosed with multiple sclerosis. Tell me more about those feelings specifically."
	3. Focusing	C. "Sometimes when patients are involved in an accident, they have flashbacks or bad dreams. Has that been happening?"

2. *Match nontherapeutic responses with their examples. Nontherapeutic responses are in alphabetical order.*

Answer	Example	Nontherapeutic Response
	1. "Don't worry. It will be all right."	**A.** Biased questions
	2. Come from several sources: equipment, other patients, colleagues, pagers, and cell phones.	**B.** Changing the subject
		C. Sympathy
	3. The nurse documents "trouble swallowing" but asks patients about "dysphagia."	**D.** False reassurance
		E. Technical language
	4. Feeling what a patient feels from the viewpoint of the nurse.	**F.** Distractions
		G. Unwanted advice
	5. Usually from the nurse's perspective, not the patient's.	
	6. When the patient says, "I'm feeling a bit nauseous," the nurse may reply, "What did you have to drink?"	
	7. "You don't use drugs, do you?"	

3. *Match nonverbal communication skills with the examples.*

Answer	Nonverbal Communication Skill	Example
	1. Physical appearance	**A.** Relaxed, professional, and eye level
	2. Posture and positioning	**B.** Professional dress, grooming, and hygiene
	3. Facial expression	**C.** "Is it okay if I examine your abdomen?"
	4. Voice	**D.** Calm, with appropriate inflections
	5. Touch	**E.** Relaxed, caring, and interested

Activity C SHORT ANSWER

1. How would you use nonverbal communication skills when interviewing a patient? Provide rationale.

_____

_____

_____

_____

2. What health beliefs, factors, and experiences do you have that might help in understanding intercultural nursing?

_____

_____

_____

_____

3. List and explain types of nontherapeutic responses used in the clinical setting.

_____

_____

_____

_____

_____

4. Explain nonprofessional involvement.

_____

_____

_____

_____

_____

5. Discuss briefly the four phases of the interview process.

_____

_____

_____

_____

6. Explain intercultural nursing. Briefly explain how you can be more culturally aware.

_____

_____

_____

_____

7. Define communication etiquette.

_____

_____

_____

_____

Activity D **MULTIPLE CHOICE**

1. While assessing a patient, the nurse is asking questions that help the patient express how she is feeling. What is this called?

   A. Sympathy

   B. Therapeutic communication

   C. Empathy

   D. Caring

2. During the patient interview, the nurse summarizes the main themes of the conversation. What is this called?

   A. Empathy

   B. Caring

   C. Reflection

   D. Restatement

3. The nurse is conducting a patient interview and responds to the patient in a way that encourages him to more completely describe his problems. What is this called?

   A. Encouraging elaboration

   B. Restatement

   C. Focusing

   D. Clarification

4. A student is following a home health nurse for a day. The nurse is using gestures when communicating with a specific patient. Purposeful gestures are used

   A. because the nurse thinks that the patient does not understand what is being said

   B. to illustrate points

   C. all of the above

   D. neither of the above

5. One technique of therapeutic communication is silence. What does silence allow the patient to do?

   A. Learn to trust the nurse

   B. Change topics if he or she wants

   C. Communicate nonverbal concern

   D. Decide how much information to disclose

6. When gathering information to assess the patient's health status and to provide therapeutic communication as indicated, what is the nurse doing?

   A. Encouraging elaboration

   B. Interviewing

   C. Summarizing

   D. Identifying themes

7. A nurse is interviewing a new patient on the unit. The nurse is interpreting what the patient is saying from the nurse's point of view. This nontherapeutic response to the patient is called what?

   A. Sympathy

   B. Empathy

   C. Restatement

   D. Summarizing

8. While interviewing a patient, the nurse asks, "What happens when you have low blood glucose?" This type of response to the patient is used for what purpose?

   A. To summarize the conversation

   B. To restate what the patient has said

   C. To encourage elaboration

   D. To clarify

ALTERNATIVE CASE STUDY SCENARIOS

In Chapter 2 of _Nursing Health Assessment_, you learned about Mr. Rowan, a 36-year-old Caucasian man who resides in an assisted-living facility and was diagnosed with AIDS 2 years ago. Consider how things might be different if he had been more adherent to his antiretroviral medication regimen. Review the following alternative situations. Based on the changes outlined below, _consider what interview techniques would be useful with this patient._

Alternative A

Mr. Rowan comes to the nurse's station for his medicine. He mentions that he has developed a cough and is not feeling very well.

- What questions might the nurse ask to elicit more information from Mr. Rowan?

- How could the nurse phrase a statement that would show empathy for this patient?

Alternative B

Mr. Rowan has returned from the clinic after a routine checkup. He is very angry because his viral load has increased dramatically since his last checkup. He says to the nurse, "I don't see any point in taking all these medicines. They aren't helping. I am going to die anyway."

- What are potential health-promotion and teaching needs for Mr. Rowan based on this information?

- How will the nurse engage Mr. Rowan in therapeutic communication?

- Identify two potential nontherapeutic responses to Mr. Rowan's statements that the nurse should avoid.

The Health History

OBJECTIVE SUMMARY

The purpose of this chapter is to help build a foundation for collecting health history data from patients. *Subjective data* are based on the signs and symptoms that the patient reports; they may not be perceived by observers. Additionally, the nurse collects an individual and family history to obtain data about past and current medical problems, surgeries, and risks for disease. Discussion also includes information on health behaviors and activities that promote health. In many settings, patients complete comprehensive forms that the nurse reviews and then asks questions about to add detail during the interview.

READING ASSIGNMENT

Read Chapter 3 in Jensen's *Nursing Health Assessment: A Best-Practice Approach.*

VOCABULARY/TERMINOLOGY

- **Activities of daily living:** Self-care activities such as eating, dressing, and grooming.
- **Functional health patterns:** Areas assessed by nurses that are based on groupings that focus on one specific segment and how the effects of health or illness influence a patient's quality of life.
- **Primary data:** Information gathered directly from the individual patient.

- **Reliable historian:** A historian who provides information consistent with existing records and comprehensive in scope.
- **Review of systems:** A series of questions about all body systems that helps to reveal concerns or problems as part of a comprehensive health assessment.
- **Secondary data:** Data gathered from the patient's chart and family members.
- **Signs:** Objective information that the nurse assesses during the physical examination.
- **Subjective data:** Data based on the signs and symptoms that the patient reports; they may not be perceived by observers.
- **Symptoms:** Subjective sensations or feelings of patients.

STUDY GUIDE

Answer the following questions, which assist you in identifying the most important information from Chapter 3 of Jensen's *Nursing Health Assessment.*

Activity A FILL IN THE BLANK

1. Identify the components of the health history.

   A. The patient explains his or her symptoms

   _____

   B. Environmental data about exposure to contagious diseases

   _____

C. The subjective sensations or feelings of patients

_____

D. Objective information that the nurse assesses during the physical examination

_____

2. Identify important elements to assess for the presenting symptom using the mnemonic OLDCARTS.

A. _____

B. _____

C. _____

D. _____

E. _____

F. _____

G. _____

H. _____

Activity B **MATCHING**

1. *Match the elements with the correct part of the health history.*

Answer	Element	Part of Health History
	1. Genogram	**A.** Growth and development
	2. Assessment of physical activities, fine and gross motor skills	**B.** Family history
	3. General health state	**C.** Review of systems

2. *Match the area of focus with the appropriate potential findings.*

Answer	Assessment Focus Area	Potential Findings
	1. Nutrition and hydration	**A.** Tremors, memory loss, numbness or tingling, loss of sensation, or coordination
	2. Thorax and lungs	

3. Abdominal-gastrointestinal

4. Abdominal-urinary

5. Endocrine and hematologic system

6. Neurological

7. Peripheral vascular

B. Polydipsia, polyuria, unexplained weight gain or loss, changes in body hair and body fat distribution, intolerance to heat or cold, excessive bruising, lymph node swelling. Result of last blood glucose

C. History of high blood pressure, thrombophlebitis, peripheral edema, ulcers, circulation, claudication, redness, pain, tenderness

D. Nausea, vomiting, normal daily intake, weight and weight change, dry skin, fluid excess with shortness of breath, or edema in the feet and legs

E. Pain, change in urine, dysuria, urgency, frequency, nocturia, incontinence. For children, toilet training, bed wetting

F. Cholelithiasis, liver failure, hepatitis, pancreatitis, colitis, ulcer or gastric reflux, appetite, nausea, vomiting, diarrhea

G. Wheezing, cough, sputum, dyspnea, last chest x-ray, last tuberculin skin test

3. *Match the assessment question with the part of assessment in which it is asked.*

Answer	Assessment Question	Part of Assessment
	1. Describe any changes that you have had in your mood or feelings	**A.** Human violence
	2. Sometimes your mom or dad might get angry with you. What happens when your mom or dad gets mad?	**B.** Sexual history and orientation
	3. What is your religious preference?	**C.** Review of systems
	4. Do you have any family history of prostate cancer?	**D.** Social, cultural, and spiritual assessment
	5. How many sexual partners have you had in the past year?	**E.** Mental health

Activity C SHORT ANSWER

1. Discuss how a nurse would make a genogram and why.

_____

_____

_____

_____

2. Nurses assess activities such as feeding, bathing, toileting, dressing, grooming, mobility, home maintenance, shopping, and cooking. What is the purpose of these assessments?

_____

_____

_____

_____

3. List and explain the areas of a functional health assessment.

_____

_____

_____

_____

4. What does a complete review of systems include?

_____

_____

_____

_____

5. List the elements assessed during the history of the present illness.

_____

_____

_____

6. Explain where a nurse would gather primary and secondary data.

_____

_____

_____

_____

7. Briefly compare and contrast a focused assessment with a comprehensive assessment.

_____

_____

_____

_____

Activity D MULTIPLE CHOICE

1. The nurse is assessing the duration of a patient's pain. What does this assessment include?

A. Whether the pain is constant or intermittent

B. Whether the pain is related to an internal organ

C. Whether the pain is neurologic

D. Whether the pain is bone-related

2. What is the nurse assessing when asking the patient "What things seem to make it better?"

A. Duration

B. Aggravating/alleviating factors

C. Functional goal

D. Pain goal

3. When the nurse questions patients about sitting, rising from a chair, standing for periods, climbing stairs, shopping, driving, and participating in sports, what is he or she assessing?

A. Pain goal

B. Quality

C. Functional goal

D. Duration

4. The nurse is taking a comprehensive health history on a new patient. Why would it be essential for the nurse to obtain a complete description of the present illness?

A. To assess if the patient is a reliable historian

B. To obtain primary data

C. To obtain demographic data

D. To establish an accurate diagnosis

5. The admitting nurse is assessing a new patient. What would be the best type of assessment to perform?

A. Focused assessment

B. Comprehensive assessment

C. Acute assessment

D. Symptomatic assessment

6. A patient comes to the ED complaining of a severe cough and difficulty breathing. This would be considered

A. Subjective secondary data

B. Subjective primary data

C. Objective secondary data

D. Objective primary data

7. The nurse is conducting an environmental assessment on a 51-year-old man who works in a coal mine. What would this environmental assessment include?

A. History of pulmonary thrombosis

B. Family history

C. Type of exposure

D. Summary of work history

8. A father brings his 6-year-old son to the ED. The child says that his forearm hurts and rates the pain as an 8/10. The father tells the nurse that the boy fell from a tree yesterday and would not stop crying over his arm, so the father decided to bring him to the ED. On examination, the nurse notes bruises in various stage of healing over the patient's back and abdomen. The nurse also notes that the boy cringes when his father touches him and will not meet the nurse's eye when asked direct questions. The father refuses to leave the room even when the boy has his arm x-rayed. What should the nurse suspect with this patient?

A. School violence

B. Sexual abuse

C. Neglect

D. Physical abuse

ALTERNATIVE CASE STUDY SCENARIOS

In Chapter 3 of *Nursing Health Assessment*, you learned about Emma Anderson, a 9-year-old African American girl who was diagnosed with asthma when she was 3 years old. Consider how things might be different if Emma lived in an apartment complex that was newer and did not have mold, cockroaches, and dust and if her school was newer and did not have old carpets and a rodent infestation.

Alternative A

Emma comes to the school nurse stating that because of the wind she is having an asthma exacerbation and she thinks her inhaler is empty.

• What part of the health assessment should the nurse reassess to help Emma?

• What information would the nurse try to elicit from Emma in the Human Violence section of the health assessment?

Alternative B

Emma is taken by her mother to her physician for a routine checkup. The physician asks when Emma's last asthma exacerbation was and if her rescue inhalers are working well for her. Emma responds that her last exacerbation was "back in October" and the rescue inhalers work rapidly and well when she has to use them.

• Would the physician consider Emma a reliable historian?

• What kind of data is the physician obtaining from Emma?

4

Techniques of Physical Examination and Equipment

An accurate and complete health history provides information about which physical assessment data health care providers should collect. Nurses combine objective data from the physical assessment with subjective data from the health history to form a more complete assessment database, as well as to develop an impression of the underlying etiology of any health problems. The four techniques of inspection, palpation, percussion, and auscultation form the basis for physical assessment.

READING ASSIGNMENT

Read Chapter 4 in Jensen's *Nursing Health Assessment: A Best-Practice Approach*.

VOCABULARY/TERMINOLOGY

- **Auscultation:** One of the techniques used for conducting a physical assessment by which the nurse listens for movements of air or fluid in the body.
- **Dull:** A tone of a sound during physical assessment that is high in pitch, sounds like a thud, and is heard over the liver.
- **Flat:** A tone of sound during physical assessment that is high in pitch, sounds dull, and is heard over bone.

- **Hand hygiene:** Practices that include the use of alcohol-based hand rubs, handwashing, and use of gloves.
- **Hyperresonant:** A tone of a sound during physical assessment that is very loud, boom-like in quality, of long duration, and heard over emphysematous lungs.
- **Inspection:** A technique used in a physical assessment by which the nurse observes the patient for general appearance and any specific details related to the body system, region, or condition under examination.
- **Ophthalmoscope:** A handheld system of lenses, lights, and mirrors that enables visualization of the interior structures of the eye.
- **Otoscope:** An instrument that directs light into the ear to visualize the ear canal and tympanic membrane.
- **Palpation:** An assessment technique by which the nurse uses the hands to feel the firmness of body parts, such as the abdomen.
- **Percussion:** An assessment technique by which the nurse uses tapping motions with the hands to produce sounds that indicate solid or air-filled spaces over the lungs and other areas.
- **Resonant:** A tone of a sound during physical assessment that is very loud, hollow in quality, of long duration, and heard over healthy lungs.

- **Standard precautions:** A set of guidelines from the Centers for Disease Control and Prevention that exist to help prevent disease transmission during contact with nonintact skin, mucous membranes, body substances, and bloodborne contacts (eg, needlestick injury).

- **Tuning fork:** A piece of equipment used with two body systems: to determine vibration sense in the neuromuscular system and to determine conductive versus sensorineural hearing loss in the ears.

- **Tympanic:** Refers to the membrane that separates the outer ear from the middle ear. It can also describe a loud, high-pitched, drum-like sound of moderate duration heard during the physical assessment.

STUDY GUIDE

Answer the following questions, which assist you in identifying the most important information from Chapter 4 of Jensen's *Nursing Health Assessment*.

Activity A FILL IN THE BLANK

1. Identify the techniques used by the nurse while conducting a physical assessment.

   A. Uses the stethoscope to hear movements of air or fluid over the lungs and abdomen

   _____

   B. Makes tapping motions with the hands to produce sounds that indicate solid or air-filled spaces over the lungs and other areas

   _____

   C. Uses the hands to feel the firmness of body parts, such as the abdomen

   _____

   D. Observes the patient for general appearance and any specific details related to the body system, region, or condition under examination ———————————

2. Identify in the correct order the five sequential steps of patient-to-patient transmission of pathogens.

   A. _____

   B. _____

   C. _____

   D. _____

   E. _____

Activity B MATCHING

1. *Match the tone with the quality of the sound.*

Answer	Tone	Quality
	1. Tympanic	**A.** Dull
	2. Flat	**B.** Hollow
	3. Hyperresonant	**C.** Drumlike
	4. Dull	**D.** Boom-like
	5. Resonant	**E.** Thud

2. *Match the assessment with the type of palpation used.*

Answer	Assessment	Type of Palpation
	1. Spleen	**A.** Deep
	2. Texture	**B.** Moderate
	3. Bladder	**C.** Light

Activity C SHORT ANSWER

1. Describe respiratory hygiene/cough etiquette.

   _____

   _____

   _____

   _____

2. Discuss preventative actions for latex allergy.

   _____

   _____

   _____

   _____

3. Describe what a nurse can do to minimize the adverse effects of repeated hand washing.

   _____

   _____

   _____

   _____

4. Describe how health care providers can transmit pathogens among patients in health care settings?

   _____

   _____

   _____

   _____

5. List and describe the four techniques of physical assessment.

_____

_____

_____

_____

6. Describe the intention of standard precautions.

_____

_____

_____

_____

Activity D **MULTIPLE CHOICE**

1. The nursing instructor is discussing standard precautions with her students. What else should the instructor talk about to prevent the transmission of pathogens?
   A. Use of alcohol-based hand cleaner
   B. Respiratory/cough hygiene
   C. How to recycle personnel protective equipment
   D. How to clean patient equipment

2. The student nurse is caring for a patient with emphysema. What sound would the student nurse expect to hear when percussing the patient's lungs?
   A. Resonant
   B. Tympanic
   C. Hyperresonant
   D. Flat

3. When the nurse observes the patient for overall characteristics including age, gender, and level of alertness, what is the nurse doing?
   A. Palpating
   B. Interviewing
   C. Inspecting
   D. Auscultating

4. A new graduate nurse is having trouble charting the details of a shift assessment on a patient. The preceptor of the new nurse explains to her that accurate descriptions are essential for
   A. information on the patient
   B. a reliable history of the patient
   C. obtaining accurate assessment information
   D. legal documentation

5. The admitting nurse in the ED is assessing a new patient. What would be the best order to perform the techniques of assessment?
   A. Auscultation; inspection; percussion; palpation
   B. Inspection; auscultation; percussion; palpation
   C. Auscultation; inspection, palpation, percussion
   D. Inspection; auscultation; palpation, percussion

6. Light palpation is appropriate to assess the
   A. appendix
   B. bladder
   C. inflamed areas of skin
   D. liver

7. A nurse, new to the hospital, is attending orientation with the nurse educator. The educator is discussing the use of deep palpation when assessing a patient. What assessment would the nurse leave out of her lecture?
   A. Appendix
   B. Enlarged spleen
   C. Inflamed intestine
   D. Enlarged liver

ALTERNATIVE CASE STUDY SCENARIOS

In Chapter 4 of *Nursing Health Assessment*, you learned about Chris Chow, a 6-year-old boy visiting the clinic today with a fever and "stuffy nose." He came in with his mother who took the day off from work to stay home with him. His temperature is 38.6°C tympanic, pulse 110, respirations 20 breaths/min, and blood pressure 108/66 mm Hg. Chris is meeting developmental milestones, though his height and weight are below the 25th percentile on the growth chart as indicated on the documentation from his well-child visit 2 months ago. Chris has a history of cystic fibrosis. He is being seen by an Advanced Practice Registered Nurse Practitioner (APRN) who has recommended that he be admitted to the hospital for IV antibiotics and steroids.

Alternative A

Chris is directly admitted to the pediatric floor with a diagnosis of left lower lobe pneumonia. The nurse admitting him is conducting a focused assessment.

- What assessment technique would be a priority in Chris's physical assessment?

- Why would it be important to teach Chris and his family respiratory/cough etiquette?

Alternative B

Because of Chris' frequent hospitalizations he has developed a latex allergy.

- What precautions would Chris's nurse take because of Chris' latex allergy?

5

Documentation and Interdisciplinary Communication

OBJECTIVE SUMMARY

Prompt reporting and recording of patient assessment data are essential to ensuring safe and efficient delivery of care. Communication occurs both verbally and in writing. Documentation involves entering patient information into the written or computerized patient record. The patient clinical record contains recorded information from all health care encounters.

READING ASSIGNMENT

Read Chapter 5 in Jensen's *Nursing Health Assessment: A Best-Practice Approach*.

VOCABULARY/TERMINOLOGY

Key Terms

- **Audit:** Review of a health care facility by an agency or outside group to determine whether that facility is providing and documenting certain standards of care.

- **Batch charting:** Waiting until end of shift or until all patients have been assessed to document findings from all of them.

- **Charting by exception:** Use of predetermined standards and norms to record only significant assessment data.

- **Confidentiality:** Keeping information private.

- **Flowsheet:** Efficient and standardized form that assembles the collected information in a way that permits easy comparison among assessment data to detect trends or a sudden change in status.

- **Handoff:** Transfer of care for a patient from one health provider to another.

- **Point of care documentation:** Occurs when nurses document assessment information as they gather it, often using a portable computer.

- **Reporting:** Occurs at handoffs, during patient rounds, during patient and family care conferences, and when calling or text-paging a provider to report a change in status or provide requested information.

Common Abbreviations

Review the following abbreviations that you may encounter in the clinical setting. Think about how you may incorporate these abbreviations into your documentation as you progress through the course.

CPOE: Computerized provider order entry

HIPPA: The Health Insurance Portability and Accountability Act

OASIS: Outcome and Assessment Information Set

SBAR: Situation, Background, Assessment, Recommendation

SOAP: Subjective, Objective, Assessment, Plan

STUDY GUIDE

Answer the following questions, which assist you in identifying the most important information from Chapter 5 of Jensen's *Nursing Health Assessment*.

Activity A FILL IN THE BLANK

1. Identify the type of charting.

   A. Uses predetermined standards and norms to record only significant assessment data

   _____

   B. Its goal is to incorporate the plan of care into the progress note

   _____

   C. Focuses on a single problem

   _____

   D. Usually, the organizing structure is time rather than an identified problem

   _____

2. Identify assessments generally found on flowsheets:

   A. _____
   B. _____
   C. _____
   D. _____

Activity B MATCHING

1. *Match the information recorded with the form on which it is recorded.*

Answer	Information Recorded	Form
	1. Individualize patient's goals, outcomes, and interventions	A. Clinical pathway
	2. A multidisciplinary tool that identifies a standard plan for a specific patient population	B. Progress notes
		C. Resident assessment instrument
		D. Plan of care
		E. SBAR

3. Coordinates the efforts of all members of the health care team to optimize the resident's quality of care and quality of life

4. Situation, background, and assessment are all based on the collection of complete and accurate assessment data. The last piece, recommendations, encompasses the nurse's suggestions for the next interventions

5. Multiple health team members document the patient's progress toward recovery

2. *Match the definition with the correct term.*

Answer	Term	Definition
	1. Audit	A. Electronically communicating orders to the laboratory, pharmacy, and nursing personnel
	2. Accrediting agency	B. A review of the records of a health care facility to determine whether that facility is providing and documenting certain standards of care
	3. eMAR	C. Establishes standards and audits patient records to evaluate the quality of care provided
	4. CPOE	D. Electronic medication administration record

Activity C **SHORT ANSWER**

1. The medical record serves multiple purposes. List what they are.

   _____

   _____

   _____

   _____

2. List the advantages of a computerized medical record.

   _____

   _____

   _____

   _____

3. Explain for what a Risk Assessment Report provides risk scores.

   _____

   _____

   _____

   _____

4. Discuss the penalties possible for health care providers who violate HIPPA.

   _____

   _____

   _____

   _____

5. As nurses are learning health assessment techniques they should also focus on what?

   _____

   _____

   _____

   _____

6. During interdisciplinary rounds what nursing issues can the nurse discuss?

   _____

   _____

   _____

   _____

Activity D **MULTIPLE CHOICE**

1. The nurse is caring for a patient with a terminal illness. What would be the purpose of convening a patient care conference?

   A. To agree on when care begins

   B. To coordinate schedules

   C. To determine what assessment data to include in a report

   D. To coordinate care

2. Why are accurate and effective verbal communication and documentation most important?

   A. They keep patients safe.

   B. They are legal documentation.

   C. They ensure safe delivery of information to other health team members.

   D. They educate other nurses.

3. During a Joint Commission visit it is found that some patient care standards are not being met. Where would problem solving occur in this instance?

   A. Unit level

   B. Systems level

   C. Department level

   D. Facility level

4. A nurse is explaining to other nurses on the unit about DRGs. What do insurance companies use to base their payment approval/disapproval on?

   A. Medical diagnosis

   B. Laboratory tests

   C. Diagnosis codes

   D. Documentation

5. A new nurse is not familiar with the electronic charting that her institution uses. What positive attribute of electronic charting could the nurse's preceptor explain to this new nurse?

   A. It maximizes compliance issues.

   B. It disables the graphing of trends in vital signs or assessment data.

   C. It allows several health team members to view the patient record simultaneously.

   D. It automatically corrects both spelling and grammar.

6. What statement about batch charting is most accurate?

   A. It provides clear documentation.

   B. It makes the chart available to multiple users.

   C. It contributes to many potential errors.

   D. It facilitates completion in a timely manner.

7. A nurse, new to the hospital, is attending orientation with the nurse educator who is discussing the documentation of patient care. The institution uses PIE charting. How would the nurse educator best describe PIE charting?

   A. Problem, Interventions, and Evaluation

   B. Position, Interaction, and Evaluation

   C. Position, Intervention, and Exit note

   D. Problem, Interventions, and Exit note

ALTERNATIVE CASE STUDY SCENARIOS

In Chapter 5 of *Nursing Health Assessment*, you learned about Mr. Chavez, 29 years old, who was admitted to the hospital with a fractured humerus following a motor vehicle collision (MVC) in which he was a passenger wearing his seatbelt. His younger cousin, the driver, was declared dead at the scene.

Mr. Chavez was born in Mexico; English is his second language, which he understands and speaks well. His temperature is 37.8°C (100°F) orally, pulse 110, respirations 20 breaths/min, and blood pressure 122/66. Current medications include patient-controlled analgesia (PCA) with morphine for pain, an antibiotic, a multivitamin, a stool softener, and medications to be taken as needed for symptoms such as itching and nausea. Initial assessment was in the emergency department (ED); an admitting assessment occurred 4 hours ago upon transfer to acute care. The nurse there is caring for him at the beginning of shift.

Alternative A

During the shift Mr. Chavez's temperature elevated to 39°C (102°F); pulse 115, respirations 21 breaths/min, and blood pressure 114/58. The nurse telephones the physician.

- When calling the physician the nurse knows that her call needs to be what?

Alternative B

The nurse is giving a verbal shift report for Mr. Chavez to the oncoming nurse.

- What could influence the completeness of this report?

General Survey and Vital Signs Assessment

OBJECTIVE SUMMARY

This chapter explores the assessment techniques required to perform the general survey and take vital signs. The general survey begins during the interview phase of health assessment. While collecting subjective data, nurses observe patients, develop initial impressions, and formulate plans for collecting objective data from the physical examination. An accurate and thorough physical examination requires keen observational skills. During the physical assessment, nurses use the senses of vision, hearing, touch, and smell. Vital signs, encompassing temperature, pulse, respirations, and blood pressure (BP), are important indicators of the patient's physiological status and response to the environment.

READING ASSIGNMENT

Read Chapter 6 in Jensen's *Nursing Health Assessment: A Best-Practice Approach*.

VOCABULARY/TERMINOLOGY

- **Afebrile:** Condition of being without fever.
- **Apnea:** The absence of spontaneous respirations for more than 10 seconds.
- **Asystole:** The absence of a pulse.
- **Auscultatory gap:** A period in which there are no Korotkoff's sounds during auscultation.
- **Blood pressure:** The measurement of the force exerted by the flow of blood against the arterial walls.
- **Bradycardia:** A heart rate less than 60 beats/min.
- **Bradypnea:** Persistent respiratory rate greater than 12 breaths/min.
- **Celsius:** A scale for measuring temperature.
- **Circadian cycle:** A roughly 24-hour cycle in the biochemical, physiological, or behavioral processes of living entities.
- **Cyanosis:** A blue coloration of the skin and mucous membranes that results from more than 5 g/dL deoxygenated hemoglobin in blood vessels near the skin surface.
- **Diastolic blood pressure:** The lowest pressure in blood pressure, which occurs when the left ventricle relaxes between beats.
- **Diurnal cycle:** Refers to patterns within an approximately 24-hour period that typically recur each day.
- **Dyspnea:** Difficulty breathing.
- **Eupnea:** Normal respiratory rate, rhythm, and effort.
- **Expiration:** Breathing out (exhaling). The intercostal muscles and diaphragm relax,

decreasing the space in the pleural cavity and passively pushing air out of the lungs.

- **Fahrenheit:** A temperature scale used mostly in the United States.

- **General survey:** An assessment that begins with the first moment of the encounter with the patient and continues throughout the health history, during the physical examination, and with each subsequent interaction. It is the first component of the assessment, when the nurse makes mental notes of the patient's overall behavior, physical appearance, and mobility.

- **Hyperpnea:** Resting respiration that is deeper and more rapid than normal.

- **Hypertension:** A blood pressure greater than 140/90.

- **Hyperthermia:** Temperature greater than 100°F (37.8°C).

- **Hyperventilation:** Deep, rapid respirations.

- **Hypotension:** Systolic blood pressure less than 90 mm Hg.

- **Hypothermia:** Core temperature less than 95°F (35°C).

- **Hypoventilation:** Shallow, slow respirations.

- **Inspiration:** Breathing in (inhaling). Occurs when the intercostal muscles and diaphragm contract and expand the pleural cavity, creating a negative pressure for air to flow actively into the lungs.

- **Orthostatic hypotension:** When going from a supine or sitting position to a standing position, a drop in systolic blood pressure of 15 mm Hg or greater, drop in diastolic blood pressure of 10 mm Hg or greater, or increased heart rate.

- **Oxygen saturation:** A relative measure of the amount of oxygen dissolved or carried in a given medium.

- **Pulse:** The throbbing sensation that can be palpated over a peripheral artery or auscultated over the apex of the heart.

- **Pulse deficit:** The difference that exists between apical and peripheral pulses.

- **Pulse oximetry:** A noninvasive technique to measure oxygen saturation of arterial blood.

- **Pulse pressure:** The difference between the systolic and diastolic blood pressures; reflects the stroke volume.

- **Respiration:** The act of breathing.

- **Sphygmomanometer:** The instrument used to measure blood pressure.

- **Systolic blood pressure:** Maximum pressure on the walls of the arteries with contraction of the left ventricle at the beginning of systole.

- **Tachycardia:** A heart rate greater than 100 beats/min in an adult.

- **Tachypnea:** A rapid, persistent respiratory rate greater than 20 breaths/min in an adult.

- **Temperature:** A measurement of the body's thermostat.

- **Vital signs:** Important indicators of the patient's physiological status and response to the environment. They encompass temperature, pulse, respirations, and blood pressure.

STUDY GUIDE

Answer the following questions, which assist you in identifying the most important information from Chapter 6 of Jensen's *Nursing Health Assessment*.

Activity A FILL IN THE BLANK

1. Identify the following descriptors of the pulse.
   A. The strength of the pulse

   _____

   B. The smooth, straight, and resilient feel of the normal artery

   _____

   C. The difference between apical and peripheral pulses

   _____

   D. The interval between beats

   _____

2. List the things that increase respiratory rate.
   A. _____

   B. _____

   C. _____

   D. _____

Activity B   MATCHING

1. *Match the normal temperature range with the route used for measurement.*

Answer	Normal Range	Site for Measurement
	1. 35.9°C–38°C	**A.** Rectal and temporal artery
	2. 35.8°C–37.3°C	**B.** Axillary
	3. 36.4°C–38.5°C	**C.** Oral

2. *Match the finding with the appropriate part of the general survey in which the nurse would make the assessment.*

Answer	Finding	Assessment Component
	1. Patient has a flat affect.	**A.** Overall appearance
	2. Patient does not make eye contact.	**B.** Hygiene and dress
	3. Face and body are symmetrical.	**C.** Body structure and development
	4. Patient appears jaundiced.	**D.** Behavior
	5. Dress is appropriate for age.	**E.** Facial expression
	6. Patient responds to questions quickly and easily.	**F.** Level of consciousness
	7. Patient is anxious and confused.	**G.** Skin color
	8. Patient stands erect with no signs of discomfort, and arms relaxed at the sides.	**H.** Speech
	9. No joint abnormalities are noted.	**I.** Mobility

3. *Match the term with its correct definition.*

Answer	Term	Definition
	1. Systolic BP	**A.** Factor that influences variation
	2. Diastolic BP	**B.** Difference between systolic and diastolic BPs; reflects the stroke volume
	3. Mean arterial pressure	**C.** Maximum pressure exerted on the walls of the arteries
	4. Ethnicity	**D.** Lowest pressure
	5. Pulse pressure	**E.** Calculated by adding one third of the systolic BP and two thirds of the diastolic BP

Activity C   SHORT ANSWER

1. List the indicators of an acute situation.

   _____

   _____

   _____

   _____

2. Discuss anthropometric measurements.

   _____

   _____

   _____

   _____

3. List patients for whom oral temperature is inappropriate and give rationale.

   _____

   _____

   _____

   _____

4. Explain how to perform a thigh BP and what a normal finding would be.

   _____

   _____

   _____

   _____

5. Explain how you would teach a patient to weigh himself or herself.

   _____

   _____

   _____

   _____

6. Explain what would be important to teach a patient undergoing surgery.

   _____

   _____

   _____

   _____

7. List the JNC 7 recommendations to help maintain BP.

   _____

   _____

   _____

   _____

Activity D   MULTIPLE CHOICE

1. The nurse is having trouble obtaining the pulse and BP in patient who is in shock. What device would the nurse use to obtain the needed vital signs?
   A. Vital signs monitor
   B. Sphygmomanometer
   C. Doppler
   D. Pulse oximeter

2. A patient arrives in the emergency department in diabetic ketoacidosis. What assessment finding would the nurse expect in this patient?
   A. Sweet-smelling breath
   B. Hypoglycemia
   C. Bradycardia
   D. O_2 saturation of less than 90%

3. The nurse is conducting a general survey of a patient new to the clinic. In what part of the survey would the nurse assess the hair distribution on the patient's body?
   A. When assessing the body structure and development
   B. When assessing the posture
   C. When assessing the range of motion
   D. When assessing the skin

4. What are various measurements of the human body, including height and weight, called?
   A. Datum
   B. Vital measurements
   C. Anthropomorphic
   D. Anthropometric

5. During an initial assessment of a new patient, the nurse notes that the patient's weight is 210 lb and his height is 6'0". What is the patient's body mass index (BMI)?
   A. 28.0
   B. 28.5
   C. 29
   D. 29.5

6. Students are touring the hospital before starting their clinical rotations. The instructor points out that the type of thermometer used in this facility is noninvasive, safe, efficient, and quick. What type of thermometer is the instructor describing?
   A. Tympanic
   B. Temporal artery
   C. Oral
   D. Axillary

7. A nurse is taking a rectal temperature on an unconscious patient. What reading would reflect temperature within the normal range?
   A. 96.8°F to 100.8°F
   B. 97°F to 101°F
   C. 97.7°F to 101.5°F
   D. 98°F to 101°F

8. A nurse on the pediatric unit is caring for a 12-year-old boy. What BP would this child have normally?
   A. 95/57
   B. 102/61
   C. 112/64
   D. 120/80

ALTERNATIVE CASE STUDY SCENARIOS

In Chapter 6 of *Nursing Health Assessment*, you learned about Mr. Sanders, a 55-year-old Caucasian man, who was admitted to the intensive care unit (ICU) following an episode of rapid heart rate and dizziness. He was monitored on the telemetry unit for 2 days because he had atrial fibrillation (a cardiac dysrhythmia that causes a fast and irregular heartbeat). He was placed on medication to decrease his heart rate; he also is taking an antihypertensive drug for high BP. Mr. Sanders started complaining of chest pain radiating down his left arm.

Alternative A

Mr. Sanders is transferred to the medical intensive care unit (MICU). He is diaphoretic, appears very anxious, and is clutching his chest.

- What vital signs would be most important to obtain on this patient when he is admitted?
- What part of the general survey would be done at this time?

Alternative B

Mr. Sanders' atrial fibrillation is stable and he is scheduled to go home in the morning.

- What would be appropriate areas for discharge teaching with this patient?

DOCUMENTATION

Form for Use in Practice

Patient Name _____   Date _____

Date of Birth _____

Physical Appearance

Age_____   Gender_____

Facial features _____

Symmetry _____

Hygiene and dress _____

Skin color _____

Body structure and development _____

Behavior

Facial expressions _____

Level of consciousness _____

Speech _____

Mobility

Posture _____

Range of Motion _____

Gait _____

Measurements

Height _____   Weight _____   BMI _____

Vital Signs

Temperature _____   Site _____

Pulse

    Rate _____   Rhythm _____

Amplitude _____   Elasticity _____

Respirations _____

Oxygen Saturation _____

Blood pressure _____   Site _____

Guide for Use in Practice

Technique	Normal Findings	Abnormal Findings
Assess overall appearance.	Patient appears stated age. Facial features, movements, and body are symmetrical.	Patient appears younger or older than chronological age or manifests facial asymmetry or obvious deformities.
Inspect hygiene and dress.	Dress is appropriate for age, gender, culture, and weather. Patient is clean and well kempt. No odors are noted.	Clothes are poorly kempt. Patient has bad or sweet-smelling breath or body odor, or is disheveled. Makeup or dress is eccentric.
Observe for even skin tones and symmetry and the amount, texture, quality, and distribution of hair.	Skin is even-toned, with pigmentation appropriate for genetic background and no obvious lesions or color variations. Hair is smooth, thick, and evenly distributed.	Skin shows pallor, erythema, cyanosis, jaundice, or lesions.
Note body structure and development.	Physical and sexual development is appropriate for age, culture, and gender. No joint abnormalities are noted.	Patient shows evidence of delayed puberty, markedly short or tall stature, disproportionate height and weight, obesity, or emaciation.
Note behavior.	Patient is cooperative and interacts pleasantly.	Patient is uncooperative or has flat affect, unusual elation, or severe anxiety.
Assess the face for symmetry and expressions while at rest and during speech.	Expression is relaxed, symmetrical, and appropriate for setting and circumstances. Patient maintains eye contact appropriate for age and culture.	Unexpected findings include inappropriate affect, inattentiveness, impaired memory, inability to perform activities of daily living, flat or mask-like expression, drooping of one side of the face, and exophthalmos.
Continually assess mental status and level of consciousness.	Patient is awake, alert, and oriented to person, place, and time (A&O × 3). He or she attends and responds to questions appropriately.	Problems include confusion, agitation, drowsiness, or lethargy.
Listen to speech pattern. Assess for fluency in language and need for an interpreter.	Patient responds quickly and easily. Volume, pitch, and rate are appropriate. Speech is clear and articulate, flowing smoothly. Word choice is appropriate.	Speech is slow and slurred, rapid, or overly loud. Patient shows difficulty finding words or uses words inappropriately.
Note how the patient sits and stands.	Posture is upright while sitting, with limbs and trunk proportional to height. Patient stands erect with no signs of discomfort, and arms relaxed at the sides.	Posture is slumped or hunched. Limbs are long in proportion to the body. Patient assumes a tripod position when sitting.
Assess range of motion.	Patient moves freely in the environment.	Motion is asymmetrical or limited. Patient has any paralysis.
If ambulatory, observe the patient's movement around the room.	Gait is steady and balanced, with even heel-to-toe foot placement and smooth movements. Other movements are smooth, purposeful, effortless, and symmetrical.	Abnormalities include tics, paralysis, ataxia, tremors, uncontrolled movements, shuffling gait, or a slow, unsteady gait.
Use a height bar to measure height of patients older than 2 years with them standing.	Findings are within normal range for age according to standardized charts.	Height is decreased from previous readings; growth is excessive or deficient.
Weigh the patient.	Findings are within normal range for age according to standardized charts.	Weight loss or gain is excessive and unexplained.
Calculate the BMI.	For adults, BMI falls from 18 to 24.9.	BMI is <18 or >24.9.

Take the temperature.	Oral temperature ranges from 35.8°C to 37.3°C (96.4°F–99.1°F).	Temperature is <35°C (95°F) or >38.5°C (101.5°F).
Assess the pulse.	For an adult the pulse is 60–100 beats/min and occurs at evenly spaced intervals. Strength is 2+. The artery feels smooth, straight, and resilient.	Pulse is >100 or <60 beats/min. Rhythm is irregular. Strength is decreased or bounding.
Count respirations for 30 s and multiply by two to obtain breaths per minute.	Normal rate for adult is 12–20 breaths/min and regular.	Respiratory rate is rapid, persistent, and >20 breaths/min in an adult. Persistent respiratory rate is <12 breaths/min.
Observe for rhythm, depth, and quality of respirations.	Regular respiratory rhythm has even intervals. Breathing is diaphragmatic with no retractions.	Hyperventilation is deep, rapid respirations. Hypoventilation is shallow, slow respirations. Patient uses accessory muscles or shows signs of cyanosis, retractions, or audible sounds such as wheezing or congestion.
Measure oxygen saturation.	Oxygen saturation is 92% or above.	Oxygen saturation is <92%.
Assess BP.	Reading is 120/70.	On two or more readings, BP is above 120, 70, or both. Systolic BP is <90 mm Hg.

CHAPTER 7

Pain Assessment

OBJECTIVE SUMMARY

This chapter covers the assessment of pain using reliable and valid pain assessment scales. It presents the basic elements of pain assessment, as well as background information on pain, pain transmission, and assessing pain in difficult-to-assess populations.

READING ASSIGNMENT

Read Chapter 7 in Jensen's *Nursing Health Assessment: A Best-Practice Approach*.

VOCABULARY/TERMINOLOGY

- **A-delta fibers:** Large nerve fibers covered with myelin; they conduct pain impulses rapidly.

- **Acute pain:** Pain that results from tissue damage, whether through injury or surgery.

- **C fibers:** Small unmyelinated nerve fibers that conduct pain impulses diffusely and slowly.

- **Central sensitization:** Excitatory process involving spinal nerves and produced by continued pain stimuli; it can persist even after peripheral stimulation is no longer present.

- **Chronic pain:** Pain that lasts beyond the normal healing period and has no role.

- **Cutaneous pain:** Derives from the dermis, epidermis, and subcutaneous tissues. It is often burning or sharp, such as with a partial thickness burn.

- **Gate control theory:** The theory of pain with the widest acceptance; it posits that the body responds to a painful stimulus by either opening a neural gate to allow pain to be produced or creating a blocking effect at the synaptic junction to stop the pain.

- **Mild pain:** Pain considered in the 1 to 3 range on a scale from 0 to 10.

- **Moderate pain:** Pain considered in the 4 to 6 range on a scale from 0 to 10.

- **Modulation:** Inhibitory and facilitating input from the brain that eases or influences sensory transmission at the level of the spinal cord.

- **Neuronal plasticity:** Ability of the nervous system to change or alter its function.

- **Neuronal windup:** Enhanced response to pain stimulus produced by prolonged pain production.

- **Neuropathic pain:** A condition that follows constant stimuli and sensitization, in which nonpainful touch or pressure becomes painful.

- **Nociception:** The perception of pain by sensory receptors located throughout the body.

- **Nociceptors:** Specialized peripheral A and C nerve fibers that carry the pain signal to the central nervous system.

- **Opioid hyperalgeisa:** An altered physiologic response to the pain stimulus in which repeated use of opioids causes a person to become more sensitive to pain.

- **Pain:** An uncomfortable feeling transmitted along pain fibers to the central nervous system.

One of the most common reasons patients seek help from health care professionals.

- **Perception:** The impulses being transmitted to the higher areas of the brain are identified as pain.

- **Peripheral sensitization:** Result of inflammatory process that creates hypersensitivity to touch or pressure.

- **Referred pain:** Originates from a specific site, but the person experiencing it feels the pain at another site along the innervating spinal nerve.

- **Severe pain:** Considered in the 7 to 10 range.

- **Somatic pain:** Originates from skin, muscles, bones, and joints. Patients usually describe somatic pain as sharp.

- **Transduction:** Noxious stimuli create enough of an energy potential to cause a nerve impulse perceived by nociceptors (free nerve endings).

- **Transmission:** The neuronal signal moves from the periphery to the spinal cord and up to the brain.

- **Visceral pain:** Originates from abdominal organs and is often described as crampy or gnawing.

STUDY GUIDE

Answer the following questions, which assist you in identifying the most important information from Chapter 7 of Jensen's *Nursing Health Assessment*.

Activity A FILL IN THE BLANK

1. Identify the types of pain.

   A. Patients usually describe this pain as sharp.

   _____

   B. This pain is often referred to as burning or sharp.

   _____

   C. Also referred to as persistent pain.

   _____

   D. Patient feels the pain at another site along the innervating spinal nerve.

   _____

2. List six pain behaviors that indicate pain in patients who cannot verbalize.

   A. _____

   B. _____

   C. _____

   D. _____

   E. _____

   F. _____

Activity B MATCHING

1. *Put the steps of the gate theory in the correct order.*

Correct Order	Step
	A. The pain stimulus passes up through and across the dorsal horn.
	B. In the cerebral cortex the stimulus is identified as pain and a response is created.
	C. Continued painful stimulus on a peripheral neuron causes the "gate" to open.
	D. The pain stimulus then passes from the peripheral nervous system at a synaptic junction.

2. *Match the pain assessment tool with its description.*

Answer	Tool	Description
	1. Numeric Pain Intensity Scale	A. 100-mm line with "no pain" at one end and "worst possible pain" at the other
	2. One-dimensional Pain Scale	B. A set of structured questions to assess pain quickly in patients with chronic pain
	3. Visual Analog Scale	C. A set of verbal descriptors used to capture the sensory aspect of the pain experience

4. Verbal Descriptor Scale
5. McGill Pain Questionnaire
6. Brief Pain Inventory
7. Brief Pain Impact Questionnaire
8. Multidimensional Pain Scale

D. Consists of a pain intensity scale, a body diagram to locate the pain, a functional assessment (general activity, mood, walking, employment, housework, relationships, sleep, and enjoyment of life), and questions about the efficacy of pain medications

E. Measures one element of the pain experience—intensity

F. Combines indices that measure pain intensity, mood, pain location (via body diagram), verbal descriptors, and questions about medication efficacy

G. Uses words such as "mild," "moderate," and "severe" to measure pain intensity

H. 11-point Likert-type scale, 0 means "no pain" and 10 means "worst possible pain"

Activity C SHORT ANSWER

1. List the four steps in nociception.

2. Explain why it is difficult to assess pain in older adults.

3. Explain why patients with a history of opioid tolerance pose difficult challenges to nurses when assessing their pain.

4. Briefly discuss the re-assessment of pain.

5. Studies have shown that nurses have difficulty accepting the patient's report of pain as valid and credible. Briefly explain why this is.

6. List differences in pain by gender.

7. Explain risks faced by surgical patients and patients with a crush-type injury. Include signs and symptoms.

8. Explain why the assessment of pain in children is complex and challenging.

Activity D **MULTIPLE CHOICE**

1. The nurse is caring for an older patient who is refusing postoperative pain medication. What question might the nurse consider asking?
   A. Can the patient afford the prescribed medication?
   B. Are effects such as pain relief causing the patient to refuse pain medications?
   C. Does the patient have positive biases about taking pain medication?
   D. Will the patient take the medication if she better understands what it is for?

2. The nursing class is learning about pain assessment. What behavior does the nurse assess when assessing pain in a patient?
   A. Repositioning
   B. Rocking
   C. Sitting up
   D. Ambulating

3. In addition to pain intensity, what is another basic element of a pain assessment?
   A. Quality
   B. Focused goal
   C. History
   D. Preferred assessment tool

4. The nurse is caring for a patient who has just returned from surgery. This patient has a history of chronic pain. What would not be an indicator of pain in this patient?
   A. Grimacing
   B. Moaning
   C. Rocking
   D. Increased respirations

5. What element is not released during the stress response?
   A. Epinephrine
   B. Norepinephrine
   C. Dopamine
   D. Cortisol

6. A multidimensional pain assessment tool combines indices that measure pain intensity, mood, pain location (via body diagram), verbal descriptors, and questions about medication efficacy. Which of these tools is a multidimensional pain assessment tool?

A. McGill Pain Questionnaire
B. Visual Analog Scale
C. Numeric Pain Intensity Scale
D. Combined Thermometer Scale

7. The nurse is working on a pediatric unit caring for a 4 year old who is recovering from the surgical repair of the humerus. When assessing the patient's pain what is the most appropriate pain assessment tool for the nurse to use?
   A. Face, Legs, Activity, Cry, Consolability Scale
   B. Visual Analog Scale
   C. FACES Pain Scale
   D. Numeric Pain Intensity Scale

ALTERNATIVE CASE STUDY SCENARIOS

In Chapter 7 of *Nursing Health Assessment*, you learned about Mrs. Bond, 42 years old, who is visiting the clinic for follow-up care for musculoskeletal pain related to fibromyalgia. She was diagnosed 5 months ago and still has not been able to control her pain to a desirable goal. Her temperature is 37°C orally, pulse 88, respirations 16, and blood pressure 112/68. Current medications include a selective serotonin reuptake inhibitor for depression, a benzodiazepine for muscle spasm, and an analgesic for pain. She had a comprehensive assessment documented 5 months ago that showed her functional abilities had decreased. Mrs. Bond has been seen twice since for pain control.

Alternative A

Mrs. Bond is referred to a pain control specialist for a comprehensive assessment of her pain.

- What pain assessment tools are most appropriate for Mrs. Bond?

- What other assessments should the nurse make?

Alternative B

Mrs. Bond is found to have adequate pain control since the medication Lyrica was added to her medication regimen.

- What teaching would the nurse include in your care planning for Mrs. Bond?

CHAPTER Second

Nutrition Assessment

OBJECTIVE SUMMARY

Nurses are involved intimately in all aspects of assessing nutritional status for patients. Determining adequate and appropriate caloric and nutrient intake occurs by analyzing data to identify actual and potential nutritional problems. Nurses must be aware of nutrients in whole foods to accurately complete nutritional assessments. When completing a nutritional assessment, the nurse considers a broad range of influences on the patient's food choices. A complete nutrition assessment includes a history of food intake, weight and height calculations, laboratory data, and use of specific nutritional tools when indicated.

READING ASSIGNMENT

Read Chapter 8 in Jensen's *Nursing Health Assessment: A Best-Practice Approach*.

VOCABULARY/TERMINOLOGY

- **Adequate intake:** The amount of a nutrient needed to keep the human healthy.

- **Albumin:** A prime ingredient of blood oncotic pressure and a carrier protein for many body and pharmacologic substances.

- **Body mass index:** A guide for maintaining ideal weight for height. It is also used as a benchmark for obesity or protein-caloric malnutrition.

- **Cachexia:** A highly catabolic state with accelerated muscle loss and a chronic inflammatory response. It is a distinct syndrome separate from anorexia with production of proinflammatory cytokines that contribute to breakdown of fat and muscle protein, causing loss of both muscle mass and fat stores.

- **Calorie count:** A tool that counts every calorie a patient takes in during a 24-hour period.

- **Carbohydrate:** A primary nutrient that provides the body's main source of energy.

- **Electrolytes:** Elements (eg, sodium, potassium) needed by the body to maintain functioning.

- **Food frequency questionnaire:** A tool to identify the number of times a person eats a specific food in a designated period.

- **Food pathogens:** Disease-causing microbes that live in the food supply.

- **Hydrogenation:** The chemical processing of animal fats used by food manufacturers to extend the shelf life of products susceptible to rancidity, such as cookies and crackers.

- **Intake and output:** Food and fluid taken into the body and urine expelled from the body.

- **Lipids:** Fats, which include triglycerides (fats and oils), sterols (eg, cholesterol), and phospholipids (eg, lecithin).

- **Mid upper arm muscle circumference/ midarm muscle areas:** Indicators of muscle and body protein reserves.

- **Percentage of ideal body weight:** Calculation based on the ideal and current weight according to the formula: *Percentage of ideal body weight = current weight/ideal weight × 100.*

- **Percentage of usual body weight:** Calculation following the formula: Percentage of usual body weight = Current weight/usual weight × 100.

- **Percentage of weight change:** Calculation following the formula: (Usual weight = present weight)/usual weight × 100.

- **Prealbumin:** A circulating protein in the blood.

- **Primary nutrients:** Nutrients essential for optimal body function—carbohydrates, proteins, fats, vitamins, minerals, water, and major electrolytes.

- **Proteins:** Macronutrients that serve important functions in cell structure and tissue maintenance.

- **Three-day food diary:** A diary kept by the patient that reviews 3 days worth of food intake.

- **Transferrin:** A serum protein with a half-life of 9 days.

- **Triceps skinfold:** A measurement of skinfold thickness. Not representative of adipose tissue throughout the body.

- **24-hour recall:** A tool used to quantify the amount of food taken in over a 24-hour time period.

- **Waist circumference:** The measurement around the waist. An indicator of accumulated body fat in the abdomen; a high circumference places people at increased risk of obesity-related diseases and early mortality.

- **Weight for height calculations:** Reference standards for height and weight.

STUDY GUIDE

Answer the following questions, which assist you in identifying the most important information from Chapter 8 of Jensen's *Nursing Health Assessment.*

Activity A FILL IN THE BLANK

1. The USDHHS and USDA jointly publish guidelines for healthy eating that are revised every 5 years.

   A. Changes in recommendations aim at promoting

   _____

   B. Emphasis, when using My Pyramid, is on

   _____

   C. Pregnant and lactating women need an extra

   _____

   D. The best bioavailable sources of vitamins and minerals are

   _____

2. Identify in alphabetical order the herbs most likely to cause herb–drug interactions.

   A. _____

   B. _____

   C. _____

   D. _____

Activity B MATCHING

1. *Match the nutrient with its description.*

Answer	Nutrient	Question
	1. Cholesterol	A. Plays a key role in the metabolism of most nutrients
	2. Carbohydrate	
	3. Vitamin	B. Plays an important role in maintaining the myelin sheath around nerves
	4. Lipid	
		C. Best absorbed from animal sources
		D. Distribution range in the normal healthy diet is 45%–65% of calories

5. B$_{12}$
6. Protein
7. Iron

E. Involved in many essential body functions such as regulating fluid and electrolyte balance and transporting molecules and other substances through the blood

F. Help to maintain body functions

G. Essential to cellular maintenance and repair

2. *Match the religion with the food restriction practiced.*

Answer	Religion		Food Restriction
	1. Catholicism	A.	Avoid consuming milk and meat in the same meal
	2. Hinduism		
	3. Mormon	B.	Substitute soy products for meat
	4. Seventh Day Adventist	C.	Avoid beef and pork
	5. Judaism	D.	Avoid pork and birds of prey
	6. Islam	E.	Many are lacto-ovo-vegetarians
	7. Buddhism	F.	Avoid coffee and tea
		G.	Avoid meat on Fridays

Activity C SHORT ANSWER

1. Briefly discuss what can happen if potassium levels become too high or too low.

_____

_____

_____

_____

2. Malnutrition and dehydration are common among residents of long-term care facilities. Explain what nurses can do to help maintain adequate nutrition in older adults.

_____

_____

_____

_____

3. "Increase food security among U.S. households and in so doing reduce hunger" is a goal of *Healthy People*. Explain what resources might be available to nurses/families to meet this goal.

_____

_____

_____

_____

4. Folate is an important vitamin considered essential to metabolism and cell synthesis. Name sources of folate, the U.S. Public Health Service recommendation for folate, and groups at risk for folate deficiency.

_____

_____

_____

_____

5. List and discuss the variations for adequate intake of water, which is essential for life.

_____

_____

_____

_____

6. Explain why more and more people are seeking and eating organic food.

_____

_____

_____

_____

7. Explain the necessity of including psychosocial information in a comprehensive nutritional assessment. Include questions that would be asked and the information such questions would elicit.

_____

_____

_____

_____

8. List and discuss the common symptoms of altered nutrition. Include questions the nurse would ask to assess symptoms.

_____

_____

_____

_____

Activity D   MULTIPLE CHOICE

1. The nurse is caring for an 88-year-old man hospitalized with a fractured hip and asks for a dietary consult because assessment findings indicate that the patient is malnourished. In conducting a comprehensive dietary assessment, what would be the method of choice for determining this patient's dietary intake?

   A. A 3-day food diary

   B. Food-frequency questionnaires

   C. 24-hour recall

   D. Direct observation

2. A nurse is teaching a nutrition class to patients with obesity. What would be an appropriate topic to teach these patients?

   A. Decreasing intake of foods with low nutrient density

   B. Diets with food restrictions

   C. Increasing intake of foods with low nutrient density

   D. The American Dietetic Association Diet

3. A nurse is caring for four patients whose weight has changed by 10% in the last 3 months. For which patient would the nurse have the most nutrition-related concerns?

   A. A 33-year-old athlete on steroids

   B. A 42-year-old patient with kidney disease

   C. A 39-year-old who has been in remission from cancer for 4 years

   D. A 27-year-old woman with morbid obesity

4. A patient has been diagnosed with stomach cancer and is scheduled for surgery in the morning. What would be appropriate to include in this patient's discharge teaching?

   A. Which foods are nutrient dense

   B. To weigh self at 2 PM every day

   C. To eat a high-calorie diet

   D. To increase fruit and vegetable intake

5. A nurse is conducting a comprehensive nutritional assessment on a patient with suspected malnutrition. Why would it be important to assess this patient's ability to cook?

   A. Determine if the patient is interested in preparing nutritious food.

   B. Assess if the patient has the ability to obtain or prepare food.

   C. Understand whether the patient wants to learn how to cook.

   D. Evaluate the patient's food preferences.

6. A nursing student is caring for a male patient who has been comatose for 14 days. For what signs of malnutrition would the student observe?

   A. Bleeding of the gums and eyes

   B. Increased size of genitalia

   C. Cranium that appears larger in proportion to body

   D. Decreased size of liver

7. Cachexia means a highly catabolic state with accelerated muscle loss. What is the other component of cachexia?

   A. Anemia

   B. Psychological desire for attention

   C. Chronic inflammatory response

   D. Nausea and vomiting

8. The nurse is doing a research project on the frequency with which certain foods are eaten during the last trimester of pregnancy. What would be the most appropriate tool to use in this research?

   A. Three-day food diary

   B. 24-hour recall

   C. Direct observation

   D. Food-frequency questionnaires

ALTERNATIVE CASE STUDY SCENARIOS

In Chapter 8 of *Nursing Health Assessment*, you learned about Karen Pitoci, 15 years old and 88 lb, who was recently discharged from the hospital with a diagnosis of anorexia nervosa. This hospital stay was the most recent of three in the past year. Her mother, a full-time homemaker, is very involved in Karen's school and social activities.

Karen is seeing a psychiatrist twice a week on an outpatient basis as well as being physically assessed by a home health nurse.

Alternative A

Karen is found to have gained 4 lb in a period of 4 weeks. She tells the nurse that she is "getting fat."

- What nutritional assessment tool might the home health nurse ask Karen to complete?

- What would be an appropriate response by the nurse to Karen's statement?

Alternative B

Karen has just been diagnosed with lactose intolerance and has been placed on a lactose-free diet.

- What supplement might Karen have to take as she continues to grow and develop?

- When teaching Karen about her new diet, what foods would the nurse teach Karen to avoid and which foods would Karen be able to eat?

DOCUMENTATION

Form for Use in Practice

Patient Name _____ Date _____

Date of Birth _____

Initial Survey

Reason for seeking health care: _____

History of present illness

- Location.

- Intensity.

- Duration.

- Description.

- Aggravating factors.

- Alleviating factors.

- Functional impairment.

- Pain goal.

Vital signs: T (route)_____   P (with site)_____   R_____   BP (site)_____   SpO$_2$_____

General appearance (posture, pursed lips, nasal flaring, LOC, skin color): _____

Height: _____   Weight: _____   BMI: _____

Respiratory movement (inspiration: expiration ratio, rate, pattern): _____

General level of distress (accessory muscles, retractions): _____

History/Interview:

- Family history of nutritional problems:

- History of malnutrition or eating disorders:

- Medications and supplements:

- Smoking history:

- Recreational drugs:

- Allergies:

- Influenza or pneumococcal vaccine:

Common Symptoms

Symptom	Yes	No	Additional Data
Sudden or gradual changes in body weight			
Change in eating habits			
Changes in skin, hair, or nails			
Decreased energy level			

Physical Assessment

Assess for evidence of diabetes or hypertension.
Assess for history of problems related to nutrition or weight.
Inspect mouth and nose.
Assess for gastrointestinal diseases.
Assess hydration (look at food and fluid intake patterns).
Assess dietary lifestyle changes.
Assess for alcohol and drug use.
Inspect skin, hair, and nails.
Assess for signs/symptoms of malnutrition.

Signature_____ Date _____

Guide for Use in Practice

Technique	Normal Findings	Abnormal Findings
Observe body type, which is noted as small build, average build, or large build.	*A wide variety of body types fall within the normal range; however, note that muscle tone and mass decrease with age. Aging also causes fat distribution to change. Fat is lost from the face and neck, while it tends to increase in the arms, abdomen, and hips.*	Obesity; lack of subcutaneous fat with prominent bones, abdominal ascites, and pitting edema; amenorrhea; cachexia.
Observe general appearance.	*A healthy adult appears energetic, alert, and erect. Skin, hair, and nails look healthy.*	Clinical findings of malnutrition can occur in many places throughout the body. Visible signs include muscle wasting, particularly in the temporal area, muscle weakness and decreased muscle size, tongue atrophy, and bleeding or changes in the integrity or hydration status of the skin, hair, teeth, gums, lips, tongue, eyes, and, in men, genitalia.
Observe the patient's ability to swallow.	*Swallowing is smooth, with no problems with the ingestion of food.*	Difficulty swallowing, known as *dysphagia*, is common in *stroke* and *neuromuscular diseases*.

Inspect urine, emesis, and stool.	*No unusual features.*	Emesis refers to vomited contents from the gastrointestinal tract. The amount should be described and measured.
Calculate BMI as follows: BMI = weight in kilograms or weight in pounds/height in meters^2 or height in inches^2 × 703.	*BMI of 18.5–24.9 is healthy or normal.*	BMI <18.5 or >24.9 is abnormal and a health risk. Adults with a BMI <17.5 or children and adolescents with a BMI less than the fifth percentile meet the criteria for an eating disorder.
Calculate the percentage of ideal body weight based on the ideal and current weight: *Percentage of ideal body weight = current weight/ideal weight × 100.*		*Mild malnutrition*: 80%–90% of ideal weight *Moderate malnutrition*: 70%–80% of ideal weight *Severe malnutrition*: <70% of ideal weight
Carefully assess circumstances surrounding any change in weight to determine causes. Cluster weight and weight change with other data to analyze if the change is from fluid, muscle mass, or fat stores. After collecting the usual weight from the history and current weight on a scale, calculate the percent weight change (percentage loss of usual weight). (Usual weight – present weight)/usual weight × 100.	*Weight has not changed significantly.*	Weight has changed by >10%.
Calculate the percentage of usual weight: Percentage of usual body weight = current weight/usual weight × 100.		*Mild malnutrition*: 85% to 95% of usual body weight *Moderate malnutrition*: 75%–84% of usual body weight *Severe malnutrition*: <75% of usual body weight
Use waist circumference to evaluate the amount of abdominal fat in men and women.	*Waist circumference <40 in (102 cm) in men or <35 in (88 cm) in women*	Waist circumference >40 in (102 cm) in men or >35 in (88 cm) in women
Assess waist-to-hip ratio to determine body fat distribution. Waist-to-hip ratio = waist circumference/hip circumference (largest point).	*The value is <1.0 in men or <0.8 in women.*	A ratio >1.0 in men or >0.8 in women indicates upper body (android) obesity, which puts the patient at risk for increased mortality and heart attack.
Measure skinfold thickness to indicate subcutaneous fat reserves.	*Normal findings are according to standardized tables that adjust for age and gender.*	Patients above the 95th or below the 5th percentiles are at risk for altered nutritional status.
Measure mid upper arm muscle circumference (MAMC) around the arm, midway between the elbow and shoulder.	*Normal findings are according to standardized tables that adjust for age and gender.*	A higher number on the arm circumference indicates both fat and muscle stores. Findings below the 10th percentile are abnormal, indicating loss of muscle. Trends that decrease over time are also significant.
Measure MAMC and the mid upper arm muscle area (MAMA): MAMC = MAC − (π × TSF). MAMA = (MAC − MAMC)^2/4π.	*Normal findings are according to standardized tables that adjust for age and gender. A higher number indicates more muscle.*	Findings below the 10th percentile are abnormal indicating loss of muscle. Trends that decrease over time are also significant.

Assessment of Developmental Stages

This chapter summarizes important information about growth and development across the life span. The content serves as a foundational context to support nurses when assessing patients of all age groups and their families. Nurses provide information, anticipatory guidance, role modeling, and protection to individuals, families, and communities to enable optimal, healthy growth and development for children and adults.

READING ASSIGNMENT

Read Chapter 9 in Jensen's *Nursing Health Assessment: A Best-Practice Approach.*

VOCABULARY/TERMINOLOGY

- **Autonomy versus shame and doubt:** Erikson's task for the toddler, who must master two simultaneous sets of social modalities: holding on and letting go.

- **Cognitive development:** Qualitative changes in a person's thinking and intellectual skills. Begins at birth and continues until adulthood—the person uses experience to move from stage to stage as thinking becomes more sophisticated and complex in interaction with his or her environment.

- **Concrete operational:** Piaget's stage of cognitive development that lasts from approximately ages 7 to 11 years, in which the child becomes capable of performing *operations,* or internalized sets of actions that people do mentally instead of physically. Examples of concrete operations include conservation and categorization.

- **Development:** Qualitative changes in a person over time, particularly in the areas of motor skills, language, psychosocial skills, and cognition.

- **Formal operations:** The last stage in Piaget's cognitive theory; hallmarks include abstract reasoning and the ability to discuss theoretical concepts.

- **Generativity versus stagnation:** The seventh stage in Erikson's model, faced by adults in middle age, in which the hallmark concern is feeling needed by others.

- **Growth:** Quantitative physical changes in a person over time.

- **Identity versus role confusion:** Erikson's task for adolescents, who begin to face adult tasks and roles and become concerned with how others evaluate them as compared with who they believe themselves to be.

- **Industry versus inferiority:** Erikson's task for the school-age child, who must learn to use the tools that adults commonly use within the specific society or environment. As the child spends more time in the school culture, prepared by teachers for the literate world, the influence of other adults dilutes the role of parents in the child's life.

- **Initiative versus guilt:** Erikson's task for the preschooler, who is actively engaged in making plans, setting goals, and accomplishing them.

- **Intimacy versus isolation:** Erikson's sixth psychosocial task, occurring in early adulthood, in which the person who has successfully navigated the search for personal identity is willing to fuse with the identity of others.

- **Preoperational stage:** The second stage of Piaget's cognitive model, which lasts from approximately ages 2 to 7 years, during which the child forms stable concepts, begins to develop mental reasoning, and constructs magical beliefs.

- **Psychosocial development:** The individual's development in interaction with the immediate environment.

- **Sensorimotor:** Piaget's first stage of cognition, experienced by infants and young toddlers.

- **Trust versus mistrust:** Erikson's first task faced in infancy, in which the baby learns that physiologic regulation is linked to a caregiver's provision of comfort.

STUDY GUIDE

Answer the following questions, which assist you in identifying the most important information from Chapter 9 of Jensen's *Nursing Health Assessment.*

Activity A FILL IN THE BLANK

1. Erikson's model includes eight stages across the lifespan. Please identify them.

   A. Infant _____

   B. Toddler _____

   C. Preschooler _____

   D. School-age child _____

   E. Adolescent _____

   F. Early adult _____

   G. Middle adult _____

   H. Late adult _____

2. Finish these statements on development.

   A. Physical growth takes place in an_____

   B. Individuals develop at_____

   C. Growth refers to changes in _____

   D. Development refers to changes in_____, _____, _____, and _____

Activity B MATCHING

1. *Match the life stage with the cognitive development in Piaget's theory.*

Answer	Life Stage	Cognitive Development
	1. Infancy	**A.** Cognitive expertise
	2. Toddlerhood and preschool	**B.** Formal operations
	3. School age	**C.** Wisdom
	4. Adolescence and young adulthood	**D.** Concrete operations
	5. Middle adulthood	**E.** Sensorimotor
	6. Older adulthood	**F.** Preoperational

2. *Match the nursing diagnosis with the appropriate intervention.*

Answer	Nursing Diagnosis	Intervention
	1. Risk for delayed child development	**A.** Offer parent the opportunity to express childhood experiences.
	2. Readiness for enhanced family processes	**B.** Provide adequate nutrition.
	3. Risk for impaired attachment	**C.** Encourage family meals.

Activity C SHORT ANSWER

1. Explain briefly the two elements of language.

   _____

   _____

   _____

   _____

2. Nurses promote healthy lifestyles. Explain what parents need to make decisions about healthy lifestyles for their children and what adults need to maintain healthy lifestyles.

   _____

   _____

   _____

   _____

3. Explain the expected growth of an infant, toddler, and preschooler.

_____

_____

_____

_____

4. Explain the growth of adolescents.

_____

_____

_____

_____

5. Explain memory functions and whether they are affected by aging.

_____

_____

_____

_____

6. Explain Uri Bronfenbrenner's theory of development.

_____

_____

_____

_____

7. Explain what Erikson meant by "ego integrity."

_____

_____

_____

_____

8. Explain differences in Piaget's stage of formal operations for young adults versus adolescents.

_____

_____

_____

_____

Activity D MULTIPLE CHOICE

1. Crystallized intelligence is also called what?
   A. Fluid intelligence
   B. Cognitive pragmatics
   C. Cognitive mechanics
   D. Expertise

2. A nurse is caring for a 22-year-old man and a 75-year-old man. If the nurse gave both patients the same simple comparison task, how much faster would the nurse expect the 22 year old to finish it than the 75 year old?
   A. 20%
   B. 30%
   C. 40%
   D. 50%

3. A growth and development professor is explaining language development to students. The professor explains that the understanding of spoken or written words and sentences is
   A. receptive language
   B. productive language
   C. primary language
   D. secondary language

4. A mother brings her 6 month old to the clinic for a well-baby checkup. She tells the nurse that she is concerned that her baby is not crawling yet. What would be important for the nurse to explain to this mother?
   A. Infants should be crawling by age 6 months.
   B. The mother should not worry because most infants start crawling after 6 months.
   C. Individuals develop at variable rates.
   D. The infant is not getting enough opportunities to crawl.

5. A nurse is discussing memory with students. What type of memory would the nurse be explaining if he was talking about retrieval of facts, vocabulary, and general knowledge?
   A. Sensory memory
   B. Semantic long-term memory
   C. Episodic long-term memory
   D. Working memory

6. The nurse is assessing a child's language development. How old would the nurse expect the child to be if she was using her first word and had a receptive vocabulary of 50 words?

    A. 6 months

    B. 8 to 12 months

    C. 10 to 15 months

    D. 18 months

7. A child who is 10 months old would be at what stage of language development?

    A. Gesturing such as showing and pointing

    B. Babbling

    C. Using two-word utterances (telegraphic speech) such as "more milk"

    D. Using first words, with a receptive vocabulary of 50 words

8. The instructor is discussing Uri Bronfenbrenner. The instructor explains that Bronfenbrenner's theory of development is based on the approach that development is what?

    A. Most important during childhood

    B. Passive

    C. Occurring in stages

    D. Continuous

ALTERNATIVE CASE STUDY SCENARIOS

In Chapter 9 of *Nursing Health Assessment*, you learned about Amber and Michael Carr, who have just become first-time adoptive parents to three biological siblings: Emily, 2 months; Jacob, 2 years; and Madeline, 5 years. Amber, a 31-year-old real-estate broker, will be leaving her job to care for the children. Michael, a 35-year-old tax accountant, is enthusiastic about fatherhood but worries about providing for the family's needs with only one income. Both Amber's and Michael's parents, who are in their late 50s and early 60s, are thrilled. They look forward to spending time with their grandchildren and teaching them about outdoor activities, such as camping and hiking.

Alternative A

Amber and Michael take the children into the clinic for the first time. The nurse performs developmental testing on Emily and Jacob and finds that Jacob is showing a significant delay in his developmental stage.

- What would be appropriate for the nurse to explain to Amber and Michael?

- What might be a reason for Jacob to be showing delays in his developmental stage?

Alternative B

The Carr family is having financial difficulties, and the decision is made for Amber to return to work part-time. Amber's and Michael's parents are going to share child care responsibilities while Amber works.

- What disciplinary issues would need clarification with this arrangement?

- What additional stressors might this cause in Amber and Michael's nuclear family?

DOCUMENTATION

Form for Use in Practice

Patient Name _____ Date _____

Date of Birth _____

Initial Survey

Reason for seeking health care:_____

History of present illness

- Duration:

- Description:

- Aggravating factors:

- Alleviating factors:

- Functional impairment:

Vital signs: T (route)_____   P (with site)_____   R_____   BP (site)_____

General behavior:_____

History/Interview:

- Family history of developmental problems:

- History of congenital problems:

- Medications and supplements:

- Smoking history:

- Recreational drugs:

- Occupational and environmental exposure:

- Allergies:

Physical Assessment:

Height:
Weight:
Motor development:

Signature_____ Date _____

Guide for Use in Practice

Technique	Normal Findings	Abnormal Findings
Perform initial survey	Posture relaxed and upright. Facial expression relaxed. Patient alert, cooperative, and oriented to time, place, and person	Kyphosis, scoliosis, or lordosis. Tripod position or leaning forward. Anxious facial expression. Disorientation
Observe behavior	Appropriate for age	Interacts with environment in a manner that is appropriate for a younger age range
Assess language	Appropriate for age	Language skills are appropriate for a younger age range

CHAPTER 10

Mental Health Assessment

OBJECTIVE SUMMARY

Mental health is an integral part of a patient's well-being. A nurse is often the first health care practitioner that a patient sees in any health care setting. The patient may be seeking care for a physical problem and thorough assessment by the nurse uncovers an underlying mental health problem. Many patients live with a mental health condition for a long time without realizing that they have a problem. Some patients self-medicate with alcohol or other substances to feel better. Nursing assessment of mental health consists of screening for preexisting, as well as current, mental health conditions for all age groups. This chapter presents assessment techniques that nurses can use to identify risk factors, assess mental status and mental health, and guide patients in planning care.

READING ASSIGNMENT

Read Chapter 10 in Jensen's *Nursing Health Assessment: A Best-Practice Approach*.

VOCABULARY/TERMINOLOGY

- **Anxiety:** A feeling of apprehension or worry, especially about the future.
- **CAGE:** An assessment tool for alcohol and substance abuse. Questions are: Have you ever felt the need to Cut down on drinking? Have you ever felt Annoyed by criticism of drinking? Have you ever had Guilty feelings about drinking? Have you ever taken a drink first thing in the morning (Eye-opener)?
- **Delusion:** False belief kept despite nonsupportive evidence.
- **Depression:** A term that can refer to a wide variety of abnormal variations in an individual's *mood*. If mood changes are persistent and cause distress or impairment in functioning, then a *mood disorder* may be present. Individuals with mood disorders experience extremes of emotions, for example sadness, that are higher in intensity and longer in duration than normal.
- **Geriatric depression scale:** A tool to assess for risk of depression in older adults.
- **HOPE:** A tool to assess for spirituality.
- **Mental status examination:** As assessment to tell the mental state of the patient.
- **Mini mental status examination:** A tool to quickly assess level of cognitive function.
- **Paranoia:** A disturbed thought process characterized by excessive anxiety or fear, often to the point of irrationality and delusion. Paranoid thinking typically includes persecutory beliefs concerning a perceived threat.
- **Psychosis:** Disorderly mental state in which the patient has difficulty distinguishing reality from internal perceptions.
- **Suicide:** The taking of one's own life.

STUDY GUIDE

Answer the following questions, which assist you in identifying the most important information from Chapter 10 of Jensen's *Nursing Health Assessment*.

Activity A   FILL IN THE BLANK

1. Fill in the blanks with elements of the role of the nurse in the mental health assessment.

   A. The mental health assessment is based on _____ of the patient.

   B. The nurse determines the extent of the questions based on the _____ and ongoing assessment of the patient's needs.

   C. The nurse performs a mental health assessment while considering the patient within the context of his or her own _____.

   D. The nurse determines whether there is a need to _____ _____ _____ in more depth.

2. Name four common factors that may influence mental health:

   A. _____

   B. _____

   C. _____

   D. _____

Activity B   MATCHING

1. *Match the associated term with its definition.*

Answer	Term	Definition
	1. Suicide ideation	A. Thoughts of, or a plan for, taking one's own life
	2. Homicide ideation	
	3. Aggressive behavior	B. Acts of verbal, physical, or sexual force, confrontation, or assault
	4. Mania	C. Hearing things that are not really there
	5. Auditory hallucinations	D. Desire to harm or kill another person or persons
		E. Elated mood and affect

6. Visual hallucinations
7. Other hallucinations

F. Feeling touch when no one or nothing is there; smelling things that others do not

G. Seeing things that are not really there

2. *Match the abnormal finding with the mood disorder.*

Answer	Mood Disorder	Abnormal Finding
	1. Blunted affect	A. Excessive sense of emotional and physical well-being inappropriate to the actual situation or environmental stimuli
	2. Depersonalization	
	3. Ambivalence	
	4. Euphoria	B. A feeling of apprehension or worry, especially about the future
	5. Anxiety	
	6. Lability	C. No emotional tone or reaction
	7. Flat affect	D. Quick change of expression of mood or feelings
		E. Having two opposing feelings or emotions at the same time
		F. Severe reduction in emotional expressiveness
		G. Feeling that oneself or one's environment is unreal

Activity C   SHORT ANSWER

1. Briefly discuss what findings you would expect in a patient diagnosed with Parkinsonism.

   _____

   _____

   _____

   _____

2. Discuss when an acute mental health assessment is necessary and what it includes.

_____

_____

_____

3. Assessing mental health is an art as well as a science. Explain what this statement means.

_____

_____

_____

_____

4. Explain how the objective data in a mental health assessment are usually organized.

_____

_____

_____

_____

5. Discuss what abnormal findings during assessment of hygiene and grooming might mean.

_____

_____

_____

_____

6. What areas would be the focus during assessment of the patient's attention span?

_____

_____

_____

_____

7. Explain the differences among dementia, confusion, delirium, and depression.

_____

_____

_____

_____

Activity D MULTIPLE CHOICE

The nurse assesses a 67-year-old man new to the mental health clinic. The following is the nurse's documentation of the encounter:

Patient appears stated age and normal weight; no obvious deformity. Posture erect and relaxed. Movements symmetrical, voluntary, deliberate, coordinated, smooth, and even. Gait steady and even. Activity moderate and relaxed. Well-groomed patient with no unusual body odors. Clothing clean and appropriate. Patient awake, alert, calm, and expressive, responding appropriately to voice cues. Converses with eyes closed and no eye contact. Facial expressions congruent with subjects. Speech of slow pace and low volume, with few fluctuations; it is unorganized and incongruent with behavior and nonverbal communication. Words slurred and indistinct. A&O × 3. Patient follows conversation and events; normal attention span. Short- and long-term memory intact. Mini-mental status examination (MMSE) completed with no deficits. Patient takes responsibility for actions. Thought processes easy to follow, logical, and relevant.

1. With which of the following is the documentation most consistent?

   A. A patient who has had a recent stroke

   B. A patient with dementia

   C. A patient with depression

   D. An aggressive patient

2. The nurse is admitting a 23-year-old woman to the acute care mental health unit. Physical examination reveals vertical cuts on the patient's forearms approximately 6 in long bilaterally. On the care plan, the nurse enters a nursing diagnosis of Risk for Self Mutilation. What would be the most immediate nursing intervention for this patient?

   A. Place patient on 1:1 nurse/patient care.

   B. Treat medical injuries.

   C. Use only plastic eating utensils.

   D. Place in a private room.

3. A patient with a nursing diagnosis of sensory-perceptual alterations would be expected to exhibit what behaviors?

   A. Visual or auditory hallucinations, agitation, normal concentration

   B. Poor concentration, irritability, violence

   C. Poor concentration, irritability, agitation, change in behavior

   D. Agitation, change in behavior, extreme anxiety

4. A patient has been diagnosed with stomach cancer and has a comorbidity of depression. For what would it be important to assess in this patient?

   A. Malnutrition

   B. Violence

   C. Suicide

   D. Noncompliance

5. The nurse is conducting a MMSE on a 77-year-old woman brought to the emergency department by her daughter. What is one of the first questions the nurse would ask this patient?

   A. Who is your best friend?

   B. What color is the sky?

   C. Who is the president?

   D. What day of the week is it?

6. The nursing student is caring for a male patient who has Korsakoff's syndrome. What behavior might the patient exhibit?

   A. Confabulation

   B. Neologisms

   C. Hypochondriasis

   D. Circumstantiality

7. An 84-year-old patient has been brought to the emergency department by ambulance after being found on the bedroom floor by a family member. The patient is found to have compromised speech. What would the nurse note?

   A. Patient is paraphasic.

   B. Patient is verbigerous.

   C. Patient is mute.

   D. Patient is aphasic.

8. The nurse is caring for four patients on the psychiatric/medical ward. Patient A exhibits echolalia; Patient B exhibits word salad; Patient C exhibits thought blocking; and Patient D exhibits perseveration phenomena. The nurse knows that all these behaviors are abnormal manifestations of

   A. socialization

   B. verbalization

   C. thought processes

   D. mood

ALTERNATIVE CASE STUDY SCENARIOS

In Chapter 10 of *Nursing Health Assessment*, you learned about Mr. Hart, a 75-year-old white man, who arrives at the community health care walk-in clinic to have his blood pressure checked. He has been to the clinic several times in the last few weeks for the same purpose. His temperature is 37°C orally, pulse 86 beats/min, respirations 16 breaths/min, and blood pressure 146/82 mm Hg. Current medications include a multivitamin, an antihypertensive, and an antidepressant (citalopram).

Alternative A

Mr. Hart tells the nurse he is afraid he is going to have a stroke, and that he lives alone. He paces the length of the examining room as he talks to the nurse.

- What do Mr. Hart's behaviors tell the nurse?

- What interventions by the nurse would be appropriate for this patient?

Alternative B

Mr. Hart is brought to the emergency department by ambulance, accompanied by his wife. The EMT reports to the nurse that Mr. Hart's facial expressions are not symmetrical; his grip is unequal; his verbalization is slurred; and he is not oriented to time or place.

- What other assessments would the nurse make in an acute assessment?

- What mental health risks is Mr. Hart facing?

DOCUMENTATION

Form for Use in Practice

Patient Name _____ Date _____

Date of Birth _____

Initial Survey

Reason for seeking health care:_____

History of present illness

- Location:
- Intensity:
- Duration:
- Description:
- Aggravating factors:
- Alleviating factors:
- Functional impairment:
- Pain goal:

Vital signs: T (route)_____   P (with site)_____   R_____   BP (site)_____ SpO_2_____

General appearance (posture, facial symmetry, mobility, ROM):_____

Weight: _____   Height: _____   BMI: _____

Mini-mental status exam:_____

General mood/behavior (agitated, afraid, anxious):_____

History/Interview:

- Family history of mental health problems:
- Medications and supplements:
  - Psychiatric medications:
  - Alternative treatments, herbs, or other substances:
- Smoking history:
- Recreational drugs:
- Occupational and environmental risk factors:
- Allergies:
- Changes noticed:
- Patient's perspective on problem:
- Typical day:
- Recent weight loss or gain:
- Sleeping habits:
- Past health history
  - Surgeries? If so, list when and why.
  - Previous mental health problem?
  - Previous treatment for a mental health problem?
  - Previous hospitalization for a mental problem?
  - History of physical, sexual, or emotional abuse?

- Support system:
- Significant others:
- Recent loss:
- Recent stressors:
- Living arrangements:
- Employment:
- Recent legal problems:
- Religious beliefs/spirituality:

Common Symptoms:

Symptom	Yes	No	Additional data
Suicide ideation			
Homicide ideation and aggressive behavior			
Altered mood and affect			
Auditory hallucinations			
Visual hallucinations			

Signature_____ Date _____

Guide for Use in Practice

Technique	Normal Findings	Abnormal Findings
Observe overall physical appearance including noticeable physical deformities, weight, and asymmetrical movements.	*Patient appears stated age, is normal weight, and shows symmetrical movements without obvious deformity*	Evidence of cutting or self-harm; physical problems such as stroke or dementia; cradle cap around the face of adults
Assess posture.	*Erect but relaxed*	Rigid (indicates *anxiety*) or slouching (indicates *withdrawal*)
Assess baseline and additional movements. Observe pace, range, and character.	*Movements are voluntary, deliberate, coordinated, smooth, and even*	Immobility (or tremor); frequent walking or pacing; tics or tardive dyskinesia
Assess gait for steadiness and rhythm.	*Steady and even*	Limping, fast or slow speed, pacing, shuffling, stiffness
Observe activity level.	*Activity moderately paced and relaxed*	Hypoactive, hyperactive, rigid, restless, agitated, gesturing, posturing, with inappropriate mannerisms, hostile/combative, or unusual
Note hair, nails, teeth, skin, and, if present, beard. Observe hygiene and grooming, including body odor and hair. Compare one side of the body with the other.	*Patient well groomed with no unusual body odors*	Poor hygiene; lice; poor grooming; excessive fastidiousness; one-sided neglect
Observe for makeup and how it is worn.	*Makeup appropriate to weather, age, gender, culture, and social situation*	Garish makeup with bold colors and outside the lines

Observe the hands for coloration, cleanliness, tremors, pill rolling, or clubbing of the nail bed. Look for any signs of itching or scratching.	*Hands clean; no tremors, pill rolling and clubbing; no signs of itching or scratching*	Clubbing, itching, scratching, signs of self-harm
Observe how the patient is dressed.	*Clothing clean and appropriate for culture and weather*	Unfastened or incorrectly worn clothes; slovenly, unkempt, overly meticulous, disheveled, inappropriate, provocative, unusual, inappropriate for weather, or multiple layers of clothes
Assess if the patient is awake, alert, or arousable.	*Patient awake and alert, responding appropriately to voice cues*	Drowsy, hyperalert, somnolent, intermittent alertness, or stupor. If the patient is not arousable, assess for breathing, stupor, or psychosis
Assess eye contact.	*Patient converses with eyes open and maintains eye contact*	Eyes closed, avoiding eye contact, staring, looking vacantly ahead, or twitching to side when discussing a traumatic event. Looking away frequently. Poor eye contact
Observe facial expressions at rest and when the patient is interacting with others.	*Patient calm, alert, and expressive; facial expressions are congruent with subjects*	Perplexed, stressed, tense, dazed, grimacing, and lacking in expression
Assess speech: Rate	*Moderately paced*	Slow, fast, latent, pressured, monotone, or disturbed
Rhythm	*Normal fluctuations*	Rhyming, slurring, mumbling, or unusual rhythm
Loudness	*Audible with moderate loudness*	Barely audible or too loud
Fluency	*Fluent*	Lengthy pauses, hesitancy, stuttering
Quantity	*A flow of conversation with pauses*	Too much or too little speech
Articulation	*Words clear and distinct*	Difficulty expressing self or finding words
Content	*Organized and congruent with behavior/nonverbal communication*	Disorganized, nonsensical, judgmental, religiously preoccupied, or sexually preoccupied speech
Pattern	*Exchange in conversation*	Fragmented sentences, circuitous speech (talks in circles and cannot answer questions), confabulation (makes up answers to cover for loss of memory), or intellectualization (uses intellectual analysis to avoid dealing with emotions); frequent or inappropriate laughter
Assess orientation.		

Tell me what day of the week, month, and year it is now.
  Where are you right now?
  What is your name (first and surname)?
  Why are you here right now?
	Alert and oriented, A&O × 3. It is also written as A&O × 4 indicating the additional information that the patient is aware of current situation (eg, why hospitalized)	Inconsistencies regarding orientation

Assess if the patient follows the conversation or is easily distractible.	*Patient follows conversation and events*	Altered attention span; restlessness, poor focus

Assess memory using the Mini Mental Status Examination.	*Short-term and long-term memory intact*	Memory lapses or problems
Assess judgment.	*The patient makes good judgments and takes responsibility for own actions*	Illogical responses, irresponsibility, lack of accountability, blaming
Assess thought processes.	*They are easy to follow, logical, coherent, relevant, goal directed, consistent, and abstract*	Illogical, incoherent, irrelevant, wandering, inconsistent, or concrete thought processes
Assess level of cognitive function by using the MMSE.	*Score of 24–30*	Score of 23 or lower

CHAPTER 11

Assessment of Social, Cultural, and Spiritual Health

Many health care professionals already understand the importance of social, cultural, and spiritual assessments or are actively pursuing educational opportunities to enhance their knowledge. This chapter presents basic principles of conducting social, cultural, and spiritual assessments and ways to incorporate findings into plans of care for patients.

READING ASSIGNMENT

Read Chapter 11 in Jensen's *Nursing Health Assessment: A Best-Practice Approach.*

VOCABULARY/TERMINOLOGY

- **Biomedical model:** The most prominent model of health, which views health as the absence of disease.

- **Community as partner assessment model:** An assessment model designed to help nurses thoroughly assess the demographics of a given community, including its values, beliefs, and history. The model also focuses on how resources (ie, recreation, physical environment, education, safety and transportation, politics and government, health and social services, communications, and economics) affect and influence the community.

- **Community level:** The scope of social assessment focusing above the individual to identify community resources, constraints, and high-priority health concerns.

- **Complementary and alternative medicine:** Therapies used instead of (*alternative*) or with (*complementary*) conventional treatments to restore health.

- **Cultural assessment:** Systematic assessment of individuals, families, and communities regarding their health beliefs and values.

- **Eudaimonistic model of health:** Model that posits that wholeness of the individual is essential to maintaining good health. Basic dimensions of wholeness include biopsychosocial and spiritual well-being. In this model, health enables the person to achieve happiness and joy, in which he or she uses aspirations as a measure of the value of each human act.

- **Roy's adaptation model:** Model posited by Sister Calista Roy, which refers to health as the patient's ability to adapt, compensate, manage, and adjust to physiologic–physical health-related setbacks. The adaptation model holds that a person is a set of parts connected to function as a whole.

- **Social assessment:** Assessment that identifies the social context influencing the patterns of health and illness for individuals, communities, and societies. Basic variables include gender, age, ethnicity, race, marital status, occupational class, shelter, employment status, and education level.

- **Societal level:** The scope of social assessment focussing above the individual and the community to inform healthy public policy and broad health-promotion initiatives.

- **Spirituality:** In the most fundamental sense, this term pertains to matters of the human soul, be it a state of mind, a state of being in the world, a journey of self discovery, or a place outside the five senses.

STUDY GUIDE

Activity A FILL IN THE BLANK

> biomedical model; complementary and alternative medicine model; eudaimonistic model of health; Gordon's functional health model; primary building blocks; Roy's adaptation model; social assessment; social assessment of the community; social assessment of the individual

1. Write the correct term in the box above next to the description of the health model and/or its elements. Choices are listed alphabetically.

   A. Views health as the absence of disease

   _____

   B. Emphasizes the interconnectedness of physical, psychosocial, and spiritual dimensions of health for individuals, communities, and populations studied

   _____

   C. Intends primarily to inform nurses about the patient's physical and mental health as related to the patient's existing resources, constraints, and demands

   _____

   D. Focuses on formal institutions in the area

   _____

   E. Gathers data to identify community resources, constraints, and high-priority health concerns

   _____

F. Posits that wholeness of the individual is essential to maintaining good health

_____

G. Considers people healthy if they can fulfill their social roles by contributing to family and society in meaningful ways

_____

H. Explores the complex interplay of mind, body, and spirit and offers opportunities to explore ways to facilitate healing

_____

I. Means the patient's ability to adapt, compensate, manage, and adjust to physiologic–physical health-related setbacks

_____

2. The specific aim of cultural assessment is to provide an all-inclusive picture of the patient's culture-based health care needs by

   A. _____

   B. _____

   C. _____

   D. _____

Activity B MATCHING

1. *Match the nursing diagnosis associated with social and spiritual domains with the appropriate nursing intervention.*

Answer	Diagnosis	Intervention
	1. Social isolation related to alterations in mental status	A. Role play situations.
	2. Spiritual distress related to challenged belief and value system	B. Offer choices of activities.
	3. Impaired social interaction related to knowledge/skill deficit	C. Assess spiritual or religious preferences.
	4. Readiness for enhanced spiritual well-being	D. Assess sources of support and make appropriate referrals.

2. *Match the population with the health characteristic.*

Answer	Population	Health-related Characteristic
	1. Hispanic men and women are less likely to die from it than Whites.	**A.** Infant mortality
	2. African Americans have almost 50% of cases.	**B.** Insurance coverage
	3. Asian adults are less likely to die from it than Whites.	**C.** Stroke
	4. American Indians are twice as likely to die from it.	**D.** HIV/AIDS
	5. Asian Americans have three times the incidence.	**E.** Cancer
	6. American Indians have 1.4 times the rate as Whites.	**F.** Diabetes
	7. About 50% of African Americans have this.	**G.** Heart disease

Activity C **SHORT ANSWER**

1. Briefly discuss spirituality and what is involved in a spiritual assessment.

_____

_____

_____

_____

2. Discuss the philosophical basis for Western medical care.

_____

_____

_____

_____

3. Florence Nightingale proposed that healing requires a special environment. Discuss this environment, including its parts and why they are needed for healing to take place.

_____

_____

_____

_____

4. Explain Roy's adaptation model, including the set of parts that make a whole.

_____

_____

_____

_____

5. Gordon developed a model of health based on functional health patterns. What are these and why are they necessary for healing?

_____

_____

_____

_____

6. Explain a social assessment and its basic variables. Discuss what the knowledge obtained from a social assessment is used for by a nurse.

_____

_____

_____

_____

7. Explain the difference between a social assessment of an individual and a social assessment of a community and why they are both important in nursing.

_____

_____

_____

_____

8. Explain the concept of primary, secondary, and potential building blocks. Give examples of each.

_____

_____

_____

_____

Activity D **MULTIPLE CHOICE**

1. A patient has a nursing diagnosis of impaired social interaction. What is a defining characteristic of this diagnosis?

A. Insufficient quantity or quality of social exchange

B. Low eye contact

C. Poor listening skills

D. Loneliness experienced as a negative state

2. Infant mortality is part of a cultural assessment. What group has 1.4 times the number of infant deaths than Whites and is more likely to begin prenatal care in the third trimester?

A. Asian Americans

B. African Americans

C. Puerto Ricans

D. American Indians

3. What group of people have a lower HIV/AIDS rate than Whites and are less likely to die from it?

A. Hispanic Americans

B. Native Americans

C. Asian Americans

D. African Americans

4. Federal mandates for culturally and linguistically appropriate services in health care exist. Which standard is most appropriate for culturally competent care?

A. Standard 3

B. Standard 5

C. Standard 7

D. Standard 9

5. One's spirituality is often considered what?

A. A part of community identification

B. Necessary for healing

C. Source of inner strength

D. Another way of expressing a connection to a church

6. What is considered an outcome related to social, cultural, and spiritual issues?

A. The patient will express meaning and purpose in life.

B. The patient will engage in interactions with others.

C. The patient will express a sense of oneness with self and others.

D. The patient will engage in church services weekly.

ALTERNATIVE CASE STUDY SCENARIOS

Mr. El-Kebbi, a 54-year-old Somalian Muslim immigrant, is being seen in an outpatient clinic for follow-up care related to his type 2 diabetes. He works in maintenance at a local hospital during the day and also has a part-time job selling used goods at auction in the evening. He takes an oral hypoglycemic, Metformin, for diabetes, and is otherwise healthy. A focused assessment was documented during his last clinic visit 6 months ago.

Alternative A

Mr. El-Kebbi has recently lost his wife and only child in an automobile accident where he was the only survivor.

- Why would a social assessment of the individual be important for this patient?

- Explain why a spiritual assessment of this patient would be important.

Alternative B

Mr. El-Kebbi was seriously injured when a boiler blew up at work. He lost an arm in the accident and is now leaving the hospital to finish recovering at home.

- What might Mr. El-Kebbi's concept of health have been before the accident?

- What might Mr. El-Kebbi's concept of health be after the accident?

- Why would it be important to assess support systems for Mr. El-Kebbi?

- Why would a community assessment be appropriate for this patient?

DOCUMENTATION

Form for Use in Practice

Patient Name _____ Date _____

Date of Birth _____

Initial Survey

Reason for seeking health care:_____

History of present illness

- Location:
- Intensity:
- Duration:
- Description:
- Aggravating factors:
- Alleviating factors:
- Functional impairment:
- Pain goal:

Vital signs: T (route)_____ P (with site)_____ R_____ BP (site)_____ SpO$_2$_____

Weight: _____ Height: _____ BMI: _____

History/Interview:

- Family history:
- History of major health problems:
- Medications and supplements:
- Smoking history:
- Recreational drugs:
- Occupational and environmental exposure:
- Allergies:
- Influenza or pneumococcal vaccine:
- Travel outside of United States in last 6 months:

Health Care Practices Assessment:

1. In what prevention activities do you engage to maintain your health?
2. Who in your family takes responsibility for your health?
3. What over-the-counter medicines do you use?
4. What herbal teas and folk medicines do you use?
5. For what conditions do you use herbal medicines?
6. What do you usually do when you are in pain?
7. How do you express your pain?
8. How are people in your culture viewed or treated when they have mental illness?
9. How are people with physical disabilities treated in your culture?
10. What do you do when you are sick? Stay in bed, continue your normal activities, etc.?

11.	What are your beliefs about rehabilitation?
12.	How are people with chronic illnesses viewed or treated in your culture?
13.	Are you averse to blood transfusions?
14.	Is organ donation acceptable to you?
15.	Are you an organ donor?
16.	Would you consider having an organ transplant if needed?

Spiritual Assessment:

1.	What is your religion?
2.	Do you consider yourself deeply religious?
3.	How many times a day do you pray?
4.	What do you need in order to say your prayers?
5.	Do you meditate?
6.	What gives strength and meaning to your life?
7.	In what spiritual practices do you engage for your physical and emotional pain?

Signature_____ Date _____

Assessment of Human Violence

This chapter provides basic information on human violence related to assessment, safety, prevention, and recovery. It describes many different types of violence, their prevalence rates, and physical and psychological effects. The chapter explores important screening and assessment techniques, such as observation for signs and symptoms of violence and interview strategies, both of which are used to collect subjective and objective data. The last part of the chapter provides information on nursing interventions related to safety, recovery, and healing.

READING ASSIGNMENT

Read Chapter 12 in Jensen's *Nursing Health Assessment: A Best-Practice Approach.*

VOCABULARY/TERMINOLOGY

- **Bullying:** Verbal and physical violence common among school-age and adolescent populations. Behaviors can range from teasing to physical assault.

- **Child maltreatment:** A wide range of abusive and neglectful behaviors toward children.

- **Elder abuse:** Maltreatment of older adults in the form of abuse, neglect, financial exploitation, or abandonment. Abuse includes intentional actions by a caregiver or other person who stands in a trust relationship to a vulnerable elder that cause harm or create a serious risk to him or her. Examples include kicking, punching, slapping, or burning.

- **Family violence:** All types of violent crime committed by an offender who is related to the victim either biologically or legally through marriage or adoption.

- **Hate crime:** Crime in which a victim is selected based on a characteristic such as race, ethnicity, sexual orientation, age, and the like and for which the perpetrator provides evidence that hate prompted him or her to commit the crime.

- **Human trafficking:** The recruitment, transportation, transfer, harboring, or receipt of people by threats, force, coercion, or deception.

- **Intimate partner violence (IPV):** Behaviors between spouses or nonmarital partners involving threatened or actual physical or sexual violence, psychological/emotional abuse, and/or coercive tactics when there has been prior physical or sexual violence.

- **Protective influences:** Factors in the environment that serve as protection against violence for the patient.

- **Punking:** Verbal and physical violence, humiliation, and shaming, usually done in public or with an audience.

- **Reframing:** A communication technique that changes the way others view something or someone.

- **Safety plan:** A formalized plan made by the victim of human violence to provide for personal safety and the safety of any children.

- **Sexual violence:** Forced sex in dating and marital relationships, gang rape, sexual harassment, inappropriate touching or molestation, sex with a patient, or forced prostitution and/or exposure to sexually explicit behavior.

- **Sibling violence:** Violence between and among siblings.

- **Victimization:** To make another person a victim.

- **War/combat violence:** Witnessing the killing of human beings, including friends and fellow service-people, intentionally killing and injuring other humans, and being intentionally injured or potentially killed by another human.

- **Youth violence:** Violence in and around schools and neighborhoods.

STUDY GUIDE

Activity A FILL IN THE BLANK

> bullying; child maltreatment; elder abuse; family violence; hate crimes; intimate partner violence; school violence; sibling violence; violence against adults with disabilities.

1. Write the correct term from the box above next to the description of the human violence it identifies. Choices are listed alphabetically.

   A. Abuse of children by parents

   _____

   B. Abuse in which the victim is biologically related to the offender or is or was related to him or her through marriage, adoption, or legal guardianship

   _____

   C. Abuse that includes intentional actions by a caregiver

   _____

   D. Violence among the most common type that children experience

   _____

   E. Daily nonfatal crimes such as theft and simple assault, as well as serious violent crime

   _____

F. Abuse in the form of verbal violence common among middle- and high-school girls

_____

G. Violent behaviors between spouses or nonmarital partners

_____

H. Group more likely to experience severe and long-term abuse, be victims of multiple violent episodes, and be abused by many perpetrators

_____

I. Psychological and emotional violence as the most common forms

_____

2. List common entry points, as described in the text, for assessment of victims of human violence:

   A. _____

   B. _____

   C. _____

   D. _____

Activity B MATCHING

1. *Match the nursing diagnosis associated with human violence with the appropriate nursing intervention.*

Answer	Diagnosis	Intervention
	1. Risk for post-trauma syndrome related to sibling abuse	**A.** Know and follow policies and procedures concerning violence.
	2. Risk for violence directed at others	**B.** Assess maternal depression.
	3. Impaired parenting related to abuse	**C.** Acknowledge the emotions experienced during stressful times.
	4. Rape-trauma syndrome related to sibling abuse	**D.** Determine any cuts, bruises, bleeding, lacerations, or other signs of injury.
	5. Dysfunctional family processes related to child neglect	**E.** Document according to forensic standards.

2. *Match the goals with the patient education topics.*

Answers	Goals		Patient Education Topics

Goals

1. Reduce the proportion of persons living in homes with loaded and unlocked firearms.

2. Reduce firearm-related deaths.

3. Reduce non-fatal firearm-related injuries.

4. Reduce maltreatment and maltreatment fatalities of children.

5. Reduce the rate of physical assault by current or former intimate partners.

6. Reduce the annual rate of rape or attempted rape.

7. Reduce physical assaults.

8. Reduce physical fighting among adolescents.

9. Reduce sexual assault other than rape.

10. Reduce weapon-carrying by adolescents on school property.

Patient Education Topics

A. Assess for physical assault, controlling behaviors, and isolation. Teach about safety and healthy relationships.

B. Assess for depression, suicide, domestic violence, and community violence.

C. Assess for safety and red flags of physical abuse. Teach about healthy communication and safety plans.

D. Assess for signs of bullying and punking. Teach about healthy communication skills, bullying, and safety.

E. Assess safety. Teach about gun violence and safety. Report cases of weapons in schools

F. Teach firearm safety.

G. Assess individual and family firearm use. Teach firearm safety.

H. Assess for human violence and neglect. Assess individual and family weapons use.

I. Assess for sexual assault or rape. Teach about healthy boundaries, relationships, communication skills, and safety planning.

J. Assess for red flags that may indicate child sexual abuse. Teach children about safe touch, healthy relationships, and safety.

Activity C SHORT ANSWER

1. Briefly discuss common psychological red flags that mask human violence.

_____

_____

_____

_____

2. Briefly explain the statement "Assessment findings are similar and different among violence survivors."

_____

_____

_____

_____

3. Discuss documentation of assessed violence in a patient. Include insight into needed subjective and objective data.

_____

_____

_____

_____

4. Explain mandated reporting.

_____

_____

_____

_____

5. Why is it necessary to assess for human violence from a cultural perspective?

_____

_____

_____

_____

6. Explain the need for safety planning. Include the basic components of a safety plan.

_____

_____

_____

_____

7. Discuss poly-victimization. Include the percentage of children involved and the definition of the term.

_____

_____

_____

_____

8. Explain why female immigrants are especially vulnerable to IPV.

_____

_____

_____

_____

Activity D   MULTIPLE CHOICE

1. When assessing for human violence in patients, it is important for the nurse to
   A. assess only older adults
   B. only assess male patients
   C. reexamine assumptions and stereotypes
   D. become familiar with research on immigrants

2. A nurse is working in the emergency department and a 6 month old is brought in by ambulance. The child is unresponsive. The mother is distraught. What symptom should make the nurse suspect shaken baby syndrome?
   A. Black eye(s)
   B. Bruising of extremities
   C. Sternal fracture
   D. Retinal hemorrhages

3. A class is working on a project focused on femicide. What would the class report about statistics related to male perpetrators of femicide?
   A. 99%
   B. 97%
   C. 93%
   D. 91%

4. What is the main reason for human trafficking?
   A. Sexual exploitation
   B. Forced marriage
   C. Cheap labor
   D. Sweatshop factories

5. Who are people who have experienced war violence?
   A. Infants born in nonparticipative nations
   B. Those who escaped war
   C. Older adults whose grandchildren are in the armed services
   D. Those who emigrate before the fighting starts

6. The risk factors for violence identified by *Healthy People* include what?
   A. Being male
   B. Long work hours
   C. Discrimination
   D. College education

7. When assessing a patient for human violence, what basic technique would the nurse need to review?
   A. Demonstrate compassion.
   B. Use a close family member of the patient as an interpreter.
   C. Speak slowly and softly, but with authority.
   D. Position self below the patient's eye level.

ALTERNATIVE CASE STUDY SCENARIOS

Sue Brown is a 24-year-old, middle-class Caucasian woman being interviewed by a psychiatric nurse practitioner at a day-treatment substance-abuse program. Sue, who tells the nurse that she prefers to be called by her first name, is dependent on opiates to treat chronic back pain from a car accident. When Sue was a child, her father traveled for work frequently; her mother stayed at home. Sue was an athlete in high school and attended 1 year of college before dropping out. She has seen health care professionals throughout her life for routine examinations, injuries, sexually transmitted infections (STIs), and dental care. Sue lives with her parents and brother and works part time as a grocery checker.

Alternative A

Sue has been declared disabled within the last 6 months because her back problems are worsening and she can no longer do gainful employment.

- Why would a human violence assessment be important for Sue?

- For what types of human violence is Sue at risk?

Alternative B

Sue has been married for 2 years and has an infant son. Sue brings the infant to the pediatrician's office several times because he has "fallen off the bed," "climbed out of his highchair," or "climbed out of his stroller."

- The nurse should suspect what with this child?

- What documentation is necessary to place in this patient's chart?

- What action is the nurse required to take by law?

DOCUMENTATION

Form for Use in Practice

Patient Name _____ Date _____

Date of Birth: _____

Initial Survey

Reason for seeking health care:_____

History of present illness:

- Location:

- Intensity:

- Duration:

- Description:

- Aggravating factors:

- Alleviating factors:

- Functional impairment:

- Pain goal:

Vital signs: T (route)_____   P (with site)_____   R_____   BP (site)_____   SpO$_2$_____

Weight: _____   Height: _____   BMI: _____

History/Interview:

- Family history:

- History of major health problems:

- Medications and supplements:

- Smoking history:

- Recreational drugs:

- Occupational and environmental exposure:

- Allergies:

- Influenza or pneumococcal vaccine:

Common Indicators of Possible Abuse or Neglect

Symptom	Yes	No	Additional data
Injuries not consistent with the story of their cause			
Sexual activity in a child younger than 14 years			
Inadequate supervision			
Serious injury			
Failure to seek timely medical care			
Multiple hospital or clinic visits for injuries			
Multiple previous fractures			
Bruises in multiple stages of healing			

Guide for Use in Practice

If any indication of any kind of abuse is suspected or assessed during the subjective or objective assessment of the patient, ask him or her to answer the following questions:

1. **Within the last year,** have you been hit, slapped, kicked, or otherwise physically hurt by someone? YES/NO
   If YES, by whom? _____
   Total number of times _____

2. **Since you've been pregnant,** have you been hit, slapped, kicked, or otherwise physically hurt by someone? YES/NO
   If YES, by whom? _____
   Total number of times _____

3. **Within the last year,** has anyone forced you to have sexual activities? YES/NO
   If YES, by whom? _____
   Total number of times _____

Score each of the following incidents according to the following scale. If any of the descriptions for the higher number apply, use the higher number.

1 = Threats of abuse, including use of a weapon
2 = Slapping, pushing; no injuries and/or lasting pain
3 = Punching, kicking, bruises, cuts and/or continuing pain
4 = Beating up, severe contusions, burns, broken bones
5 = Head injury, internal injury, permanent injury
6 = Use of weapon; wound from weapon

Developed by the Nursing Research Consortium on Violence and Abuse. Readers are encouraged to reproduce and use this assessment tool.

CHAPTER 13

Skin, Hair, and Nails Assessment

OBJECTIVE SUMMARY

This chapter reviews the normal anatomy and physiology of the skin, hair, and nails; common variations of normal integumentary findings; and findings related to systemic disorders. It outlines data collection strategies related to common skin lesions, alterations in skin integrity, risk factors for skin cancer, current health-promotion practices, and wound assessment. It presents a systematic method for skin assessment, and strategies for interweaving assessment of the skin with the examination of other systems. This chapter discusses strategies for accurately documenting subjective and objective findings of the skin, hair, and nails, and presents information relating to health promotion and disease prevention, such as skin self-assessment, dry skin care, pressure ulcer prevention, and skin protection.

READING ASSIGNMENT

Read Chapter 13 in Jensen's *Nursing Health Assessment: A Best-Practice Approach.*

VOCABULARY/TERMINOLOGY

- **ABCDE of melanoma detection:** Asymmetry; Border irregularity; Color; Diameter of more than 6 mm; Evolution of lesion over time.

- **Apocrine glands:** Glands in the axillae and genital area that open into hair follicles and become activated at puberty. They secrete a thick, milky sweat into hair follicles that, once mixed with bacterial skin flora, produce a characteristic musky odor.

- **Brawny skin:** Skin that is dark and leathery.

- **Bulla:** Fluid-filled lesion greater than 1 cm in circumference.

- **Café-au-lait macules:** Flat pigmented skin lesions.

- **Clubbing of the nails:** Finding in the nails that indicates chronic hypoxia.

- **Crust:** Dried secretions from a primary skin lesion.

- **Cyanosis:** Gray or blue skin color, indicating lack of oxygen.

- **Dermis:** The second layer of the skin, which acts to support the epidermis.

- **Dysplastic nevus:** An atypical mole.

- **Ecchymosis:** Bruise or bruising.

- **Eccrine glands:** Glands that cover most of the body, with the exception of the nailbeds, lip margins, glans penis, and labia minora. They are most numerous on the palms and soles, open directly onto the skin surface, and secrete a weak saline solution (*sweat*) in response to environmental or psychological stimuli.

- **Epidermis:** Outermost layer of the skin.

- **Erosion:** Loss of the epidermis, usually not extending into the dermis or subcutaneous layer.

- **Erythema:** Redness.

- **Excoriation:** Lesion resulting from scratching or excessive rubbing of the skin or a discrete lesion.

- **Fissure:** Linear break in the skin surface, not related to trauma.

- **Flushing:** Turning red, as with fever.

- **Jaundice:** Yellowish discoloration of the skin and conjunctiva caused by a buildup of bilirubin in the body.

- **Keloid:** Excessive fibrous tissue replacement, resulting in an enlarged scar and deformity.

- **Lanugo:** Fine hair that may cover the newborn.

- **Lichenification:** Accentuation of normal skin lines resembling tree bark, commonly caused by excessive scratching.

- **Linea nigra:** A dark line that appears on the pregnant woman, usually disappears after childbirth, and extends from umbilicus to pubis.

- **Macule:** Flat, distinct, colored area of skin that is less than 10 mm in diameter and does not include a change in skin texture or thickness.

- **Malar rash:** Red macular lesions distributed over the forehead, cheeks, and chin, resembling the pattern of a butterfly.

- **Melanoma:** The most serious type of skin cancer, which develops in cells that produce melanin.

- **Melasma:** A blotchy discoloration on the face of pregnant women; also called "mask of pregnancy."

- **Nails:** Epidermal appendages that arise from a nail matrix in the epidermis, near the distal portions of each finger and toe.

- **Nodule:** Solid palpable lesion greater than 1 cm in diameter, often with some depth.

- **Pallor:** Paleness of the skin.

- **Papule:** Raised, defined lesion of any color, less than 1 cm in diameter.

- **Photoallergy:** Reaction to the sun, often caused by a medication, that manifests with blisters and redness on exposed skin and occurs only after repeated exposure to offending substance. It persists for some time after removal of the offending substance, UV exposure, or both.

- **Photosensitivity:** Rash that appears after exposure to the sun.

- **Phototoxicity:** Reaction caused by a drug's molecules absorbing energy from a particular UV wavelength and then damaging surrounding tissues. The result is marked and severely tender sunburn.

- **Plaque:** Raised, defined lesion of any color, greater than 1 cm in diameter.

- **Pressure ulcer:** Loss of skin surface, extending into dermis, subcutaneous tissue, fascia, muscle, bone, or all of these.

- **Primary lesions:** Reddened lesions that arise from previously normal skin and include maculae, papules, nodules, tumors, polyps, wheals, blisters, cysts, pustules, and abscesses. May be further described as nonelevated, elevated-solid, or fluid-filled.

- **Pruritis:** Itching.

- **Purpura:** Red or purple skin discolorations that do not blanch when pressure is applied. They are caused by bleeding underneath the skin. Purpura measure 0.3 to 1.0 cm.

- **Pustule:** Purulent fluid-filled raised lesion of any size.

- **Scale:** Rapid turnover of epidermal layer, resulting in accumulation and delayed shedding of outermost epidermis.

- **Scar:** Fibrous replacement of lost skin structure.

- **Sebaceous glands:** Glands located throughout the body, except the palms and soles, that open into hair follicles and secrete *sebum* (oil-like substance that assists the skin in moisture retention and friction protection).

- **Secondary lesions:** Skin changes that appear following a primary lesion (eg, formation of scar tissue, crusts from dried burn vesicles).

- **Self-skin examination:** An examination of the skin that the patient himself or herself performs to identify potentially problematic lesions.

- **Subcutaneous layer:** Innermost skin layer; provides insulation, storage of calorie reserves, and cushioning against external forces. Composed mainly of fat and loose connective tissue, it also contributes to the skin's mobility.

- **Sunblocks:** Substances applied to the skin to deflect rays from absorption.

- **Sunscreens:** Substances applied to the skin to absorb harmful UV rays. They need to be applied every 2 hours for maximum protection.

- **Tenting:** A persistent pinch.

- **Terminal hair:** Darker and coarser hair than vellus hair. It varies in length and is generally found on the scalp, brows, and eyelids. In postpubertal people, terminal hair is found on the axillae, perineum, and legs; on postpubertal males, it also appears on the chest and abdomen.

- **Turgor:** Skin's ability to change shape and return to normal (elasticity). Used to assess the status of fluid loss or dehydration in the body.

- **Ultraviolet light index:** The scale that rates exposure to ultraviolet light.

- **Uremic frost:** Precipitation of renal urea and nitrogen waste products through sweat onto the skin.

- **Vellus hair:** Fine, short, hypopigmented hair located all over the body.

- **Vernix:** Cheese-like substance comprised of shed epithelial cells and sebum; can cover the skin of a newborn.

- **Vesicle:** Fluid-filled lesion less than 1 cm in diameter.

- **Vitiligo:** Skin condition characterized by areas of no pigmentation.

- **Wheal:** Raised, flesh-colored or reddened edematous papules or plaques, varying in size and shape.

STUDY GUIDE

Activity A FILL IN THE BLANK

1. Finish these statements about the epidermis.
   A. The stratum germinativum contains _____ and _____.
   B. Keratinocytes are chiefly composed of keratin, a tough _____ providing the epidermis with resistance to friction and trauma.
   C. Larger amounts of _____ produce darker skin and hair, whereas larger amounts of _____ are responsible for lighter skin and lighter hair.

D. Thickness of the epidermis remains constant throughout the _____ and across _____.
E. As the skin's outermost layer, the epidermis functions as the body's first line of defense against _____, _____, and _____.

2. Finish these statements about the hair and nails.
   A. _____ muscles attached to each hair follicle contract in response to environmental and nervous stimuli, causing the hair and follicle to be erect.
   B. The shape of the hair shaft determines the curliness of hair, with oval shape producing _____ hair than rounded shape.
   C. The nails arise from a nail matrix in the _____ of the skin, near the distal portions of each finger and toe.
   D. The nail bed is _____ and visible as a _____ through the transparent nail plate.

Activity B MATCHING

1. *Match the wound classification with its description.*

Answer	Wound Classification	Description
	1. Proliferative phase	A. Begins within 30 minutes of injury and lasts approximately 2–3 days
	2. Infected	
	3. Clean-contaminated	B. Wounds made under sterile conditions and not at risk for infection
	4. Inflammatory phase	
	5. Clean	C. Begins at end of inflammatory phase and may last up to 4 weeks
	6. Infected	
	7. Remodeling phase	D. Begins at end of proliferative phase and may last as long as 2 years
		E. Wounds that have been exposed to contaminants

F. Wounds that have been exposed to contaminants or exhibit evidence of infection prior to surgery

G. Wounds made under sterile conditions but involve the respiratory, gastrointestinal, genital, or urinary tracts without unusual contamination

2. *Match the intervention with the nursing diagnosis.*

Answer	Intervention	Nursing Diagnosis
	1. Document wound assessment.	**A.** Risk for infection
	2. Provide alternatives such as distraction, breathing, and relaxation.	**B.** Impaired skin integrity
	3. Apply appropriate dressing.	**C.** Impaired tissue integrity
	4. Protect wound with dressing.	**D.** Pain related to tissue injury and treatments

Activity C LABELING

1. For each photo, identify the type of skin lesion.

A.

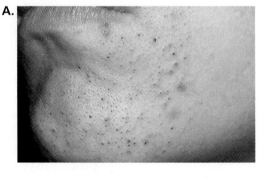

B.

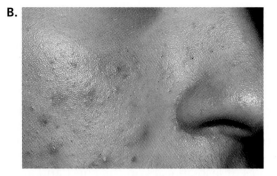

C.

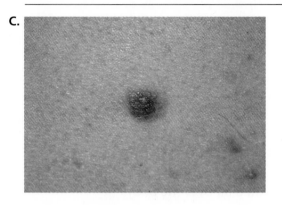

D.

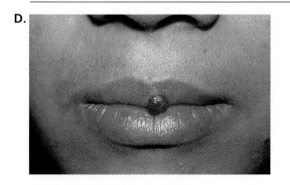

E.

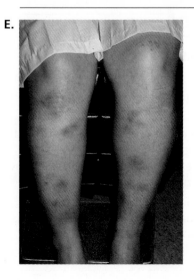

F.

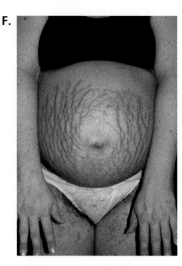

_____

Activity D **SHORT ANSWER**

1. Explain the Braden Scale for assessing skin breakdown.

   _____
   _____
   _____
   _____

2. Identify two common nursing diagnoses associated with skin problems.

   _____
   _____
   _____
   _____

3. Discuss the basics of performing a skin evaluation, including normal and possible abnormal findings.

   _____
   _____
   _____
   _____

4. Explain the categorization of skin lesions as primary or secondary. Give examples of each.

   _____
   _____
   _____
   _____

5. Discuss the risks of tattooing.

   _____
   _____
   _____
   _____

6. When does the nurse have a perfect time to assess the need for and provide patient education teaching? Include the main focus of patient teaching for the integumentary system.

   _____
   _____
   _____
   _____

7. Explain the need for an acute assessment of the skin.

   _____
   _____
   _____
   _____

Activity E **MULTIPLE CHOICE**

1. The nurse is admitting a 79-year-old man for outpatient surgery. The patient has bruises in various stages of healing all over his body. Why is it important for the nurse to report these findings to the surgeon?

   A. The patient may have been abused.

   B. The patient is elderly.

   C. The patient may have a clotting disorder.

   D. The patient may have suffered frequent falls.

2. A new nurse on the long-term care unit is learning how to assess a patient for skin breakdown. What would be the most likely instrument this nurse would use?

   A. Newton scale

   B. Blackden scale

   C. Norton scale

   D. Braden scale

3. A nurse in a dermatology clinic cares for adolescent patients with multiple purulent fluid-filled lesions on their faces, shoulders, backs, and chests. What is the most likely medical diagnosis for these patients?

   A. Cystic acne

   B. Pustular acne

   C. Bullous impetigo

   D. Chicken pox

4. When documenting that a patient has freckles, the appropriate term to use is

   A. macules

   B. patches

   C. vesicles

   D. bullae

5. A patient with a zosteriform rash has a rash that

   A. has lesions distributed over a large body area

   B. appears with a single lesion in close proximity to a larger lesion, as if "orbiting" the larger lesion

   C. is distributed along a dermatome

   D. is distributed equally on both sides of the body

6. A mother brings her 4-year-old daughter to the clinic and reports that the child has developed a rash that she is constantly scratching on her abdomen. On examination, the nurse finds that the rash is serpiginous. The nurse would know that the rash is most probably caused by

   A. scabies

   B. lice

   C. ticks

   D. allergies

7. A community health nurse is planning an educational event for the parent-teacher association of the local elementary school. In discussing chicken pox, how would the nurse describe the rash?

   A. Fluid-filled lesions greater than 1 cm in diameter

   B. Purulent fluid-filled raised lesions of any size

   C. Raised, reddened edematous papules or plaques, varying in size and shape

   D. Fluid-filled lesions less than 1 cm in diameter

ALTERNATIVE CASE SCENARIOS

Remember Mr. Stoli, the 65-year-old Russian immigrant, who is currently hospitalized with a venous ulcer. He has been on the acute care unit since yesterday and is scheduled to have a wound vacuum applied later today. Current medications include a thiazide diuretic for high blood pressure, platelet inhibitor for peripheral vascular disease (PVD), and insulin for type 2 diabetes mellitus. The nurse documented assessment findings for Mr. Stoli last shift. The patient's temperature was 37.4°C orally, pulse 92 beats/min, respirations 16 breaths/min, and blood pressure 142/78 mm Hg.

Alternative A

Mr. Stoli calls the nurse and tells her he has developed a rash on his abdomen. On inspecting Mr. Stoli's abdomen, the nurse finds a serpentine rash. Mr. Stoli complains of urticaria. The nurse suspects scabies.

- What nursing diagnosis do you propose based on the data above?

- How will the nurse validate this diagnosis?

- What interventions might be indicated based upon the suspected diagnosis?

Alternative B

Mr. Stoli has been transferred to a long-term care facility. His venous ulcer is healing nicely and he is scheduled to go home in 2 days. He gets up during the night to go to the bathroom and he falls, striking his lower left leg on the bedside commode, causing a 1-inch laceration. When Mr. Stoli sees his physician for a routine follow-up, he is found to have an area of swelling, redness, warmth, and tenderness.

- What would be an appropriate nursing diagnosis for this patient?

- What nursing interventions would you propose to use for this patient?

DOCUMENTATION

Form for Use in Practice

Patient Name _____ Date _____

Date of Birth _____

Initial Survey

Reason for seeking health care:_____

History of present illness

- Location:
- Intensity:
- Duration:
- Description:
- Aggravating factors:
- Alleviating factors:
- Functional impairment:
- Pain goal:

Vital signs: T (route)_____ P (site)_____ R_____ BP (site)_____ SpO$_2$ _____

Weight: _____ Height: _____ BMI: _____

General appearance: _____

General level of distress: _____

Risk Factors and History:

- Do you have any family history of integumentary problems?
- Have you ever been diagnosed with an integumentary disease?
- Are you taking any medications for integumentary problems?
- Are you taking any natural supplements or over-the-counter medications?
- Do you smoke cigarettes or use other tobacco products?
- Has anyone ever told you that you have high blood pressure?
- Has anyone ever told you that you have high blood cholesterol?
- Do you have a history of diabetes mellitus?
- What is your usual weight? What is your height?
- What is your usual level of physical activity?
- What is your typical diet?
- How much alcohol do you usually drink per day? Week? Month?
- Do you use any recreational drugs such as cocaine?

Common Symptoms:

Symptom	Yes	No	Additional data
Pruritis			
Rash (multiple lesions)			
Single lesions or wounds			

Physical Assessment:

Inspect all body areas. Begin at the crown of the head, part the hair to visualize the scalp, and progress caudally to the feet.
Assess undersides of feet and separate toes. Note general skin color.
Inspect for any lesions. If observed, identify configuration, pattern, morphology, size, distribution, and exact body location.
Identify any infections, using infection-control principles.
Note any inflammatory lesions.
Assess for any infestations.
Observe for growths, tumors, or vascular or other miscellaneous lesions.
Inspect any wounds or incisions. If observed, note shape; measure length, width, and depth with a ruler.
Describe any wounds related to trauma. Assess status of blood supply to the skin, making note of any bleeding or ecchymosis (bruising).
Identify risk for skin breakdown (especially in hospitalized or inactive patients).
Classify wound as partial or full thickness; if a pressure ulcer is present, identify the stage.
Document ulcer features: Size: Margins: Surrounding tissues: Any varicosities or telengectasias: Granulation tissue: Drainage, odor, or necrotic tissue: Amount, color, consistency, odor of exudate: Location: Pain:
Assess for nonpressure ulcers; note the characteristics of the wound.
Classify any burns based on depth of tissue destruction and percentage of total body surface area (TBSA) affected.
Inspect each fingernail and toenail. Assess for color, thickness, and consistency.
Assess the nail angle.
Inspect the hair. Color: Consistency: Distribution: Hair loss: Hair shaft:
Note areas of decreased or absent hair. Note any lesions or color changes there. Observe hair shafts near the root for lice or nits.
Using the dorsal surface of the hands, assess skin temperature.

Using the palmar surface of the fingers and hands, assess for skin moisture and texture.
Assess skin turgor.
Assess for vascularity by applying direct pressure to the skin surface with the pads of your fingers.
Palpate lesions for tenderness, mobility, and consistency.
Palpate each fingernail and toenail.
Palpate the hair. Grasp 10–12 hairs and gently pull.

Signature_____ Date _____

Guide for Use in Practice

Technique	Normal Findings	Abnormal Findings
Inspect all body areas, beginning at crown of head, parting hair to visualize scalp, and progressing caudally to feet. Assess undersides of feet; separate toes. Note general skin color.	*Pigmentation consistent throughout the body. Patients with darker skin may normally have hypopigmented skin on the palms and soles.*	Changes in pigmentation in any areas. Vitiligo, flushing, erythema, cyanosis, pallor, rubor, brawny, jaundice, uremic frost.
Inspect for any lesions. If observed, identify configuration, pattern, morphology, size, distribution, and exact body location.	*Freckles, birth marks, skin tags, moles, and cherry angiomas*	Configuration of lesions: annular, arciform, iris, linear, polymorphous, punctuate, serpiginous, nummular/discoid, umbilicated, filiform, verrucaform. Pattern: asymmetric, confluent, diffuse, discrete, generalized, grouped, localized, satellite, symmetric, or zosteriform.
Identify any infections.	*None*	Acne, cellulitis, impetigo, German measles, herpes simplex, measles, pityriasis rosea, roseola, warts, candida, tinea corporis, and tinea versicolor.
Note any inflammatory lesions.	*None*	Psoriasis, eczema, contact dermatitis, urticaria, allergic drug reaction, insect bites, or seborrhea.
Observe for growths, tumors, or vascular or other miscellaneous lesions.	*None noted*	Moles or nevi, skin tags, lipoma, lentigo, actinic keratosis, basal cell cancer, squamous cell cancer, malignant melanoma, Kaposi's sarcoma, vascular lesions (eg, hemangiomas, nevus flammeus, spider or star angiomas, venous lake).
Inspect any wounds or incisions.	*Patient has no wounds or a wound is healing, as evidenced by pink to red tissue.*	Partial-thickness wounds; full-thickness wounds; yellow, white, brown, or black (eschar) necrotic tissue. Pale tissue. Surrounding area inflamed and red or pale with poor circulation.
Describe any wounds related to trauma. Assess status of blood supply to the skin, making note of any bleeding or ecchymosis (bruising).	*None*	Petechiae, purpurae, ecchymoses, hematomas, lacerations, abrasions, puncture wounds, or avulsions.

Identify risk for skin breakdown.	*Patient scores 14 or above on Norton scale or 18 or above on Braden scale.*	Score <14 on the Norton scale and 14–18 on the Braden scale.
Assess for nonpressure ulcers; note wound characteristics.	*No evidence of this finding*	Neuropathic, venous (vascular), or arterial ulcers.
Inspect each fingernail and toenail. Assess for color, thickness, and consistency.	*Nails smooth, translucent, and consistent in coloration and thickness. Longitudinal ridging is common in aging patients. Longitudinal pigmentation in dark-skinned patients is normal.*	Splitting of nail tips; thickened nails; discoloration of the nailbed.
Assess nail angle.	*Diamond-shaped opening is visible between the two fingernails, indicating a nail angle of at least 160 degrees.*	Clubbing of the nails (angle of the nail to the finger is more than 160 degrees).
Inspect hair, noting color, consistency, distribution, areas of hair loss, and condition of the hair shaft.	*Hair is equally and symmetrically distributed across the scalp. Shafts are smooth, shiny, of even consistency, and without evidence of breakage.*	Hair in the beard area, abdomen, upper back, shoulders, sternum, and inner upper thighs on female patients.
Note areas of decreased or absent hair. Note any lesions or color changes of the scalp. Observe hair shafts near the root for lice or nits.	*Scalp skin is of consistent color with rest of the body.*	Brittle or broken hair shafts. Lice or their nits (eggs) on the hair shaft. Excessive dryness and scaling of the scalp.
Using the dorsal surface of the hands, assess skin temperature.	*Temperature is consistently warm or cool, and appropriate for environment.*	Increased temperature, lesions, swelling, color changes.
Using the palmar surface of the fingers and hands, assess for skin moisture and texture.	*Moisture is consistent throughout, with evenly smooth skin texture.*	Excessive dryness. Excessive moisture. Cracked or fissured skin.
Assess skin turgor.	*Skin promptly recoils to its normal position.*	Skin is persistently pinched (tenting).
Assess for vascularity of the skin.	*On releasing your finger, color promptly returns to normal.*	Delayed return of the skin color to normal after direct pressure. Altered circulation can result in pallor or rubor of an extremity.
Palpate each fingernail and toenail.	*Nails are smooth, nontender, and firmly adherent to the nail bed. Lateral and proximal folds are nontender and nonswollen.*	Swelling, redness, or tenderness in the lateral or proximal folds. Sponginess of the nail bed.
Palpate the hair. Grasp 10–12 hairs and gently pull.	*Hair is smooth. Just a few hairs are in your hand.*	Excessive loss of hair (more than six hairs).

Head and Neck with Lymphatics Assessment

OBJECTIVE SUMMARY

This chapter describes assessment of the head and neck regions, exploring pertinent anatomy and physiology, as well as variations based on age, gender, and culture. Methods for collecting subjective and objective data related to skull or scalp injury, lymphatic function, and thyroid function are included. Other key components of the chapter include the signs and symptoms of headache, lymphadenopathy, and parathyroid and thyroid imbalances; correct techniques for inspection and palpation of the structures of the head and neck; and descriptions of common normal and abnormal findings.

READING ASSIGNMENT

Read Chapter 14 in Jensen's *Nursing Health Assessment: A Best-Practice Approach*.

VOCABULARY/TERMINOLOGY

- **Anterior triangle:** Area of the neck between the sternocleidomastoid muscle and midline of the neck.

- **Cranium:** The collective bones of the head. The term skull is used synonymously.

- **Fontanels:** Membrane-covered spaces between the bones of the cranium in the infant.

- **Graves' disease:** Severe hyperthyroidism.

- **Lymph nodes:** Small oval structures throughout the body that filter bacteria and viruses and help to fight infection. They normally range in size from very tiny (less than 1 mm) to more than 1 cm. Lymph nodes of the head and neck region are some of the most accessible to physical examination.

- **Macrocephaly:** Enlargement of the head, usually from obstruction of the flow of cerebrospinal fluid.

- **Mandible:** Lower jaw.

- **Maxilla:** Upper jaw.

- **Microcephaly:** Smaller than normal head size, noted at birth and associated with underdevelopment of the brain and mental retardation.

- **Nasolabial folds:** Slight prominence of tissue between the nose and lips; should be symmetrical upon inspection.

- **Posterior triangle:** Area of the neck between the sternocleidomastoid muscle and trapezius muscles.

- **Salivary glands:** Three pairs of glands that secrete saliva into the mouth: parotid, sublingual, and submandibular.

- **Sternocleidomastoid muscle:** Large muscle attached to the sternum and clavicle inferiorly and mastoid process of the temporal bone superiorly. This muscle separates the anterior and posterior triangles of the neck.

- **Sutures:** Flat joints between the bones of the skull. In the infant, these sutures are not calcified, allowing for skull bone and brain growth.
- **Trapezius muscle:** Large muscle of the upper back and posterior neck connected to the occipital bone superiorly and spinous processes of the thoracic and seventh cervical vertebrae inferiorly and the shoulder.

STUDY GUIDE

Activity A   FILL IN THE BLANK

1. Finish these statements about an acute assessment of the head and neck.

   A. Patients with acute head injuries and neurologic changes must be _____ and _____ assessed by the health care team.

   B. It is essential to keep the spine _____ _____to prevent spinal cord injury, and devices should not be removed until the spine is _____ of injury.

   C. Patients with severe headaches may be unable to provide a _____ _____, but a focused _____ and _____ examination looking for neurologic changes are _____ nursing behaviors.

   D. Patients experiencing a _____ _____ may present with neck pain—so any patient with sudden onset of neck or jaw pain should be evaluated.

2. List the signs/symptoms of hyperthyroidism.

   A. _____

   B. _____

   C. _____

   D. _____

   E. _____

   F. _____

   G. _____

   H. _____

Activity B   MATCHING

1. *Match the head and neck problem with its description.*

Answer	Problem	Description
	1. Acromegaly	A. Enlarged thyroid gland; can be associated with hyperthyroidism, hypothyroidism, or normal thyroid function.
	2. Bell's palsy	
	3. Parkinson's disease	
	4. Cushing's syndrome	B. Skin is firm and loses mobility, seemingly fixed to underlying tissues.
	5. Sclero-derma	
	6. Cerebral vascular accident	C. A "brain attack."
	7. Goiter	D. With severe hypothyroidism, patients present with periorbital swelling and edema of the face, hands, and feet.
	8. Myxedema	

E. Excessive production of exogenous ACTH results in a round "moon" facies, fat deposits at the nape of the neck, "buffalo hump," and sometimes a velvety discoloration around the neck (*acanthosis nigra*).

F. Paralysis, usually unilateral, of the facial nerve (CN VII); can be transient or permanent.

G. A mask-like facial appearance, rigid muscles, diminished reflexes, and a shuffling gait.

H. Thickening of the skin, subcutaneous tissue, and facial bones and coarsening of facial features.

2. *Match the intervention with the nursing diagnosis.*

Answer	Intervention	Nursing Diagnosis
	1. Gather data to help determine if cause is physiological or psychological.	**A.** Activity intolerance
	2. Assess characteristics.	**B.** Fatigue
	3. Teach patient it may take several weeks to notice a change.	**C.** Chronic pain
	4. Refer patient to physical therapy.	**D.** Knowledge deficit

Activity C   SHORT ANSWER

1. You are caring for a 36-year-old trauma victim following a motor vehicle collision. Both computed tomography and magnetic resonance imaging show no evidence of a spine injury. What would be your next nursing action and why?

_____

_____

_____

_____

2. Explain why hypothyroidism in an older adult often lacks the classic symptoms seen in a younger person.

_____

_____

_____

_____

3. Discuss why it is important to assess for hypothyroidism in a pregnant woman and what can happen if it goes undetected.

_____

_____

_____

_____

4. Explain what the finding of facial asymmetry might mean when inspecting the head.

_____

_____

_____

_____

5. Discuss hypothyroidism, including its signs and symptoms, and when a nurse should suspect it in a patient.

_____

_____

_____

_____

6. Explain why the diagnosis of a cervical spine injury is often difficult. Include identifying the people at risk and explaining why they are at risk.

_____

_____

_____

_____

7. Explain the fontanels found in the newborn skull at birth. Include their purpose and when they are supposed to close.

_____

_____

_____

_____

Activity D   MULTIPLE CHOICE

1. An Anatomy and Physiology instructor is discussing the lymphatic system of the head and neck. Why would the instructor emphasize the importance of the drainage pattern of the lymph?

A. Nurses need to follow lymph patterns to track the course of a disease.

B. The drainage pattern can help the nurse understand why the disease is spreading.

C. Enlargement of a node may be a sign of pathology that is from a distance.

D. The drainage pattern may help pinpoint the source of the pathology near the enlarged node.

2. When assessing the head and neck, the nurse should realize that variations in skull or neck shape or size relate most to what?

   A. Height and weight

   B. Ethnic background

   C. Cultural background

   D. Gender

3. The nurse in an emergency department is caring for a minimally responsive 27-year-old victim of a motorcycle accident. The patient was not wearing a helmet. When assessing the patient's head and neck, for what would the nurse be assessing?

   A. Strain

   B. Cyanosis

   C. Pallor

   D. Bleeding

4. A nurse is caring for a patient admitted with neck pain. The patient is febrile. What is the most likely medical diagnosis for this patient?

   A. Migraine

   B. Meningitis

   C. Macule

   D. Measles

5. The nurse is caring for a patient who comes to the clinic reporting a lump by her ear. What are the symptoms of a cancerous lymph node?

   A. Node is fixed and rubbery.

   B. Node is less than 1 cm in size and feels mushy.

   C. Node is soft and moves freely.

   D. Node matches the node on the opposite side of the body.

6. One of the goals of *Healthy People* related to the head and neck is to reduce activity limitation from chronic back conditions. What nursing intervention would be most appropriate?

   A. Teach rationale for assessing thyroid level.

   B. Encourage use of seatbelts.

   C. Teach proper posture, bending, and lifting.

   D. Teach back exercises.

7. A community health nurse is attending a seminar on headaches. What would this nurse learn is a red flag for headaches?

   A. Stiff neck

   B. Pain centered behind the eyes

   C. Pain that is longstanding

   D. Pain without new symptomatology

ALTERNATIVE CASE SCENARIOS

Faye Davis-Pierce, 21 years old, is visiting her college clinic for the first time with reports of fatigue and weight gain of 20 lb over the past 3 months. She is also concerned because her hair has been falling out. Her temperature is 36.8°C orally, pulse 64 beats/min, respirations 12 breaths/min, and blood pressure 98/66 mm Hg. Her height is 5 ft 8 in, weight is 208 lb, and BMI is 31.6 (obese). Current medications include an oral contraceptive and a multivitamin.

Alternative A

Based on the changes outlined below relative to the case of Faye Davis-Pierce, *consider what other outcomes, information, and problems would affect the overall picture and shape your responses.*

Subjective: Faye reports that she has gained 20 lb. In addition to weight gain and a period 7 weeks ago, Faye discloses that she is worried that she might be pregnant. She was away from school for a weekend, forgot her oral contraceptives, and missed two doses. She reports that she also feels nauseous some mornings.

Objective: Appears anxious.

- How will these findings change the focus of the subjective data collected?

- What other objective data will the nurse collect to rule out or confirm other diagnoses?

- What health promotion and learning needs are identified?

Alternative B

Subjective: Faye says that she handles stress by eating and that this semester is especially challenging. She rewards herself by having favorite foods, especially the desserts in the dorm. She knows that she should be exercising but does not have the energy to get to the gym. Her thyroid laboratory values are normal; a pregnancy test is negative.

Objective: Appears depressed.

- How will the nurse work with Faye Davis-Pierce to promote health and reduce risk for illness?

- How are the psychosocial and physiological issues related?

- Which nursing diagnosis is highest priority and what is the rationale?

DOCUMENTATION

Form for Use in Practice

Patient Name _____ Date _____

Date of Birth _____

Initial Survey

Reason for seeking health care: _____

History of present illness

- Location:

- Intensity:

- Duration:

- Description:

- Aggravating factors:

- Alleviating factors:

- Functional impairment:

- Pain goal:

Vital signs: T (route)_____ P (with site)_____ R_____ BP (site)_____ SpO$_2$_____

Weight: _____ Height: _____ BMI: _____

General appearance: _____

General level of distress: _____

Risk Factors and History:

- Have you ever had an accident that resulted in a loss of consciousness or head injury?

- Do you wear a seat belt?

- Do you wear a bicycle helmet?

- Were you ever treated with radiation to the neck, chest, or back?

- Have you had any surgeries involving your head or neck?

- Do you have a family history of thyroid problems?

  - Who had the illness?

  - Was it hypothyroidism or hyperthyroidism?

  - When did the person have it?

  - How was it treated?

  - What were the outcomes?

- Do you take any regular medications?
    - How much alcohol do you drink?
    - Do you take any herbal products?

Common Head and Neck Symptoms

Symptom	Yes	No	Additional data
Headache			
Neck pain			
Limited neck movement			
Facial pain			
Lumps or masses			
Hypothyroidism			

Physical Assessment:

Inspect the head.
Inspect facial features for symmetry and size.

Inspect the hair.
 	
    Distribution and quantity:
 	
    Texture:
 	
    Cleanliness:

Inspect the neck. • Neck muscles: • Sternocleidomastoid: • Thyroid: • Isthmus:
Palpate the temporal artery.
Palpate the scalp.
Palpate the thyroid (anterior or posterior).
Palpate for discernable lymph nodes in the head and neck: pre-auricular, posterior auricular, occipital, submental, submandibular, tonsilar, anterior cervical chain, posterior cervical chain, and supraclavicular. For any that is palpable, note: • Location: • Size: • Consistency: • Mobility: • Delimitation:
If the thyroid is enlarged, either unilaterally or bilaterally, auscultate over each lobe using the bell of the stethoscope.

Signature_____ Date _____

Guide for Use in Practice

Technique	Normal Findings	Abnormal Findings
Inspect the head.	*Head is centered, proportional to body (1/7), erect, and without tremors, tics, or unusual movements. Skull is round without obvious deformities. Neck muscles are symmetric.*	Facial asymmetry, enlarged bones or tissues, puffy "moon" face, increased facial hair in females, periorbital edema
Inspect facial features for symmetry and size.	*Nasolabial folds are symmetric.*	Asymmetric nasolabial folds; signs of trauma; lesions
Inspect the hair for, Distribution and quantity: Texture: Cleanliness:	*Hair is evenly distributed across the scalp, extending from superior aspect of the forehead to base of the cranium and top of the ears bilaterally.*	Male-pattern baldness, unusual distribution or patterns of hair growth on the face or skull, nits, lice
Inspect the neck Neck muscles Sternocleidomastoid Thyroid Isthmus (may be visualized with tangential light and asking the patient to swallow a sip of water)	*Trachea is midline. A slight symmetric elevation may be observed in the mid-neck.*	Thyroid enlargement or masses
Palpate the temporal artery in the space above the cheek bone near the scalp line.	*Temporal artery pulse is 2–3 on a 4-point scale.*	Temporal arteritis
Palpate the scalp.	*Scalp is symmetric without tenderness, masses, lesions, or differences in firmness.*	Bulging or depression of the bony structure of the scalp, bulging or depressed fontanels in infants
Palpate the thyroid, either from the anterior or posterior approach.	*If palpable, thyroid is smooth, rubbery, nontender, and symmetrical. It is barely palpable beneath the sternocleidomastoid muscle.*	Unilateral bulging, neck masses, unusual hardness or softness, tenderness
Palpate for discernable lymph nodes in the head and neck following a systematic pattern, usually pre-auricular, posterior auricular, occipital, submental, submandibular, tonsilar, anterior cervical chain, posterior cervical chain, and supraclavicular.	*Usually no lymph nodes are palpable in the adult. If palpable, describe location, size, consistency, mobility, and delimitation.*	Palpable, tender, and warm lymph nodes; hard, rubbery, irregular, fixed, and nontender lymph nodes
If the thyroid is enlarged, either unilaterally or bilaterally, auscultate over each lobe for a bruit using the bell of the stethoscope.	*No bruits or vascular sounds are audible.*	Bruits (most often found with *toxic goiter, hyperthyroidism,* or *thyrotoxicosis*)

15

Eyes Assessment

OBJECTIVE SUMMARY

This chapter reviews anatomy and physiology pertinent to ocular and visual function, along with key variations in eye assessment related to lifespan and culture. It explores subjective data collection for eye health, including assessment of risk factors and focused history related to common symptoms. Content on objective data collection includes correct techniques for assessing vision, ocular movements, the external eye, and exterior and interior ocular structures; normal and unexpected visual and ocular findings; and appropriate documentation. Tests of visual acuity are part of screening during the complete physical examination and ongoing assessments for patients with identified ocular and visual problems or diseases.

READING ASSIGNMENT

Read Chapter 15 in Jensen's *Nursing Health Assessment: A Best-Practice Approach*.

VOCABULARY/TERMINOLOGY

- **Amblyopia:** Condition in which the vision in one eye is reduced because the eye and brain are not working together. It is the most common cause of visual impairment in children.

- **Asthenopia:** Eye strain.

- **Blepharitis:** Inflammation of the margin of the eyelid.

- **Blindness:** Inability to see; loss of vision.

- **Cataract:** Opacity of the crystalline lens of the eye, which obstructs the passage of light.

- **Chalazion:** Cyst (meibomian gland lipogranuloma) in the eyelid resulting from inflammation of the meibomian gland.

- **Conjunctiva:** Clear membrane that covers the sclera (white part of the eye) and lines the inside of the eyelids.

- **Conjunctivitis:** Inflammation or infection of the transparent membrane (conjunctiva) that lines the eyelid and part of the eyeball.

- **Cornea:** Transparent front part of the eye that covers the iris, pupil, and anterior chamber.

- **Emmetropia:** Refractive index.

- **Exophthalmos:** Bulging of the eye anteriorly out of the orbit.

- **Extraocular muscles:** Muscles that control eye movement and hold the eye in place in the socket.

- **Glaucoma:** Disease in which the optic nerve is damaged, leading to progressive, irreversible loss of vision. It is often, but not always, associated with increased pressure of the eye.

- **Hordeolum:** Stye.

- **Hyperopia:** Farsightedness.

- **Iris:** Anatomical eye structure responsible for controlling the diameter and size of the pupils and the amount of light reaching them.

- **Jaeger test:** Acuity test for near vision.

- **Lacrimal apparatus:** Physiologic system containing the orbital structures for production and drainage; consists of the lacrimal gland and its excretory ducts, lacrimal canaliculi, lacrimal sac, nasolacrimal duct, and nerve supply.

- **Lens:** Optic device with perfect or approximate axial symmetry; transmits and refracts light, converging or diverging the beam.

- **Limbus:** Border between the cornea and sclera.

- **Macula:** Structure lateral to the optic disc, the area with the greatest concentration of cones.

- **Macular degeneration:** Disease that gradually causes loss of sharp central vision, needed for common daily tasks.

- **Myopia:** Nearsightedness.

- **Ophthalmoscope:** Instrument used to visualize the inner eye and its structures.

- **Optic disc:** Also called optic nerve head; location where ganglion cell axons exit the eye to form the optic nerve.

- **Palpebral fissure:** Almond-shaped open space between the eyelids.

- **Presbyopia:** Considered a natural part of aging; a condition that results from loss of elasticity of the crystalline lens. As this happens, the ciliary muscles that bend and straighten the lens lose their power to accommodate.

- **Pupil:** Opening in the center of the iris of the eye that allows light to enter the retina.

- **Retina:** Light-sensitive tissue lining the inner surface of the eye.

- **Retinopathy:** Damage to retinal blood vessels. The two most common causes are diabetes and hypertension.

- **Sclera:** White part of the eye.

- **Snellen's test:** Test using a Snellen's chart to measure visual acuity.

STUDY GUIDE

Activity A   FILL IN THE BLANK

1. Finish these statements about the extraocular structures of the eye.

   A. _____ are loose and mobile.

   B. The _____ is the almond-shaped open space between the eyelids.

   C. The lower eyelid's margin is at the _____ _____, which is the border between the cornea and sclera.

   D. The _____ _____ protects and lubricates the cornea and conjunctiva by producing and draining tears.

2. List the extraocular muscles that control the eyes.

   A. Elevates the eye upward and adducts and rotates the eye medially

   _____

   B. Rotates the eye downward and adducts and rotates the eye medially

   _____

   C. Turns the eye downward and abducts and rotates the eye laterally

   _____

   D. Moves the eye medially

   _____

   E. Turns the eye upward and abducts and turns the eye laterally

   _____

   F. Moves the eye laterally

   _____

Activity B   MATCHING

1. *Match the intraocular structure with its definition.*

Answer	Structure	Definition
	1. Choroid	**A.** Helps to maintain the size and shape of the eye
	2. Lens	
	3. Ciliary body	**B.** Permits light to enter the eye
	4. Sclera	**C.** Covers the recessed portion of the eye
	5. Iris	
	6. Pupil	**D.** Refracts and focuses light on to the retina
	7. Cornea	
		E. Contains the muscle that controls the shape of the lens
		F. Is transparent and avascular
		G. Regulates the amount of light that enters the pupil

2. *Match the intervention with the nursing diagnosis.*

Answer	Intervention	Nursing Diagnosis
	1. Remove hazards from room, such as razors and matches.	**A.** Disturbed visual sensory perception
	2. Teach patient to clear cords and furniture from pathways, and use good lighting.	**B.** Disturbed sensory perception
	3. Converse with and touch patient frequently.	**C.** Risk for injury

3. *Match the* **Healthy People** *goal related to vision with the appropriate nursing intervention.*

Answer	Goal	Intervention
	1. Reduce uncorrected visual impairment due to refractive errors.	**A.** Assess with each patient the use of safety equipment when playing sports.
	2. Reduce blindness and visual impairment in children and teens 17 years and younger.	**B.** Review importance of maintaining blood glucose levels in the normal range to reduce eye damage.
	3. Reduce occupational eye injury and increase the use of appropriate personal protective eyewear in recreational activities and hazardous situations around the home.	**C.** Emphasize proper eye protection, which can prevent many sports-related eye injuries.
	4. Increase the proportion of public and private schools that require use of appropriate head, face, eye, and mouth protection for students participating in school-sponsored physical activities.	**D.** Assess for family history of blindness or visual impairment.
	5. Increase the proportion of adults with diabetes who have an annual dilated eye examination.	**E.** Discuss with patients the need for vision screens.
	6. Reduce visual impairment due to diabetic retinopathy, glaucoma, and cataracts.	**F.** Discuss with patients the purpose and need for a dilated eye examination to establish the health of the retina.

Activity C **SHORT ANSWER**

1. A patient comes to the emergency department with an eye injury. Explain what the nurse would assess for in an acute assessment and what would constitute the need for an emergent referral.

_____

_____

_____

_____

2. Explain the changes that occur with the eyes of older adults and how these changes affect their vision.

_____

_____

_____

3. Explain the actions of the superior and inferior rectus muscles, including where they insert into the eye.

_____

_____

_____

_____

4. Explain how culture affects the eye.

_____

_____

_____

_____

5. Explain why it is important to ask the patient about diet when assessing eyes and vision.

_____

_____

_____

_____

6. Explain what risks you would assess when doing a risk assessment for the eye and what you can do to minimize the risk.

_____

_____

_____

_____

7. Discuss the difference between high velocity injuries to the eye and blunt force injuries to the eye. Include how they are treated.

_____

_____

_____

_____

Activity D MULTIPLE CHOICE

1. The nurse is caring for a 63-year-old Asian American who can neither read nor speak English. What would be the appropriate chart to use to assess this patient's vision?

   A. Allen

   B. Snellen E

   C. Ishihara

   D. PEARLA

2. A patient has a nursing diagnosis of disturbed visual sensory perception. Which of the following is the most appropriate outcome for this patient?

   A. Patient will remain independent in own home.

   B. Patient will obtain a Seeing Eye dog.

   C. Patient will obtain contact lenses to improve self-concept.

   D. Patient will remain free from harm resulting from a loss of vision.

3. A patient has been found to have abnormal vision. What would be the nurse's next step?

   A. Refer patient to ophthalmologist.

   B. Refer patient to social services to get money for glasses.

   C. Refer patient to Lions Club to get voucher for free glasses.

   D. Refer patient to optometrist.

4. A patient comes to the clinic, reporting that he woke up this morning with a painful right eye. What would be the most appropriate response from the nurse?

   A. "It is probably just allergies. If it still hurts in the morning call me."

   B. "A painful eye happens sometimes with allergies. Do you have allergies?"

   C. "You will need to see the doctor to have your eye checked."

   D. "Did you do anything different yesterday? You may have eye strain."

5. A patient asks a nurse if any foods promote eye health. What food would the nurse include as a response?

   A. Deep-water fish

   B. Low-fat meat

   C. Foods that contain lots of water (ie, watermelon)

   D. Multigrain foods

6. A 52-year-old patient with myopia calls the ophthalmology clinic very upset. She tells the nurse, "I keep seeing spots or something floating across my vision. What is wrong with me?" What would be the most appropriate response by the nurse?

   A. "It is not an uncommon finding in people older than 40 years for this to happen. They are called 'floaters'."

   B. "Please come into the clinic right away so we can see what is wrong."

   C. "Because it is almost five o'clock, please go to the emergency department right away. This sounds very serious."

   D. "I have an opening tomorrow at 2 in the afternoon. Can you come in then?"

7. An infant has red, dry, and irritated eyes. In what part of the eye are these findings consistent with a problem?

   A. Vitreous chamber

   B. Aqueous chamber

   C. Lacrimal apparatus

   D. Sinus

ALTERNATIVE CASE SCENARIOS

Mr. Harris, a 61-year-old African American man, is in the adult medicine clinic for a routine physical examination. His temperature is 37°C, pulse 86, respirations 16, and blood pressure 118/68. Upon reviewing documentation from his last annual assessment, the nurse notes that Mr. Harris takes a blood pressure medication and cholesterol-lowering agent. The patient previously worked as a janitor for the school system and now is a school bus driver. He has a 5-year history of glaucoma, for which he uses eye drops. Today, he states that his vision seems worse than usual.

Alternative A

Subjective: Mr. Harris has clouded, blurry, and dim vision. He is having increasing difficulty with vision at night and sensitivity to light and glare. At times he sees halos around lights.

Objective: Distance vision 20/80 left, 20/100 right. Needs two times reading glasses for small print. Opacities present in the lens.

- What other symptoms might the nurse assess?

- How will the nurse work with Mr. Harris to promote health for this diagnosis?

- What effects on the patient's functional status might this impairment have?

Alternative B

Subjective: Mr. Harris complains of acute loss of vision in the center of both visual fields.

Objective: The macula of an eye has atrophy (late age-related macular degeneration). There is loss of retinal tissue, and blood vessels are visible through the area of retinal atrophy.

- Is the patient's condition stable, urgent, or an emergency?

- How will the nurse focus, organize, and prioritize the subjective and objective data collection?

- How will the nurse work with Mr. Harris to promote health and reduce risk for illness?

DOCUMENTATION

Form for Use in Practice

Patient Name _____ Date _____

Date of Birth _____

Initial Survey

Reason for seeking health care: _____

History of present illness

- Location:

- Intensity:

- Duration:

- Description:

- Aggravating factors:

- Alleviating factors:

- Functional impairment:

- Pain goal:

Vital signs: T (route)_____   P (site)_____   R_____   BP (site)_____ SpO_2_____

Weight: _____ Height: _____ BMI: _____

General appearance: _____

General level of distress: _____

Risk Factors and History:

First-degree relatives with (check all those that apply):

Myopia		Cataracts	
Hyperopia		Glaucoma	
Strabismus		Retinitis pigmentosa	
Color blindness		Retinoblastoma	

Personal History of:

	Y/N	Details		Y/N	Details
Cataracts			Thyroid disease		
Glaucoma			Eye injury		
Hypertension			Eye surgery		
Diabetes			Facial surgery		
Lens implant			LASIK		

Medications

- Artificial tears:
- Decongestants:
- Corticosteroids:
- Antibiotics:
- Antihistamines:
- Prescribed eye drops:

Allergies/Exposures

- Allergies:
- Exposure to rubella in the womb:
- Congenital syphilis:
- Occupational exposures to toxins, chemicals, infections, or allergens:
- Stress level:

Eye Health

- Last eye examination:
- Glaucoma screening results:
- Glasses:
- Contacts: Care: Type:
- Protective eyewear:
- Nutritional health:

Common Eye Symptoms:

Symptom	Yes	No	Additional data
Pain			
Trauma			
Visual change			
Blind spots, floaters, or halos			
Discharge			
Change in activities of daily living (ADLs)			

Physical Assessment:

Assess distance visual acuity with Snellen or Allen chart.
Assess near vision with the Jaeger chart or newsprint.
Assess color vision using Ishihara cards or by having the patient identify color bars on the Snellen chart.
Test static confrontation.
Test kinetic confrontation.
Assess corneal light reflex.
Perform the cover test.
Assess the cardinal fields of gaze.
Inspect eyebrows, lashes, and eyelids; note eye shape and symmetry.
Note general appearance of the eyes.
Inspect and palpate the lacrimal apparatus (if the patient reports eye fatigue or dry eyes).
Inspect and palpate the bulbar conjunctiva.
Inspect the sclera for color, exudates, lesions, and foreign bodies.
Use a penlight or ophthalmoscope split light to inspect the cornea. Observe the angle of the anterior space and the clarity and translucence of the lens.
Inspect the iris for color, nodules, and vascularity.
Examine the pupil using a direct method.
Test for accommodation (CN III).
(Advanced practice) Perform ophthalmoscopic examination. • Optic disc: • Vessels: • Fundus:

Signature_____ Date _____

Guide for Use in Practice

Technique	Normal Findings	Abnormal Findings
Assess distance visual acuity by having the patient read the Snellen or Allen chart (based on developmental age or reading ability).	*Refractive index (emmetropia) of the eye is 20/20 bilaterally.*	Leaning forward, squinting, hesitation, misidentification of more than three of seven objects, or more than a two-line difference between eyes. A larger number on the bottom (eg, 20/60) indicates diminished distance vision.
Assess near vision with a Jaeger chart or newsprint.	*Visual acuity for near vision is 14/14 bilaterally.*	Decreased ability to accommodate
Assess color vision using Ishihara cards or by having the patient identify color bars on the Snellen chart.	*Patient correctly identifies the embedded figures in the Ishiara cards or the color bars on the Snellen chart.*	Incorrect identification of embedded figures or color bars
Test static confrontation.	*Patient accurately reports number of fingers presented in all four quadrants.*	Reports of an incorrect number of fingers
Test kinetic confrontation.	*Patient sees the fingers at about the same time as the nurse if the peripheral visual field is normal in that quadrant.*	A patient who sees fingers presented on either side only on one side; patient sees only from an inferior or superior position.
Test the corneal light reflex.	*Light reflection is in exactly the same spot in both eyes.*	Discrepancy in light reflection
Perform the cover test.	*Gaze is steady and fixed.*	Refixation
Test cardinal fields of gaze.	*Eyes move smoothly and symmetrically in all nine cardinal fields of gaze.*	Nystagmus anywhere but the extreme lateral angles
Inspect eyebrows, lashes, and eyelids; note eye shape and symmetry.	*Eyebrows show no unexplained hair loss. Lashes curve outward away from the eyes and are distributed evenly along the lid margins. Eyelids open and close completely, with spontaneous blinking. Eye shape varies from round to almond but is symmetrical.*	**Eyebrows:** unexplained hair loss; with normal aging, the outer third of the eyebrow thins **Eyelashes:** curved inward away toward the eye, distributed unevenly along lid margin, or both **Eyelids:** incomplete opening or closing; no spontaneous blinking; improper positioning with respect to iris and limbus **Eye shape:** asymmetry
Note general appearance of the eyes.	*Eyes are in parallel alignment.*	Eyes not in parallel alignment; *ptosis* (drooping of the eyelids)
Inspect and palpate the lacrimal apparatus (if the patient reports eye fatigue or dry eyes).	*Lacrimal apparatus is not enlarged or tender.*	Enlarged lacrimal apparatus
Inspect the bulbar conjunctiva for color, injection (redness), swelling, exudates, or foreign bodies.	*Bulbar conjunctiva is normally transparent with small blood vessels visible.*	Erythema, cobblestone appearance, sharply defined bright red blood (*subconjunctival hemorrhage*), abnormal thickening of the conjunctiva from the limbus over the cornea (*pterygium*)
Inspect the sclera for color, exudates, lesions, and foreign bodies.	*Sclera is clear, smooth, white, and without exudate, lesions, or foreign bodies.*	Jaundice, bluing, and drainage

Use a penlight or ophthalmoscope split light to inspect the cornea. Observe the angle of the anterior space and the clarity and translucence of the lens.	*A normal angle allows full illumination of the iris. Lens is transparent.*	Narrow angle (*glaucoma*); cloudiness of the lens (*cataract*)
Inspect the iris for color, nodules, and vascularity.	*Color is evenly distributed, smooth, and without apparent vascularity. A normal variation is mosaic variant.*	Iris nevus, hyphema, blepharitis, chalazion, conjunctivitis, exophthalmos, hordeolum (stye), amblyopia (lazy eye), osteogenesis imperfecta
Examine the pupil using a direct method.	*Pupil is black, round, and equal with a diameter of 2–6 mm. Both pupils constrict directly and consensually.*	Anisocoria (unequal pupils), Horner's syndrome, Argyle Robertson pupil, Adie's pupil, key hole pupil (coloboma), miosis, mydriasis, oculomotor (CN III) nerve damage
Test for accommodation (CN III).	*Pupils constrict (accommodation) and eyes cross (converge). PERRLA.*	Pupils do not constrict or converge as expected

CHAPTER 16

Ears Assessment

OBJECTIVE SUMMARY

This chapter explores ear assessment. It reviews anatomy of the ear and physiology related to hearing and equilibrium, including key variations associated with lifespan, culture, and the environment. The section on subjective data collection covers family history, personal history, medications, and risk factors contributing to otitis media, loss of hearing, and vertigo. Information on collecting objective data describes methods for assessing anatomy, auditory perception, and equilibrium.

READING ASSIGNMENT

Read Chapter 16 in Jensen's *Nursing Health Assessment: A Best-Practice Approach*.

VOCABULARY/TERMINOLOGY

- **Air conduction:** Normal pathway by which sounds travel to the inner ear.

- **Audiogram:** Test for auditory acuity conducted by an audiologist in a soundproof room.

- **Bone conduction:** Pathway for sound transmission that bypasses the external ear and delivers sound waves/vibrations directly to the inner ear via the skull.

- **Cerumen:** Waxy substance secreted by glands in the ear.

- **Cochlea:** Part of the bony labyrinth that includes the portions of the inner ear responsible for hearing.

- **Conductive hearing loss:** Hearing loss that results when sound wave transmission through the external or middle ear is disrupted.

- **Equilibrium:** Condition of a system in which competing influences are balanced. The sense of a balance present in humans and animals.

- **Eustachian tube:** Conduit that connects the middle ear to the nasopharynx and allows for pressure regulation of the middle ear.

- **Incus:** Anvil-shaped small bone or ossicle in the middle ear that connects the malleus to the stapes. It conducts sound to the inner ear.

- **Malleus:** Also called the *hammer*; a hammer-shaped small bone or ossicle of the middle ear that connects with the incus and is attached to the inner surface of the eardrum.

- **Organ of Corti:** Also called the spiral organ; contains auditory sensory cells (hair cells) in the inner ear of mammals.

- **Otalgia:** Pain in or around the ear.

- **Otosclerosis:** Common conductive hearing loss resulting from the slow fusion of any combination of the ossicles in the middle ear.

- **Presbycusis:** Natural sensorineural loss.

- **Rinne test:** Test conducted with a tuning fork to examine the differentiation between bone conduction (BC) and air conduction (AC).

- **Semicircular canals:** Three half-circular, interconnected tubes inside each ear that are filled with a fluid called endolymph and a motion sensor with little hairs (cilia) whose ends are embedded in a gelatinous structure called the cupula. As the skull twists in any direction, the endolymph is thrown into different sections of the canals. The cilia detect when the endolymph rushes past, and a signal is then sent to the brain.

- **Sensorineural hearing loss:** Hearing loss that results from a problem somewhere beyond the middle ear, from inner ear to auditory cortex.

- **Stapes:** Also called the *stirrup*; the stirrup-shaped small bone or ossicle in the middle ear that attaches the incus to the fenestra ovalis, the "oval window" which is adjacent to the vestibule of the inner ear. It is the smallest and lightest bone in the human body.

- **Tinnitus:** Perception of buzzing or ringing in one ear or both ears that does not correspond with an external sound.

- **Tympanic membrane:** Oblique, multilayered, translucent, and pearly gray barrier between the external auditory canal and middle ear.

- **Vertigo:** Type of dizziness, where there is a feeling of motion when one is stationary.

- **Vestibular function:** Proprioception and equilibrium.

- **Vestibule:** Central part of the labyrinth, as used in the vestibular system.

- **Weber's test:** Use of a tuning fork to help to differentiate the cause of unilateral hearing loss.

- **Whisper test:** Test in which an examiner whispers a sentence and asks the patient to repeat it to evaluate loss of high-frequency sounds.

STUDY GUIDE

Activity A   FILL IN THE BLANK

1. Finish these statements about the inner ear.

   A. The inner ear is responsible for the translation of sound to _____

   B. The inner ear is the only section of the ear responsible for _____

   C. The conduits of the inner ear are known collectively as the _____

   D. The _____ includes the portions of the inner ear responsible for hearing.

   E. Vestibular function is maintained in the _____ and _____

2. List the four openings to the middle ear chamber.

   A. _____

   B. _____

   C. _____

   D. _____

Activity B   MATCHING

1. *Match the structure of the ear with its definition.*

Answer	Structure	Definition
	1. Auditory ossicle	**A.** Connects the middle and inner ear
	2. Pars tensa	**B.** The stapes rests here
	3. Eustachian tube	**C.** A small relaxed and opaque portion of the tympanic membrane
	4. Bony labyrinth	**D.** Most of the tympanic membrane
	5. Oval window	**E.** Tiny bone responsible for conducting sound waves to the inner ear
	6. Pars flaccida	**F.** Conduit of the inner ear
	7. Round window	**G.** Conduit that connects the middle ear to the nasopharynx

2. *Match the intervention with the nursing diagnosis.*

Answer	Intervention	Nursing Diagnosis
	1. Encourage adequate nutrition.	**A.** Disturbed auditory sensory perception
	2. Provide alternatives such as distraction, breathing, and relaxation.	**B.** Risk for infection
	3. Allow patient to see your face.	**C.** Pain

Activity C LABELING

1. Label the structures of the ear (from the list below) at the proper place on the figure below.

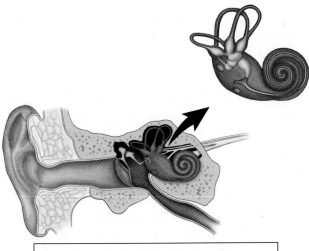

Eustachian tube, cochlea, incus, malleus, pinna, semicircular canals, stapes, tympanic membrane

Activity D SHORT ANSWER

1. Identify the location of the Eustachian tube and discuss its function.

_____

_____

_____

_____

2. Briefly explain the process of hearing.

_____

_____

_____

_____

3. Identify the most common cause of conductive hearing loss in the adult and explain why it happens.

_____

_____

_____

_____

4. Explain otosclerosis. Include the age group in which it is most often found and what it causes.

_____

_____

_____

_____

5. When assessing the ears of an older adult, what normal variations might the nurse expect to find? What accommodations for the physical examination might the nurse need to make?

_____

_____

_____

_____

6. Explain normal placement of the ear on the skull.

_____

_____

_____

_____

Activity E MULTIPLE CHOICE

1. Which of the following is an important patient teaching topic related to the ears?
   A. How to clean the ear with cotton swabs
   B. How to prevent a cholesteatoma
   C. How to prevent skin cancer
   D. What causes barotrauma

2. A patient calls the clinic and tells the nurse that the doctor told her that she has "otalgia." The patient cannot remember what the doctor explained this to be. How would the nurse most appropriately respond?
   A. "Otalgia is a dysfunction of the ear."
   B. "Otalgia is pain in the ear."
   C. "Otalgia is the beginning of hearing loss."
   D. "Otalgia is a disease of the inner ear."

3. The nurse is providing patient teaching to the mother of a 3 month old with otitis media. What would the nurse explain is a risk factor for otitis media?
   A. Being outside in the spring
   B. Cigarette residue on clothing
   C. Being taken out in crowds
   D. Being an only child

4. A patient has Darwin's tubercule. What is this?
   A. A type of skin cancer found on the ear
   B. A growth in the ear canal
   C. A growth in the bony labyrinth
   D. A small painless nodule on the helix

5. A patient comes to the clinic and reports pain when he touches his ear. With what is this finding consistent?
   A. Acoustic neuroma
   B. Otitis externa
   C. Otitis media
   D. Meniere's disease

6. Upon examination, the Advanced Practice Nurse finds that a patient has otitis media with effusion. What assessment finding is indicative of this diagnosis?
   A. A diffuse cone of light
   B. A gray tympanic membrane
   C. A perforated tympanic membrane
   D. Inflammation in the ear canal

7. A 52-year-old patient fails the Romberg's test. The nurse explains that this might indicate a dysfunction in what part of the ear?
   A. The bones of the middle ear
   B. The Eustachian tubes
   C. The pinna
   D. The vestibular portion of the inner ear

8. A nurse is writing a care plan for a patient who has been found to have a progressive hearing loss. What would be an appropriate outcome for this patient?
   A. Patient's ear canal will be free from cerumen.
   B. Patient will have normal hearing.
   C. Patient will accept the use of a hearing aid.
   D. Patient will be free from pain.

ALTERNATIVE CASE SCENARIOS

Mrs. Petino is a 25-year-old immigrant from El Salvador. She comes to the clinic today with concerns of ear pain, "buzzing" in her ears, and hearing loss. Mrs. Petino has been to the clinic five times in the last 4 months for ear concerns. She was treated once for bilateral otitis media. She currently works in a tuna-packing plant as a line custodian. Her immunizations are current. Temperature is 37.4°C orally, pulse 86 beats/min, respirations 16 breaths/min, and blood pressure 126/78 mm Hg. Current medications include 500 mg acetaminophen taken 2 hours ago.

Alternative A

Based on the changes outlined below, consider what other outcomes, information, and problems would affect the overall picture of Mrs. Petino and shape your responses.

Subjective: "I am dizzy all the time."

Objective: Mrs. Petino supports herself on the chair and examination table and moves slowly when she is changing position.

- What should the nurse do to further evaluate Mrs. Petino's vertigo?
- What nursing interventions might be appropriate for Mrs. Petino?
- What outcomes might the nurse write for Mrs. Petino? How will the nurse evaluate them?

Alternative B

Subjective: "I'm fine."

Objective: Mrs. Petino is holding her head and squinting whenever a loud noise occurs in the room.

- How does sensitivity to sound differ from hearing loss?
- How can the nurse obtain additional subjective information from Mrs. Petino? How should the nurse phrase questions?
- What nursing diagnoses might be highest priority and what is the rationale?

DOCUMENTATION

Form for Use in Practice

Patient Name _____ Date _____

Date of Birth: _____

Initial Survey

Reason for seeking health care: _____

History of present illness

- Location:

- Intensity:

- Duration:

- Description:

- Aggravating factors:

- Alleviating factors:

- Functional impairment:

- Pain goal:

Vital signs: T (route)_____   P (site)_____   R_____   BP (site)_____   SpO$_2$_____

Weight: _____   Height: _____   BMI: _____

General appearance: _____

General level of distress: _____

Risk Factors and History:

- Family history of ear or hearing problems:

- Sun exposure:

- Skin cancer:

- Previous ear infections:

- Hearing loss:

- History of tinnitus:

- History of vertigo:

- Ear surgeries:

- Noise exposure:

- Smoking history:

- Second-hand smoke exposure:

- Allergies:

Medications

- Prescription drugs (for each, document dosage, frequency, and route):

- Immunizations

Common Ear Symptoms:

Symptom	Yes	No	Additional data
Hearing loss			
Vertigo			
Tinnitus			
Otalgia			

Physical Assessment:

Assess ears:
   Inspect:
   Palpate:

Assess hearing:
   Amplitude:
   Frequency:

Conduct:
   Whisper test:
   Rinne test:
   Weber's test:

Assess equilibrium: Romberg's test:

Signature_____ Date _____

Guide for Use in Practice

Technique	Normal Findings	Abnormal Findings
Inspect the ears.	*They are symmetrical, equal in size, and fully formed.*	Microtia, macrotia, edematous ears, cartilage pseudomonas infection, carcinoma on auricle, cyst, frostbite
Inspect the face.	*Tone is uniform with the ears. Skin is intact. Small painless nodules on the helix are a variation of normal anatomy known as Darwin's tubercle.*	Broken skin, ears disproportionate to face, obvious deformities
Palpate the auricle.	*Ears are firm without lumps, lymph tissue is not palpable, ears are nontender, and no pain is elicited with palpation or manipulation of the auricle. No pain occurs with palpation of the mastoid process.*	Enlarged lymph nodes; pain with auricle movement or tragus palpation (indicates *otitis externa* or furuncle)
Perform the whisper test.	*Patient repeats the entire sentence to you without errors.*	Patient cannot repeat the sentence clearly or misses components.
Use a tuning fork to perform the Rinne test.	*AC is twice as long as BC.*	BC longer or the same as AC
Use a tuning fork to perform the Weber test.	*Patient hears the sound in both ears and at equal intensity.*	Unilateral identification of the sound

Otoscopic Examination: The RN rarely uses an otoscope to inspect the ear. An APRN completes the otoscopic examination.		
Inspect the external meatus and canal with an appropriately sized speculum.	*The canal has fine hairs; some cerumen lining the wall skin is intact, with no discharge.*	Redness, swelling of the external auditory canal, and discharge
Visualize the tympanic membrane. Visualize portions of the malleus, umbo, manubrium, and short process through the translucent membrane. A well-aerated middle ear allows visualization of part of the incus as well.	*Tympanic membrane is intact and translucent and allows visualization of the short process of the malleus. The cone of light is visible in the anterior inferior quadrant.* *A variation of normal is a tympanic membrane with white areas (sclerosis).*	Swelling or bulging of the tympanic membrane; a diffuse cone of light; a perforated tympanic membrane
Use the bulb insufflator attached to the head of the otoscope to observe tympanic membrane movement.	*The tympanic membrane moves inward when inflated and outward with release.*	Movement of the tympanic membrane is different from the normal pattern or the membrane fails to move
Assess equilibrium by using the Romberg test.	*Findings are within normal limits.*	Failure of the Romberg test may indicate dysfunction in the vestibular portion of the inner ear, semicircular canals, and vestibule.

Nose, Sinuses, Mouth, and Throat Assessment

OBJECTIVE SUMMARY

This chapter focuses on assessment of the nose, sinuses, mouth, and throat. It reviews anatomy and physiology, common normal variations, and relevant lifespan, cultural, and environmental considerations. The chapter serves as a guide to the collection of subjective data related to upper respiratory and mouth problems, which can result from occupational exposures, recreational activities (eg, smoking), family history of allergic rhinitis, systemic disorders, and head and neck cancer. It reviews nasal discharge, congestion, and obstruction; snoring; sore throat; and facial pain and pressure. Presentation of objective data collection includes examination techniques and correct documentation of normal and abnormal findings.

READING ASSIGNMENT

Read Chapter 17 in Jensen's *Nursing Health Assessment: A Best-Practice Approach*.

VOCABULARY/TERMINOLOGY

- **Allergic salute:** An upward rubbing of the external nose induced by itching; may lead to a crease or bend in the nose, most commonly in children with allergies.

- **Angular cheilitis:** Maceration of the skin at the corners of the mouth; caused by overclosure of the mouth.

- **Ankyloglossia:** A short lingual frenulum; may be congenital, restricting movement of the tongue and subsequently speech.

- **Anosmia:** Decreased smell.

- **Atopy:** Allergy.

- **Bednar aphthae:** Ulcerative abrasions on the posterior hard palate that result from hard sucking.

- **Bifid uvula:** Minor cleft of the posterior soft palate.

- **Choana:** Opening of the nose.

- **Choanal atresia:** Restriction of the bucco-nasal membrane.

- **Columella:** Anatomical structure that divides the oval nares (nostrils).

- **Deviation of septum:** Deflection of the center wall of the nose (septum).

- **Dysphagia:** Difficulty swallowing.

- **Epistaxis:** Nosebleed.

- **Epstein pearls:** Small, white, glistening, pearly papules along the median border of the hard palate and gums; a normal finding in newborns.

- **Epulis:** Localized gingival enlargement. May lead to a tumor-like mass.

- **Fordyce's granules:** Small isolated white or yellow papules on the buccal mucosa, representing insignificant sebaceous cysts or salivary tissue.

- **Geographic tongue:** Tongue appearance with creases, bends, and unusual appearance; tends to occur in people with allergic disease but has no significant pathology.

- **Gustatory rhinitis:** Clear rhinorrhea stimulated by the smell and taste of food.

- **Halitosis:** Bad breath.

- **Hemangioma:** Benign mass of blood vessels.

- **Koplik's spots:** Finding in rubeola measles; appearance resembles grains of salt on the erythematous base of the buccal mucosa opposite the first and second molars.

- **Leukoplakia:** White patches with well-defined borders found on the lips or gums.

- **Lingula frenulum:** Anatomical structure that connects the base of the tongue to the floor of the mouth.

- **Ludwig's angina:** Swelling that results from infection in the floor of the mouth and pushes the tongue up and back. It can lead to eventual airway obstruction.

- **Milia:** Small white bumps across the bridge of the nose; a common newborn finding.

- **Oral candidiasis:** White coating of the tongue. Also known as thrush.

- **Osteo-meatal complex:** The collective middle turbinate and middle meatus area.

- **Peritonsillar abscess:** Abscess in the anterior tonsillar pillar that may result from collection of fluid.

- **Petechiae:** Small red spots under the skin resulting from blood that escapes the capillaries; may occur with trauma, infection, or decreased platelet counts.

- **Pharyngitis:** Inflammation of the pharyngeal walls.

- **Polyps:** Grape-like swollen nasal membranes, may appear white and glistening.

- **Rubeola measles:** Infectious disease with symptoms of a maculopapular rash on the buccal mucosa, fever, inflammation of the nasal mucous membrane, nasal discharge (coryza), and cough.

- **Scrotal tongue:** Fissures that become inflamed with food or debris and appear in the tongue.

- **Septal perforation:** Hole in the midline septum.

- **Smooth, glossy tongue:** Tongue and buccal mucosa that appear smooth and shiny from papillary atrophy and thinning of the buccal mucosa.

- **Sucking tubercle:** In infants the formation of a small pad of tissue in the middle of the upper lip.

- **Tonsillitis:** Inflammation of the tonsils.

- **Torus palatinus:** Bony prominence in the middle of the hard palate.

- **Trismus:** Inability to open the jaw.

- **Vermillion:** Junction of the lip and facial skin.

- **Vestibule:** Anatomic name for the nares; comprised of skin and ciliated mucosa.

- **Xerostoma:** Dry mouth.

STUDY GUIDE

Activity A FILL IN THE BLANK

1. Write the medical term next to its description:

   A. Small white bumps across the bridge of the nose

   _____

   B. Congenital disorder in which the back of the nasal passage (choana) is blocked, usually by abnormal bony or soft tissue formed during fetal development

   _____

   C. Restricting movement of the tongue and subsequently speech

   _____

   D. Nonparasitic antigen capable of stimulating a type-I hypersensitivity reaction in atopic individuals

   _____

   E. Lining of the nose

   _____

   F. Anterior portion of the nasal septum, which has a rich vascular supply

   _____

   G. Opening that connects a sinus to the nasal cavity itself

   _____

H. Common site of occult nasopharyngeal malignancies

_____

I. Lymphoid tissue located in the roof of the nasopharynx

_____

J. Area that opens into the mouth in the buccal mucosa just opposite the upper second molar

_____

Activity B MATCHING

1. _Match the condition with common related assessment findings._

Answer	Condition	Findings
	1. Gingival hyperplasia	**A.** Pain at and around site
	2. Leukoplakia	**B.** Bruise-like lesions that form plaques and progress into nodular, red-purple, nonblanching firm lesions
	3. Aphthous ulcers	
	4. Torus palatinus	
	5. Kaposi's sarcoma	
		C. Foul odor, whistling sound, recurrent crusting or bleeding from the nose
		D. Enlargement of gum tissue
		E. White lesion firmly attached to mucosal surface; does not scrape off

2. _Match the nursing diagnosis with the appropriate intervention._

Answer	Diagnosis	Intervention
	1. Altered oral mucous membrane	**A.** Perform mouth care if patient is unable to do so independently.
	2. Altered breathing pattern	**B.** Elevate head of bed.
	3. Impaired swallowing	**C.** Provide fluids and mouth care.
	4. Impaired dentition	**D.** Give frequent fluids to liquefy secretions.

3. _Match the nasal/oral finding with the systemic disease._

Answer	Nasal and Oral Finding	Systemic Disease
	1. Oral ulceration, rhinorrhea, rhinalgia, aphthous ulceration of nose or nasopharynx that heals without scarring	**A.** Pemphigus-pemphigoid
	2. Copious, thick, viscous mucus that blocks airways	**B.** Wegner's granulomatosis
	3. Tertiary nasal septal swelling; may develop into perforation	**C.** Bechet's disease
	4. Blister formation on external nose or anterior septum	**D.** Syphilis
	5. Nasal crusting, mucosal ulcerations	**E.** Cystic fibrosis
	6. Kaposi's sarcoma	**F.** Tuberculosis
	7. Nasal crusting, ulcerations, epistaxis, chronic rhinosinusitis, septal perforations	**G.** AIDS

Activity C SHORT ANSWER

1. As people age, physiologic changes occur in the mouth and the tongue. Discuss these changes, including what they cause.

_____

_____

_____

_____

2. Discuss diagnostic testing for allergies.

_____

_____

_____

_____

3. While caring for a patient with nose, mouth, sinus, and/or throat problems, what are potential outcomes that would be appropriate?

_____

_____

_____

_____

4. People who are allergic usually try to avoid allergens. Explain the precautions these patients can take in their homes to control allergens.

_____

_____

_____

_____

5. Discuss techniques used to assess the nose, mouth, sinus, and throat. Identify whether the technique is common or specialty/ advanced assessment.

_____

_____

_____

_____

6. Discuss the throat. List what elements are in the throat, including lymphatic tissue.

_____

_____

_____

_____

7. Explain the function of the upper respiratory tract and mouth.

_____

_____

_____

_____

Activity D **MULTIPLE CHOICE**

1. When assessing a patient, the nurse notes a brownish ridge along the gum line. The finding is normal for this patient. From which of the following cultural backgrounds is this patient most likely?

   A. African American

   B. Native American

   C. Pacific Island American

   D. Asian American

2. A patient is found to have a smooth, glossy tongue. What might this indicate?

   A. Vitamin B_{12} deficiency

   B. Vitamin D deficiency

   C. Vitamin C deficiency

   D. Vitamin B_1 deficiency

3. A woman brings her 4-week-old son to the clinic. She is concerned about ulcerative abrasions that have developed on the posterior hard palate. What would the nurse explain that these abrasions are?

   A. Epstein pearls

   B. Bednar aphthae

   C. Koplik's spots

   D. Sucking tubercles

4. A 27-year-old woman presents at the clinic for her routine prenatal appointment. She tells the nurse that she has developed a mass on her gum and is afraid she has oral cancer. The nurse would know that this finding is most likely

   A. A sterile tooth abscess

   B. An infected parotid gland

   C. An enlarged lymph node

   D. An epulis forming on the gum

5. An anatomy instructor is discussing the nose with the prenursing class. What would the instructor explain the osteo-meatal complex as?

   A. The superior turbinate and inferior meatus area

   B. The middle turbinate and inferior meatus area

   C. The middle turbinate and middle meatus area

   D. The superior turbinate and middle meatus area

6. A staff educator from the hospital is providing an event for the hospital staff. The educator is talking about health promotion activities for people with diseases of the nose, mouth, throat, and sinuses. What would the educator include in the presentation?

   A. How to safely put an infant to bed with a bottle

   B. Delaying dental care in children until age 5 years

   C. How to reduce periodontal disease

   D. How oral cancer is diagnosed

7. A patient comes to the clinic and reports nosebleeds. What area of the nose is the bleeding most likely coming from?

   A. Thompson's plexus

   B. Koppleback's area

   C. Little's area

   D. Wharton's plexus

ALTERNATIVE CASE SCENARIOS

Mrs. Davis, an 89-year-old Caucasian woman, was admitted to the hospital 13 days ago with pneumonia. She had complications during her stay, was transferred to intensive care, and is now on the rehabilitation unit in preparation for her return home. Her temperature is 37°C orally, pulse 88 beats/min, respirations 20 breaths/min, and blood pressure 138/72 mm Hg. Current medications include a mild diuretic and beta blocker for blood pressure, an inhaler to open her airways, and an antibiotic for the pneumonia. Her assessment was documented on the previous shift.

Review the following alternative situations related to Mrs. Davis. Based on the changes outlined below, *consider what other outcomes, information, and problems would affect the overall picture and shape your responses.*

Alternative A

Subjective: "I just got a bloody nose."

Objective: Moderate amount of blood draining from right naris. Has been on oxygen from admission 2 days ago. Nares dry and red. Pulse 88 beats/min, R 20 breaths/min, BP 122/78 mm Hg.

- Is the patient's condition stable, urgent, or an emergency?

- What factors place her at risk for epistaxis?

- What additional assessment information will the nurse collect?

Alternative B

Subjective: "It hurts on my upper lip."

Objective: Clear vesicles present on upper lip with indurated base. Rates pain 2/10 at rest but increases to 4/10 with pressure, speaking, or eating. States that she has a history of cold sores when she gets stressed.

- How might the lesions be associated with the patient's other chronic and acute problems?

- What special precautions might the nurse take related to infection control?

- Which nursing diagnoses might be appropriate and what is the rationale?

DOCUMENTATION

Form for Use in Practice

Patient Name _____ Date _____

Date of Birth _____

Initial Survey

Reason for seeking health care: _____

History of present illness

- Location:

- Intensity:

- Duration:

- Description:

- Aggravating factors:

- Alleviating factors:

- Functional impairment:

- Pain goal:

Vital signs: T (route)_____   P (with site)_____   R_____   BP (site)_____   SpO$_2$_____

Weight: _____   Height: _____   BMI: _____

General appearance: _____

General level of distress: _____

History/Interview:

- Family history of nose, mouth, sinus, and throat problems:

- History of sinusitis, tonsillitis, carcinoma:

- Medications and supplements:

- Smoking history:

- Recreational drugs:

- Occupational and environmental exposure:

- Allergies:

- Last chest x-ray and TB test:

- Influenza or pneumococcal vaccine:

- Travel to high-risk areas:

Common Symptoms:

Symptom	Yes	No	Additional data
Facial pressure/pain/headache			
Snoring/sleep apnea			
Obstructive breathing			
Epistaxis (nosebleeds)			
Halitosis (bad breath)			
Anosmia (decreased smell)			
Cough			
Pharyngitis/sore throat			
Dysphagia (difficulty swallowing)			
Dental aching/pain			
Hoarseness/voice changes			
Oral lesions			

Physical Assessment:

Inspect the external nose.
(APRN) Palpate the nose.
(APRN) Inspect the internal nose with an otoscope, nasal speculum, or both.
• Observe the color of the mucous membranes.
• Inspect any mucus.
• Note the color and character of the nose.
• Assess nasal airflow.
(Optional) Ask the patient to identify common scents.
Inspect the sinus areas for redness or swelling.
(APRN) Transilluminate the sinus cavities.
Palpate and percuss the maxillary, ethmoid, and frontal sinuses.
Inspect lips.
Inspect the buccal mucosa.
Inspect the entire U-shaped area in the floor of the mouth.
Assess the parotid (Stensen's) duct.
Inspect the teeth and gums.
Note numbers and position of teeth, general appearance, signs of decay, and alignment.
Note odor of the patient's breath.
Note position of the uvula.
Inspect color and surface of the hard and soft palate.
Inspect tongue, including dorsum (top surface), sides, and underneath.
Ask the patient to stick out the tongue.
(Optional) Test the gag reflex.
Inspect Wharton's ducts.
Evaluate salivary flow.
Palpate parotid, submandibular, and sublingual glands for swelling or tenderness.
(Optional) Assess Stensen's duct and Wharton's duct for a stone, growth, or any lesions.
Visualize the pharynx, tonsils, soft palate, and anterior and posterior tonsillar pillars.
(APRN) Palpate the neck to assess inflammatory and other changes that may occur in the throat.
(APRN) Assess ability to swallow.

Signature_____ Date _____

Guide for Use in Practice

Technique	Normal Findings	Abnormal Findings
Inspect the nose.	*It appears symmetrical, midline, and proportionally shaped to facial features. Skin surface is smooth without lesions; coloration is consistent with other facial complexion.*	Asymmetry, swelling, or bruising
(APRN) Palpate the nose or sinuses with the thumb and forefinger.	*There is no pain, tenderness, or break in contour.*	Tenderness on palpation and crepitus
(APRN) Inspect the internal nose with an otoscope, nasal speculum, or both. Observe the color of the mucous membranes. Inspect any mucus. Note the color and character of the nose. Assess nasal airflow.	*Septum is midline; its mucosa is pink and moist with no prominent blood vessels or crusts. A small amount of drainage is clear. Airflow around the normal nasal structures is adequate.*	Infection and inflammation of nasal mucosa; excessive clear watery drainage; thick discolored mucus or gross pus; absence of normal structures (eg, turbinates); deviation of the nasal septum; crusting or prominence of nasal vessels; septal perforation; polyps
(Optional) Ask patient to identify common scents. Smell testing may be performed with the use of a sniff test card.	*Patient correctly identifies scents.*	Anosomia; sudden loss of smell
Inspect the sinus areas (forehead, between the eyes, and both cheeks) for redness or swelling.	*Findings are symmetrical with no redness or swelling.*	Redness and swelling over the sinuses
Palpate and percuss the maxillary, ethmoid, and frontal sinus areas.	*No tenderness or fullness is present.*	Tenderness or fullness
Inspect lips, noting color, moisture, lesions, and oral competence.	*Lips are pink and moist with no lesions.*	Dryness or cracking; lesions or aphthous ulcers; swelling or edema of lips; oral incompetence; cleft lip or inadequate repair
Fully inspect the buccal mucosa, noting color and pigmentation. Inspect the entire U-shaped area in the floor of the mouth. Note the parotid (Stensen's) duct.	*Buccal mucosa and soft and hard palates are pink with no lesions.*	Poor oral hygiene; inflamed buccal mucosa; white patches (leukoplakia); ulceration; petechiae (small red spots resulting from blood, which escapes the capillaries); redness or swelling of Stensen's duct
Inspect the teeth and gums. Note numbers and position of teeth. Note general appearance and signs of decay. Note alignment. Note the odor of the patient's breath.	*Gingiva is pink and moist without inflammation. Teeth are well aligned with no evidence of decay. Breath has no foul odor.*	Teeth may be stained or have *decay.* Swollen or red gums with bleeding may indicate *gingivitis.* Foul breath may suggest infection.
Note the position of the uvula. Have the patient say "ah," noting the rise of the uvula and function of the vagus (CN X).	*Uvula rises symmetrically with "ah."*	Swollen uvula; uvula that is bifid or has a notch or cleft; no upward movement of the uvula when the patient says "ah" (indicates dysfunction of CN X)
Inspect the color and surface of the hard and soft palate.	*Palate is intact.*	With cleft palate, nasopharyngeal incompetence and resultant nasal air leak during speech

Inspect the tongue, including the dorsum (top surface), sides, and underneath. Note papillae on the dorsum, small anterior, and large posterior. Ask the patient to stick out the tongue.	*Tongue is smooth and midline.*	Lesions or ulcers; geographic tongue; white coating of the tongue
Inspect Wharton's ducts in the floor of the mouth. Evaluate salivary flow from the submandibular salivary gland.	*Ducts are smooth without inflammation.*	Swelling or redness of Wharton's duct; *Ludwig's angina*
Palpate the parotid, submandibular, and sublingual glands for swelling or tenderness.	*There is no swelling or tenderness.*	Swelling, duct obstruction
(Optional) Place a gloved hand inside the cheek to assess Stensen's duct and Wharton's duct for a stone, growth, or any lesions.	*Ducts are smooth with no signs of stones, lesions, or growths.*	A firm area at either Stensen's or Wharton's duct; lesions of oral mucosa
Pressing down slightly with the tongue blade on the midpoint of the tongue, visualize the pharynx, tonsils, soft palate, and anterior and posterior tonsillar pillars. Note color, symmetry, enlargement, and any lesions. Grade the tonsils.	*Tissue is pink and moist with symmetrical margins. No enlargement or lesions are noted. Tonsils are absent or 1+.*	Mucosal inflammation; hypertrophy of tonsils; superficial scars or crypts; white curd-like material embedded in the tonsil mucosa; asymmetrical tonsillar enlargement; peritonsillar abscess (*quinsy*); squeezed appearance of the general proportion of the throat; red and white patches in the throat; difficulty swallowing; tender or swollen glands (lymph nodes) in the neck; red and enlarged tonsils
(APRN) Palpate the neck to assess inflammatory and other changes that may occur in the throat. Anterior and posterior cervical chain lymph nodes and submental areas are palpated as part of a normal neck examination.	*Nodes are symmetrical, soft, and nontender.*	Enlargement of the anterior, posterior, or submental lymph nodes of the neck
(APRN) Evaluate swallowing.	*Swallowing takes <1 second with no sign of aspiration.*	Dysphagia

CHAPTER 18

Thorax and Lungs Assessment

OBJECTIVE SUMMARY

This chapter assists you to identify the important vocabulary and content on respiratory assessment. Subjective information such as coughing is reviewed. Objective data include breath sounds and adventitious sounds. After the completion of this chapter, you should be able to perform the respiratory assessment including auscultation of normal breath sounds and identification of abnormal breath sounds.

READING ASSIGNMENT

Read Chapter 18 in Jensen's *Nursing Health Assessment: A Best-Practice Approach.*

VOCABULARY/TERMINOLOGY

- **Crepitus:** Crackling sensation with palpation.
- **Diaphragmatic excursion:** Distance that the diaphragm moves with inhalation.
- **Dyspnea:** Shortness of breath.
- **Fremitus:** Vibrations on the chest with talking.
- **Hemoptysis:** Sputum with blood.
- **Kyphosis:** Very bent over posture.
- **Orthopnea:** Difficulty breathing when lying flat.
- **Pallor:** Very pale skin color.
- **Paroxysmal nocturnal dyspnea:** Sudden onset of shortness of breath at night.

- **Purulent:** Sputum cloudy with bacteria.
- **Rubor:** Reddish skin color.
- **Scoliosis:** Spine that curves to one side in an area.
- **Tenacious:** Very thick sputum.

STUDY GUIDE

Activity A FILL IN THE BLANK

adventitious breath sounds; bronchial breath sounds; bronchophony; bronchovesicular breath sounds; crackles; egophony; stridor; vesicular breath sounds; wheezes; whispered pectoriloquy

1. Write the medical term from the list above next to the description of the breath sound. Choices are listed alphabetically.

   A. Breath sounds normally heard in the bases of the lungs

   _____

   B. High pitched crowing sound from the upper airway

   _____

   C. When the patient talks softly the sound is heard loudly

   _____

D. Breath sounds normally heard at the second intercoastal space anteriorly

_____

E. Fine popping noises in the lungs that are abnormal

_____

F. When the patient says "eee" the sound is "aaa"

_____

G. Term for breath sounds that are abnormal or extra

_____

H. Breath sounds normally heard over the trachea

_____

I. Whistling musical abnormal sound in the lung

_____

J. When the patient says "99" the sound is clear and loud

_____

A.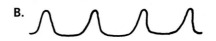

_____

B.

_____

C. Inspiration Expiration

_____

D.

_____

E.

_____

F.

Hyperpnea   Apnea

_____

G.

_____

Activity B LABELING

1. Draw in the lobes of the lungs on the diagram below and mark with an X where you will place the stethoscope when auscultating.

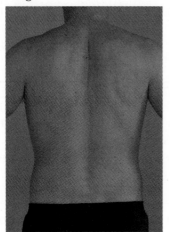

2. Using the words in the box below, write the medical term next to the pattern identified in the following pictures.

> Biot's respirations; bradypnea; Cheyne-Stokes respirations; eupnea; hyperventilation; hypoventilation; tachypnea

Activity C SHORT ANSWER

1. What are some areas for health promotion and patient teaching during the respiratory assessment?

_____

_____

_____

_____

2. Name five factors that place a client at risk for respiratory problems.

_____

_____

_____

_____

3. What characteristics of a cough and sputum should be noted in both subjective and objective data collection?

_____

_____

_____

_____

4. Explain ronchal fremitus.

_____

_____

_____

_____

5. Explain why a nurse should count newborn respirations for a full minute.

_____

_____

_____

_____

6. Describe the accessory muscles used in respiration. Where would retractions be noted?

_____

_____

_____

_____

7. Explain what information pulmonary function tests give and the elements of these tests.

_____

_____

_____

_____

8. Because older adults are at increased risk for respiratory complications during stress, explain what a nurse must pay close attention to.

_____

_____

_____

_____

Activity D **MULTIPLE CHOICE**

1. A patient has a nursing diagnosis of ineffective airway clearance. What intervention would be most appropriate?

   A. Position to decrease workload of breathing.

   B. Administer oxygen.

   C. Teach deep breathing.

   D. Increase fluids.

2. When an infant is born, changes occur in the circulatory system aiding the baby to breathe on his or her own. What is one of these changes?

   A. Opening of the ductus arteriosus

   B. Closure of the foramen ovale

   C. Entry of oxygen into the blood

   D. Production of surfactant in the lungs

3. A person with a barrel chest has a problem doing what?

   A. Taking a deep breath

   B. Coughing

   C. Maintaining oxygen saturation

   D. Breathing at a normal respiratory rate

4. A 37-year-old man presents at the emergency department complaining that he is having trouble breathing. What would the nurse include in this patient's acute assessment?

   A. Auscultating the lungs

   B. Raising the head of the bed

   C. Giving inhalers

   D. Assessing pulse

5. A patient with advanced chronic obstructive pulmonary disease (COPD) is very fatigued and on bed rest. Clustering of care has become necessary. When would the nurse auscultate this patient's lungs?

   A. When ambulating the patient

   B. When turning the patient

   C. Right after the patient's meal

   D. After bathing the patient

6. The staff educator from the hospital's respiratory unit is providing an educational event for the local Junior League. The educator is talking about health promotion activities for people with respiratory diseases or those who are at high risk for respiratory complications. What would the educator include in the presentation?

A. Encourage refinements to approaches patients already are practicing.

B. Reinforce existing healthy habits.

C. Reduce complications of existing or established diagnoses.

D. Diagnose problems at the annual physical.

7. A patient comes to the clinic complaining of waking during the night with sudden shortness of breath. She is diagnosed with paroxysmal nocturnal dyspnea. Before leaving the clinic, the patient asks the nurse what causes paroxysmal nocturnal dyspnea. What would be the nurse's best response?

A. Fluid overload from elevation of the legs

B. Congestive heart failure

C. Cardiac decompensation

D. Fluid overload related to renal failure

APPLICATION

Remember Mr. Jin, the man with COPD and congestive heart failure (CHF) discussed in Chapter 18 of Jensen's *Nursing Health Assessment*. Read through his physical assessment findings below, underline the abnormal findings, and identify two interventions that you will make based upon the assessment.

> **Inspection:** T 38°C oral, P 102 beats/min, R 24 breaths/min, BP 156/78 mm Hg, SaO_2 90%. T 38°C oral, P 102 beats/min, R 24 breaths/min, BP 156/78 mm Hg, SaO_2 90%. Alert and oriented. Patient sitting in chair with increased respiratory effort. Nasal flaring and pursed lip breathing are present. Needing to pause to take breaths in the middle of sentences. Skin color pale, using neck muscles to breathe, no retractions. Clubbing present in fingers. Coughing up moderate amounts of thick yellow sputum. Denies chest pain. Increased dyspnea and respirations 32 breaths/min when ambulating in hall.
>
> **Palpation:** Tactile fremitus increased in right base.
>
> **Percussion:** Right base dull to percussion.
>
> **Auscultation:** Few wheezes scattered through lung fields. Decreased breath sounds noted in right base. Bronchophony, egophony, and whispered pectoriloquy are present over right base.
>
> *J. Nguyen, RN*

Interventions: _____

_____

_____

_____

ALTERNATIVE CASE STUDY SCENARIOS

The following information is based upon Mr. Jin's situation, but the assessment findings are different. Based on the changes outlined below, *consider what other outcomes, information, and problems would affect the overall picture and shape your responses.*

Alternative A

Mr. Jin's temperature is 37°C. He has clear sputum production. His lungs have increased wheezes but no crackles. His oxygen saturation is 85%. He is slightly cyanotic and disoriented to date and place. He has no chest pain.

- What is causing his oxygen saturation to be so low?

- Is his condition stable, urgent, or an emergency?

- How will the nurse intervene and evaluate interventions? Should the nurse call the rapid response team?

Alternative B

Mr. Jin's temperature is 36.5°C and he has frothy sputum production. His lungs have his usual wheezes but also are reduced in the bases. His oxygen saturation is 93%. He has gained 10 lb in the last 2 days, his rings are tight, and he has run out of his thiazide diuretic so has not taken it in the last 2 days. He has neck vein distention and peripheral edema.

- What is causing Mr. Jin's sputum to be frothy?

- What other information might you collect based upon his symptoms?

- What is the relationship of his other symptoms to his breath sounds?

ROLE-PLAYING SCENARIOS

Scenario 1

Demographics: 56-year-old man, married, one child who is living away from home, employed as a plumber.

Scenario: Has been feeling fatigued over the past week, elevated temperature, coughing, "can't sleep because of cough."

Past medical history: Hypertension, hypercholesterolemia, low back pain, pneumonia 2 years ago. Taking blood pressure and high cholesterol medication, garlic tablets, and coenzyme Q10.

Behavior during interview: Appears concerned, asking if it's pneumonia. Wondering if he needs to stay home from work.

Presenting information:

- **Location:** Cough present "deep in chest."
- **Intensity:** 8/10.
- **Duration:** Continuous. Not getting better.
- **Description:** Cannot take a full breath, cough interfering with breathing, can't cough up any secretions but feels like there's "stuff" down in there.
- **Aggravating factors:** Deep breathing, lying flat.
- **Alleviating factors:** Leaning forward, staying quiet.
- **Functional impairment:** Afraid he'll need to miss work.
- **Pain goal:** 2/10.

Physical findings during assessment:
Temperature 38.6°C orally, P 102 beats/min, R 20 breaths/min, BP 166/78 mm Hg. O_2 saturation 88%. Skin color flushed. Splinting left side with coughing. Small amount sputum thick, yellow. Lungs with moderate amount of gurgles in left lower third of lung fields.
Using the above information, analyze the data and write a SOAP note that shows your thinking.

Nursing diagnosis or problem: _____

_____

_____

Signature _____

Date _____

Scenario 2

Demographics: 23-year-old woman, single, lives in apartment with roommate. College student, uninsured, works part time as waitress.

Scenario: Wheezing for 2 days that keeps her awake at night. Chest feels tight, nonproductive cough, shortness of breath.

Past medical history: Has had asthma since 8 years old, urinary tract infection last year, immunizations up to date, tonsillectomy age 6 years. Takes multivitamin and fish oil daily.

Behavior during interview: Anxious, does not want to have an asthma flare up again. Cannot miss time away from classes, already feeling behind. Cannot miss work as she needs the income to pay the rent.

Presenting information:

- **Location:** Tightness generalized over chest.
- **Intensity:** Tightness is 4/10, wheezing 6/10.
- **Duration:** Two days.
- **Description:** "I just feel like I can't catch my breath. I've started wheezing again and it won't stop." "I haven't had anything like this in 2 years."
- **Aggravating factors:** Tree pollen, dust mites.
- **Alleviating factors:** Inhalers usually work but she hasn't used one in 2 years.
- **Functional impairment:** Concerned about missing school, work.
- **Pain goal:** Wants tightness and wheezing gone.

Physical findings during assessment:
Temperature 36.8°C tympanic, pulse 124 beats/min, R 32 breaths/min, BP 108/66 mm Hg. SpO_2 is 84%. Appears pale, tired, anxious. Lips and mucous membranes pale. Bilateral coarse expiratory wheezes present throughout lung fields. Using sternomastoid accessory muscles. Supraclavicular retractions present. Dry, hacking cough that is nonproductive.
Using the above information, analyze the data and write a SOAP note that shows your thinking.

Nursing diagnosis or problem: _____

_____

_____

Signature _____

Date _____

DOCUMENTATION

Form for Use in Practice

Patient Name _____ Date _____

Date of Birth _____

Initial Survey

Reason for seeking health care: _____

History of present illness

- Location:

- Intensity:

- Duration:

- Description:

- Aggravating factors:

- Alleviating factors:

- Functional impairment:

- Pain goal:

Vital signs: T (route)_____   P (with site)_____   R_____   BP (site)_____ SpO_2_____

Weight: _____   Height: _____   BMI: _____

General appearance (posture, pursed lips, nasal flaring, LOC, skin color): _____

Respiratory movement (inspiration: expiration ratio, rate, pattern): _____

General level of distress (accessory muscles, retractions): _____

History/Interview:

- Family history of respiratory problems:

- History of asthma, bronchitis, emphysema, pneumonia:

- Medications and supplements:

- Smoking history:

- Recreational drugs:

- Occupational and environmental exposure:

- Allergies:

- Last chest x-ray and TB test:

- Influenza or pneumococcal vaccine:

- Travel to high-risk areas:

Common Symptoms:

Symptom	Yes	No	Additional data
Chest pain or discomfort			
Difficulty breathing			
Orthopnea			
Paroxysmal nocturnal dyspnea			
Cough or mucus			
Wheezing or tightness in chest			
Change in functional ability			

Physical Assessment:

Inspect color, shape, condition of patient's fingernails.
Assess muscles and external intercostals.
Inspect chest shape and configuration.
Palpate chest.
Test chest expansion (optional).
Percuss chest (optional).
Test diaphragmatic excursion (optional).
Test for fremitus (optional).

Auscultate lungs.

	Breath sounds	Amplitude	Ratio of Inspiration: Expiration	Clear or adventitious sounds*
Over trachea				
Over bronchi				
Anterior lungs	L R			L R
Posterior lungs	L R			L R

*Are they inspiratory, expiratory, or both? Do they clear with coughing or deep breathing? Where specifically do you hear them?

Test for voice sounds: brochophony (optional).
Test for voice sounds: egophony (optional).
Test for voice sounds: whispered pectoriloquy (optional).
Assess for cough.
Assess for sputum.

Signature_____ Date _____

Guide for Use in Practice

Technique	Normal Findings	Abnormal Findings
Perform initial survey.	*Posture relaxed and upright. Facial expression relaxed. Patient alert, cooperative, and oriented to time, place, and person.*	Kyphosis, scoliosis, or lordosis. Tripod position or leaning forward. Anxious facial expression. Disorientation.
Observe skin color.	*Appropriate tone for patient's racial background. Normal skin color is pink.*	Color: pallor, jaundice, flushed, cyanosis (central vs. peripheral), erythema, ruddiness, mottled.
Assess respiratory movements.	*Expiration is twice as long as inspiration. Normal rate is 12–20 breaths/minute. Rhythm is regular and breathing appears easy and quiet (eupnea). An occasional sigh is normal.*	Document measurements. Label if tachypnea, hyperventilation, bradypnea, hypoventilation, Cheyne-Stokes, Biot's, agonal, or apnea. Forced expiration, guarding or increased work of breathing.
Assess oxygen saturation.	*92%–100%*	<92% may require immediate intervention.
Inspect color, shape, condition of fingernails.	*Pink nailbeds, smooth rounded nails, 160 degrees*	Clubbing
Assess muscles and external intercostals.	*Diaphragm and external intercostals do most of the work. Retractions are absent.*	Accessory muscle use (sternomastoid, scalene, trapezius, latissimus dorsi, pectoralis major and minor, platysma, rectus abdominus, internal intercostal). Retractions (supraclavicular subcostal, intracostal).
Inspect chest shape.	*Spinous processes of the vertebrae are midline; scapulae are symmetric in each hemithorax. Chest wall is cone-shaped (narrower at the bottom than the top), symmetric, and oval (narrower from front to back than from side to side). The transverse (side to side):anterior-posterior (AP) ratio is between 1:2 and 5:7. Although ribs are not visible in most people, those that are slope at approximately 45 degrees. Chest expansion is symmetric. Normally AP to transverse ratio is 1:2.*	Increased ratio, scoliosis, kyphosis, barrel chest, pectus excavatum, pectus carnatum, asymmetry, paradoxical respirations
Palpate chest.	*Thorax is nontender without any lesions, lumps, masses, or crepitus.*	Pain, tenderness, lesions, lumps, masses, or crepitus
Test chest expansion.	*The thumbs move apart symmetrically, approximately 5–10 cm.*	Thumbs move apart asymmetrically or <5 cm.
Percuss chest.	*Healthy lung tissue sounds resonant. In patients with extremely large chests, percussion sounds may become dull secondary to the increased tissue mass.*	Percussion becomes hyperresonant with obstructive lung disease. Percussion will be less resonant over areas of consolidation or masses.
Test diaphragmatic excursion.	*Diaphragmatic excursion should be one or two rib spaces, or 3–5 cm and 7–8 cm in well-conditioned adults.*	Asymmetrical or reduced excursion occurs in neuromuscular or respiratory disease.

Test for fremitus.	*Normal variations are wide-ranging, depending on voice intensity and pitch, position of the bronchi in relation to the chest wall, and chest size. Fremitus is normally more intense between the scapulae, where the bronchi bifurcate, and less intense at the bases, where more porous tissue reduces the transmission of vibrations.*	Reduced or increased fremitus occurs with decreased ventilation or areas of consolidation.
Auscultate lungs.	*Vesicular sounds are soft, low-pitched, and found over fine airways near the site of air exchange.* *Bronchovesicular sounds are found over major bronchi, which have fewer alveoli.* *Bronchial sounds are loud, high-pitched, and found over the trachea and larynx.* *Expiration is longer than inspiration, similar to normal breathing. As auscultation progresses down to the smaller airways, it takes time for air to move in, so inspiration is longer than expiration in vesicular sounds.*	Diminished or absent breath sounds, bronchial or bronchovesicular sounds in lung periphery. Describe adventitious sounds (crackles, wheezes, gurgles, stridor). Are they inspiratory or expiratory? Do they clear with coughing? Where specifically do you hear them?
Test for voice sounds.	*Sounds are muffled and difficult to distinguish.*	The word "ninety-nine" is easily understood and louder over dense areas. This is called brochophony. In egophony, the "ee" sounds like a loud "A." Sounds are louder and clearer than the whispered sounds, as if the patient is directly whispering into the stethoscope. This is called whispered pectoriloquy.
Assess for cough.	*No cough*	Cough present. Describe as croupy, barking, brassy, dry, hacking, productive, wet, moist
Assess for sputum.	*No sputum*	Evaluate amount, color, purulent, tenacious, bloody, or frank hemoptysis.

Heart and Neck Vessels Assessment

OBJECTIVE SUMMARY

This chapter helps the nurse to identify important vocabulary and information related to cardiovascular assessment. After completion of this chapter, the nurse should be able to perform the cardiovascular assessment, including auscultation of heart sounds.

READING ASSIGNMENT

Read Chapter 19 in Jensen's *Nursing Health Assessment: A Best-Practice Approach*.

VOCABULARY/TERMINOLOGY

- **Afterload:** Pressure in the great vessels.

- **Apex:** The bottom of the heart.

- **Arrhythmias:** Abnormal heart rhythms with early (premature), delayed, or irregular beats.

- **Automaticity:** Property that enables the heart to generate its own impulses.

- **Base:** Top of the heart.

- **Bruit:** Swooshing sound similar to the sound of the blood pressure.

- **Cardiac output:** Amount of blood ejected from the left ventricle each minute.

- **Diastole:** Ventricular relaxation.

- **Dyspnea on exertion:** Shortness of breath with effort.

- **Fixed split:** During auscultation, when the two components of the cardiac cycle are heard during both inspiration and expiration. The split is wide and results from right bundle branch block or early opening of the aortic valve.

- **Flat neck veins:** Barely visible neck veins, even when lying flat.

- **Hepatojugular reflex:** A test in which the examiner presses gently on the liver to increase venous return. Pulsation increases for a few beats and then returns to normal less than 3 cm above the sternal angle.

- **Jugular venous distention:** A condition associated with heart failure and fluid volume overload. The neck veins appear full, and the level of pulsation may be greater than 3 cm above the sternal angle.

- **Murmur:** Abnormal heart sound that may result from intrinsic cardiovascular disease or circulatory disturbance. Murmurs in adults usually indicate disease.

- **Nocturia:** Urinating during the night. A common symptom associated with redistribution of fluid from the legs to the core when lying. As the fluid shifts, the kidneys are better perfused, increasing urine production.

- **Orthopnea:** Onset or worsening of dyspnea on assuming the supine position with improvement upon sitting up, most often seen in cardiac cases.

- **Palpitation:** Rapid throbbing or fluttering of the heart; may be associated with arrhythmias.

- **Paradoxical split:** Sound that occurs when the pulmonic valve closes before the aortic from left bundle branch block, right ventricular pacemaker. The sounds usually fuse during inspiration.

- **Paroxysmal nocturnal dyspnea:** Also known as cardiac asthma; sudden, severe shortness of breath at night that awakens a person from sleep, often with coughing and wheezing. It is most closely associated with congestive heart failure.

- **Point of maximal intensity:** Point where the inferior tip of the heart may cause a pulsation.

- **Preload:** Volume in the right atrium at the end of diastole.

- **Pulse deficit:** Apical pulse minus the number of missed beats.

- **Rub:** Most important physical sign of acute pericarditis. It is triple phased during midsystole, middiastole, and presystole. The scratchy, leathery quality results from the parietal and visceral pleurae rubbing together. The sound increases on leaning forward and during exhalation. It is heard best in the third left intercoastal space (ICS) at the sternal border.

- **Sinus arrhythmia:** Normal variation in heart rate in which the rate increases at the peak of inspiration and slows at the peak of expiration.

- **Snap:** Early diastolic sound associated with mitral stenosis.

- **Split heart sound:** Audible heart sound that occurs when the valves close at slightly different times.

- **Stroke volume:** How much blood is ejected with each beat or stroke.

- **Systole:** Contraction of the ventricles.

- **Wide split:** Found with right bundle branch block from delayed depolarization of the right ventricle.

STUDY GUIDE

Activity A FILL IN THE BLANK

| bruit, click, gallop, murmur, rub, snap, split |

1. Write the appropriate medical term from the box above next to the description of the sound. Choices of terms are listed alphabetically at the bottom of the question.

   A. Extra heart sound described as S3 or S4

   _____

   B. Whooshing sound that is either systolic or diastolic

   _____

   C. Double heart sound caused from valves closing at slightly different times

   _____

   D. Ejection sound in early diastole caused by stenosis

   _____

   E. Whooshing sound over large vessel caused by stenosis

   _____

   F. High-pitched, scratchy sound caused by pericardial friction

   _____

   G. Sound from stenotic atrioventricular (AV) valve, usually accompanied by a system murmur

   _____

Activity B MATCHING

1. *Match the cardiovascular term with the appropriate root. The roots are listed alphabetically.*

Answer	Term	Root
	1. Above	A. angio
	2. Veins	B. brady
	3. Blockage	C. cardio
	4. Blood vessel	D. embolo
	5. Veins	E. phlebo
	6. Heart	F. supra
	7. Slow	G. tachy
	8. Fast	H. thrombo

2. Match the assessment technique with normal findings.

Answer	Technique	Normal Findings
	1. Auscultate normal heart sounds.	A. There are usually two pulsations with a prominent descent, compared to the carotid pulse, which has one pulsation and a prominent ascent with systole.
	2. Inspect jugular venous pulse.	
	3. Inspect jugular venous pressure.	
	4. Assess carotid pulse.	B. Normal findings are up to 3 cm above the sternal angle, which is equivalent to a central venous pressure of 8 mm Hg. If exact levels are not measured, document findings as "JVP normal," "JVP not elevated," "neck veins not distended," or "no JVD."
	5. Palpate apical pulse.	
	6. Palpate precordium.	

C. Normal strength is 2+ or moderate. Pulses are equal bilaterally.

D. Normal impulses are absent or located in the fourth to fifth left ICS at the midclavicular line (MCL) with no lifts or heaves.

E. The point of maximal intensity (PMI) is usually in the fifth left ICS at the MCL when present. No pulsations are palpated in other areas.

F. S1 is greater than S2 in the mitral and tricuspid areas; S2 is greater than S1 in the aortic and pulmonic areas; S1 is equal to S2 at Erb's point.

Activity C SEQUENCING

1. Correctly order the following events in the cardiac cycle, beginning with atrial filling.

Order No.	Event
	Aortic and pulmonic valves close.
	Aortic and pulmonic valves open.
1	Atrium fills and contracts.
	Mitral and tricuspid valves close.
	Mitral and tricuspid valves open.
	Ventricles contract.
	Ventricles eject.

Activity D SHORT ANSWER

1. Explain the hereditary link to cardiovascular disease.

_____

_____

_____

_____

2. Identify what events are considered medical emergencies.

_____

_____

_____

_____

3. Describe how carotid artery pulses are assessed. State special safety precautions.

_____

_____

_____

_____

4. Describe the significance of S3, S4, and friction rub.

_____

_____

_____

_____

5. Describe the mechanism for murmurs; differentiate between systolic and diastolic.

_____

_____

_____

_____

6. Define three common nursing diagnoses associated with heart problems.

_____

_____

_____

_____

_____

Activity E MULTIPLE CHOICE

1. When asked to define the continuous rhythmic movement of blood during contraction and relaxation of the heart, what should be the student's best answer?

A. It is the cardiac circulation.

B. It is the cardiac output.

C. It is the cardiac cycle.

D. It is the cardiac workload.

2. A new nurse on the telemetry unit is reviewing information about how to correctly read electrocardiograms. The nurse is expected to know that the PR interval is

A. the spread of depolarization in the atria

B. the time from firing of the sinoatrial (SA) node to the beginning of depolarization in the ventricle

C. the spread of depolarization and sodium release in the ventricles to cause ventricular contraction

D. relaxation of the ventricles and repolarization of the cells

3. When learning about hereditary variability, the student would learn that what ethnic group has the highest number of premature deaths (younger than 65 years)?

A. Hispanic

B. African American

C. Native American

D. Pacific Islanders

4. A triage nurse is working in the emergency department of a county hospital. Four patients come in at the same time. Patient A has an arrhythmia diagnosed as atrial fibrillation; Patient B is in chronic congestive heart failure; Patient C is assessed and found to have a probable pulmonary embolism; Patient D complains of chest pain relieved by nitroglycerin and rest. Which patient would be the nurse's highest priority?

A. Patient A

B. Patient B

C. Patient C

D. Patient D

5. The nurse on the cardiac unit is caring for a patient who thinks he was having a myocardial infarction when he came to the emergency department. When reviewing laboratory data on this patient, the nurse notes that all tests are within normal limits except for the cholesterol and C-reactive protein. These are both elevated outside the normal range. The nurse knows that an elevated cholesterol and C-reactive protein

A. more than double the risk of cardiac disease

B. have no correlation with increased risk of cardiac disease

C. are both sensitive and specific to heart failure

D. are clinical proof that the patient had a coronary event

6. Statistics show that a patient who smokes is twice as likely to

A. develop venous insufficiency

B. have sudden cardiac arrest

C. develop peripheral arterial disease (PAD)

D. die before age 65 years

7. A community health nurse is planning a screening day for blood pressure and cholesterol. What kind of prevention would this be?

   A. Primary
   B. Secondary
   C. Tertiary
   D. Community

ALTERNATIVE CASE SCENARIOS

Remember Mrs. Lewis, the woman with chest pain whose case is documented throughout Chapter 19 of Jensen's *Nursing Health Assessment*. Read through her objective findings below, underline the abnormal findings, and identify five additional assessments that you will make.

> **Inspection:** Sitting with the head of the bed at 45-degree angle, appears comfortable but somewhat anxious. BP 122/62 mm Hg, P 112 beats/min, R 16 breaths/min, T 37°C, oxygen saturation 94%. Skin color pale, some diaphoresis. Chest shape symmetrical without visible apical impulse. Respirations without dyspnea. No neck vein distention.
>
> **Palpation:** Apical impulse not present. Peripheral pulses 3+ without edema.
>
> **Percussion:** Not performed.
>
> **Auscultation:** Heart rate 112 with 3 to 5 premature beats/min. Pulse deficit of 5. S1 > S2 at apex and S2 > S1 at base. No murmurs, rubs, or gallops. *G. Indigo, RN*

Additional Assessments

1. _____
2. _____
3. _____
4. _____
5. _____

Alternative A

Subjective: "I have this sharp and stabbing pain in the left side of my chest."

Objective: Rates pain as 7/10, aggravated by lying flat, deep breathing, and coughing. Reduced by sitting up and leaning forward. BP 152/86 mm Hg, P 112 beats/min and regular, R 36 breaths/min, and shallow, oxygen saturation 98%. S1 and S2 regular with no murmurs or gallops. New pericardial friction rub auscultated loudest in the fifth left ICS at the sternal border. Skin pink; patient appears anxious.

- Is Mrs. Lewis's condition stable, urgent, or an emergency?
- How is this pain different from the pain described in Chapter 19 of Jensen's *Nursing Health Assessment*?
- What additional assessments will the nurse perform?

Alternative B

Subjective: "I'm very short of breath, and it feels like my legs are tight."

Objective: BP 130/66 mm Hg, P 108 beats/min, R 32 breaths/min, oxygen saturation 84%. Heart rate and rhythm regular with a new S4. Lung sounds decreased in both bases. Very short of breath, coughing up moderate amounts of thin frothy sputum. Skin pale, appears anxious. 4+ pitting edema in legs bilaterally. No urine output since admission.

- What nursing diagnosis do you propose based on the data above?
- How will the nurse validate this diagnosis?
- What interventions might be indicated based upon the suspected diagnosis?

ROLE-PLAYING SCENARIOS

Scenario 1

Demographics: 59-year-old man

Reason for seeking care: Gets fatigued after mild activity, climbing stairs

Past medical history: Myocardial infarction (MI) 1 year ago, 3 years ago, and 10 years ago. Stent placed after second MI. Current medications include a beta blocker and an antilipidemic.

Behavior during interview: Tired, short of breath after activity.

Presenting information:

- **Location:** Chest.
- **Intensity:** 4. Gets "really bad" so has to rest after going up only 3 stairs.
- **Duration:** Intermittent. Fatigue started with stairs 3 weeks ago.

- **Description:** "Heart pounding, racing, feels like it will jump out of chest, dizzy if I don't stop."

- **Aggravating factors:** Exercise, exertion.

- **Alleviating factors:** Rest.

- **Functional impairment:** Cannot walk uphill. Cannot do normal 3-block exercise in neighborhood.

- **Goal:** Wants to be able to do normal uphill 3-block exercise in neighborhood.

Physical findings: Pulse 124 beats/min, BP 110/62 mm Hg, + jugular vein distention, grade II/IV systolic ejection murmur, crackles in lungs, 1+ edema in legs, fatigued. Low ejection fraction on echocardiogram. Does not have metabolic capacity to meet metabolic demands of the body.

Using the above information, analyze the data and write a SOAP note that shows your thinking.

Nursing diagnosis or problem:

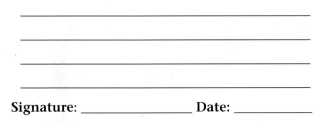

Signature: _____ Date: _____

Scenario 2

Demographics: 82-year-old man.

Reason for seeking care: Intermittent pain in chest, has had it for 5 years, takes nitroglycerine to relieve.

Past medical history: High blood pressure for 43 years, both parents with history of high blood pressure and father had MI. Bilateral knee replacements from degenerative joint disease 10 and 11 years ago. History of depression. Taking antihypertensive, antidepressant, and nitroglycerine tablets as needed for chest pain.

Behavior during interview: Alert, oriented, appropriate.

Presenting information:

- **Location:** Center of chest, approximately sixth ICS at midsternal line.

- **Intensity:** When it happens, can be a 7/10 scale.

- **Duration:** Intermittent—about once a month, lasts 10 to 15 minutes. Has been stable over the last year.

- **Description:** Clenching, squeezing, tight into throat.

- **Aggravating factors:** Activity, yard work, walking up one flight of stairs at home.

- **Alleviating factors.** Nitroglycerine, rest.

- **Functional impairment:** When pain presents, must stop activity and rest. Would like to be able to do yard work without worrying about having a heart attack and chest pain.

- **Pain goal:** No pain.

Physical findings: T 37°C oral, P 76 beats/min, R 14 breaths/min, BP 112/72 mm Hg. Urine output and nutritional intake balanced. No edema, lung sounds clear. Alert and oriented, mentation appropriate.

Using the above information, analyze the data and write a SOAP note that shows your thinking.

Nursing diagnosis or problem: _____

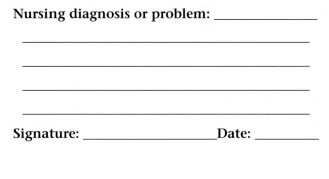

Signature: _____ Date: _____

DOCUMENTATION

Form for Use in Practice

Patient Name _____ Date_____

Date of Birth _____

Initial Survey

- Reason for seeking health care:_____

History of present illness

- Location:
- Intensity:
- Duration:
- Description:
- Aggravating factors:
- Alleviating factors:
- Functional impairment:
- Pain goal:

Vital signs: T (route)_____ P (site)_____ R_____ BP (site)_____ SpO$_2$_____

Weight: _____ Height: _____ BMI: _____

General appearance: _____

General level of distress:_____

Risk Factors and History:

- Family history of cardiovascular problems:
- Previous diagnosis with chest pain, heart attack, heart failure, or irregular rhythm:
- Medications for cardiac problems:
- Natural supplements or over-the-counter medications:
- Smoking/tobacco use:
- Cholesterol level:
- Glucose level:
- Physical activity:
- Typical diet:
- Alcohol use:
- Recreational drugs:

Common Symptoms:

Symptom	Yes	No	Additional data
Chest pain			
Dyspnea			
Orthopnea			
Cough			
Diaphoresis			
Fatigue			
Edema			
Nocturia			
Palpitations			

Physical Assessment:

- Inspect jugular venous pulse and pressure:
- Test hepatojugular reflex (optional):
- Inspect and palpate carotid pulse:
- Auscultate carotid pulse:
- Inspect precordium:
- Palpate precordium:
  - Percuss precordium (optional):
  - Auscultate precordium:
  - Apical pulse rate and rhythm (1 minute):
  - Use diaphragm and bell, compare S1 and S2, listen in systole and diastole:

Area	Compare S1 and S2	Murmur	Extra sounds
Aortic			
Pulmonic			
Erb's point			
Tricuspid			
Mitral (apical)			

Signature_____ Date _____

Guide for Use in Practice

Technique	Normal Findings	Abnormal Findings
Inspect jugular venous pulse. Record measurement.	*There are usually two pulsations with a prominent descent, compared to the carotid pulse, which has one pulsation and a prominent ascent with systole.*	Bulging, engorged or distended veins, flat veins
Inspect jugular venous pressure.	*Up to 3 cm above the sternal angle, which is equivalent to a central venous pressure of 8 mm Hg. If exact levels are not measured, document "JVP normal," "JVP not elevated," "neck veins not distended," or "no JVD."*	Greater than 3 cm above the sternal angle
Palpate for hepatojugular reflex.	*JVP up to 3 cm above the sternal angle, which is equivalent to a central venous pressure of 8 mm Hg.*	JVP above 3 cm for more than 15 seconds
Inspect and palpate carotid pulse.	*Contour is smooth with a rapid upstroke and slower downstroke. Strength is 2+ or moderate. Pulses are equal bilaterally.*	Asymmetry, diminished pulse, bounding
Auscultate carotid pulse	*No bruit*	Bruit
Inspect precordium.	*Impulses are absent or located in the fourth to fifth left ICS at the MCL with no lifts or heaves.*	PMI displaced laterally, lift or heave
Palpate precordium.	*PMI is in the fifth left ICS at the MCL when present. No pulsations are palpated in other areas.*	PMI displaced laterally, thrill
Percuss precordium.	*The left border of the heart is percussed from the apex in the fourth to fifth left ICS at the MCL.*	PMI displaced laterally
Auscultate precordium.	*S1 and S2 with regular rhythm*	Irregular rhythm, murmurs (diastolic vs. systolic), extra sounds (S3, S4, friction rub)

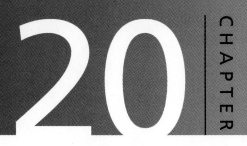

Peripheral Vascular and Lymphatic Assessment

CHAPTER 20

OBJECTIVE SUMMARY

This chapter focuses on comprehensive assessment of the peripheral vascular and lymphatic systems. Nurses must understand the independent roles of the arterial, venous, and lymphatic systems, as well as their integrated functioning as the circulatory system. Doing so enables them to develop holistic plans for circulatory well-being in their patients. A review of pertinent anatomy and physiology provides the basis for the collection of subjective and objective information. The section on subjective data collection gives details to help nurses evaluate history, risk factors, and symptoms associated with peripheral vascular health. The content on objective assessment outlines a methodical approach to assessing peripheral pulses, extremity temperature, skin condition, perfusion, and fluid status, and describes alterations from normal.

READING ASSIGNMENT

Read Chapter 20 in Jensen's *Nursing Health Assessment: A Best-Practice Approach.*

VOCABULARY/TERMINOLOGY

- **Arteriosclerosis:** Calcification of the arteries.
- **Atherosclerosis:** Thickening of the arterial walls caused by a build-up of fatty plaque. It is a progressive, systemic disease.

- **Deep vein thrombosis (DVT):** Clot that forms in a vein deep in the body; characterized by pain, edema, and warmth of an extremity.
- **Dependent rubor:** Redness that develops in an extremity that is dependent, especially as a sign of inflammation. Indicates arterial insufficiency.
- **Edema:** Swelling caused by fluid in the tissues.
- **Embolism:** Clot.
- **Intermittent claudication:** Pain brought on by exertion and relieved by rest.
- **Peripheral arterial disease (PAD):** Atherosclerosis in the peripheral arteries, causing their narrowing. Increases dramatically in the 7th and 8th decades of life.
- **Peripheral vascular disease (PVD):** Disease of the blood vessels outside the heart and brain, often a narrowing of those vessels that carry blood to the legs, arms, stomach, or kidneys. Characterized by pain, numbness or tingling, cramping, skin changes, edema, and reduced functional ability.
- **Thrombus:** Formation of a clot inside a blood vessel, causing narrowing of the arteries.
- **Varicosities:** Dilated, elongated, and tortuous veins irrespective of size.

STUDY GUIDE

Activity A   FILL IN THE BLANK

1. Fill in the blank in the following sentences:

    A. _____control blood pressure.

    B. Smooth _____cells line the inner layer of all blood vessels.

    C. The venous system is a _____system.

    D. A _____created by respiration, skeletal muscle contraction, and intraluminal valves regulates blood flow in the venous system.

    E. Veins contain _____ that prevent the retrograde flow of venous blood, thus maintaining unidirectional flow.

    F. The _____ at the junctions of the subclavian and internal jugular veins return the lymph fluid to the circulation.

2. Finish the sentences about cultural considerations in patients with peripheral vascular and lymphatic problems.

    A. Peripheral arterial disease (PAD), the most prevalent vascular disease, is highest in _____.

    B. _____ play a prominent role in atherosclerosis in addition to many of the cardiovascular risk factors.

    C. Primary varicose veins are seen more often in people older than _____ and in those with _____.

    D. _____, a disease that poses a significant risk factor for PAD, is increased in African Americans.

Activity B   MATCHING

1. **Match the definition with the diagnostic test.**

Answer	Definition	Diagnostic Test
	1. Evaluates the saphenous vein valves	A. Color change
	2. Check for arterial insufficiency	B. Manual compression
	3. Evaluates the competence of the valves	C. Venous duplex
	4. Evaluates arterial occlusion	D. Trendelenberg
	5. Evaluates venous occlusion	E. Arteriogram

2. **Match the nursing diagnosis with the appropriate intervention.**

Answer	Diagnosis	Intervention
	1. Altered arterial tissue perfusion	A. Refer to physical therapy as indicated.
	2. Altered peripheral tissue perfusion	B. Perform assessment: Pain, pulses, pallor, paresthesia, paralysis.
	3. Risk for peripheral neurovascular dysfunction	C. Assess dorsalis pedis and posterior tibial pulses bilaterally.
	4. Activity intolerance	D. Provide range-of-motion exercises twice daily.

3. **Match the abnormal findings with variations in arterial pulses.**

Answer	Abnormal Findings	Pulses
	1. Alternating small and large amplitude, regular rate	A. Weak pulses
	2. Weak on palpation and easily obliterated	B. Pulsus paradoxus
	3. Double systolic peak	C. Pulsus alternans
	4. Palpable decrease in amplitude on quiet inspiration	D. Pulsus bigeminus
	5. Increased pulse pressure, rapid rise and fall, brief systolic peak	E. Bounding pulse
	6. Alternating irregular beats; one normal beat and then one premature beat with alternating strong and weak amplitude	F. Pulsus bisferiens

4. *Read the following categories and descriptions given for each. For each category, mark with an A if the associated description applies to an arterial ulcer or with a B if the associated description applies to a venous ulcer.*

Answer	Category	Description
	Location	Ankle, medial malleolus, distal third of leg
	Borders	Regular
	Ulcer base	Pale, yellow
	Drainage	Moderate to large amount
	Gangrene	Not present
	Pain	Painful; decreased with dependency
	Skin	Stasis dermatitis, pigmentation changes
	Pulses	Decreased or absent

Activity C   SHORT ANSWER

1. Explain the purpose of the lymphatic system, including how the lymphatic system supports the vascular system.

_____

_____

_____

_____

2. Discuss the physiologic changes that occur in the older adult's peripheral vascular system.

_____

_____

_____

_____

3. Discuss the need for an acute assessment related to the peripheral vascular system. Include when to stop the assessment and get help.

_____

_____

_____

_____

4. Discuss the gathering of data to identify health-promotion areas and patient teaching needs related to the peripheral vascular system.

_____

_____

_____

_____

5. Explain the assessment of a family history related to peripheral vascular disease. Include questions that the nurse should ask.

_____

_____

_____

_____

6. Identify options for modifying risk factors and improving outcomes for patients with peripheral vascular disease.

_____

_____

_____

_____

7. Identify appropriate interventions to achieve desired outcome for patients with peripheral vascular disease.

_____

_____

_____

_____

Activity D   MULTIPLE CHOICE

1. The largest arteries of the upper extremities are the
   A. brachial arteries
   B. subclavian arteries
   C. abdominal arteries
   D. radial arteries

2. A new nurse on the vascular unit is caring for a patient with an embolus in the deep part of the peripheral vascular system. In what vessel might the embolus be?

   A. Lesser saphenous vein

   B. Ileal duct

   C. Greater saphenous vein

   D. Peroneal tibial vessel

3. A nurse is providing patient education to a group of patients entering the third trimester of pregnancy. The nurse explains to the patients that their blood volume has nearly doubled, and that this extra volume combined with pressure from the fetus can cause what?

   A. Independent edema

   B. Leg cramps

   C. Hemorrhoids

   D. Venous ulcers

4. Older patients develop an increased incidence of peripheral vascular disease beginning in what decade of life?

   A. 5th

   B. 6th

   C. 7th

   D. 8th

5. A student nurse learns that a pulmonary embolism may result from a DVT. The student knows to be alert for any signs of a pulmonary embolism including

   A. diaphoresis

   B. pain in the legs

   C. increased oxygen saturation

   D. bradycardia

6. Patients with PAD need to understand why it is important to monitor

   A. Na^+ and K^+ levels

   B. C-reactive protein levels

   C. creatinine levels

   D. triglyceride levels

7. The nurse is preparing discharge teaching for a patient diagnosed with a lymphatic disorder. What is one of the main teaching points the nurse should include?

   A. How to apply TED hose

   B. Signs and symptoms of DVT

   C. To avoid sitting for long periods

   D. To walk at least 2 miles/day

ALTERNATIVE CASE SCENARIOS

From Chapter 20 of the Jensen text, you should remember Mr. Tretski, an 88-year-old Caucasian man living in a long-term care facility. His medical diagnoses include a myocardial infarction (MI) 15 years ago, high blood pressure, high cholesterol level, chronic renal failure, and PAD. He is taking a statin for his cholesterol and an antiplatelet medication for the PAD. He also is slightly confused, with impaired recent memory.

Review the following alternative situations related to Mr. Tretski. Based on the changes outlined below, consider what other outcomes, information, and problems would affect the overall picture and shape your responses.

Alternative A

Mr. Tretski has lower leg edema, bronze-brown pigmentation with varicose veins, warm skin, capillary refill less than 3 seconds, 2+ pulses bilaterally, and no pain or claudication in his legs.

- What health-related teaching might be indicated?

- What is the cluster of symptoms indicating? What might be the medical and nursing diagnoses?

- What nursing interventions might be indicated in this situation?

Alternative B

Mr. Tretski has an abrupt onset of pain rated 8/10, paresthesia, and weakness in his left leg. His left leg is cold and paler than the right. Pulses in the left are absent, even with the Doppler. Pulses in the right are 1+.

- Is Mr. Tretski's condition stable, urgent, or an emergency?

- How will the nurse focus, organize, and prioritize subjective and objective data collection?

- How will the nurse communicate these findings to others? Draft a sample of written (SOAP note) and verbal (using SBAR) communication.

DOCUMENTATION

Form for Use in Practice

Patient Name _____ Date _____

Date of Birth _____

Initial Survey

Reason for seeking health care: _____

History of present illness

- Location:
- Intensity:
- Duration:
- Description:
- Aggravating factors:
- Alleviating factors:
- Functional impairment:
- Pain goal:

Vital signs: T (route)_____ P (site)_____ R_____ BP (site)_____ SpO$_2$ _____

Weight:_____ Height:_____ BMI:_____

General appearance: _____

General level of distress: _____

Risk Factors and History:

- Family history of cardiovascular problems:
- Past diagnosis with chest pain, heart attack, heart failure, or irregular rhythm:
- Medications:
- Natural supplements or over-the-counter medications:
- Smoking/tobacco use:
- Previous diagnosis with high blood pressure:
- Blood cholesterol level:
- Blood glucose level:
- Exercise:
- Recent trauma to any of the extremities:
- Typical diet:
- Alcohol use:
- Recreational drug use:

Common Symptoms:

Symptom	Yes	No	Additional data
Pain			
Numbness or tingling			
Cramping			
Skin changes			
Edema			
Decreased functional ability			

Physical Assessment:

Note size and symmetry of arms and hands.
Inspect color of arms and hands and for venous pattern.
Inspect nail beds for color and angle.
Note any edema of arms and hands; test for pitting.
Inspect for any ecchymoses or lesions of the upper extremities.
Palpate the arms and hands for temperature.
Assess skin texture and turgor.
Assess capillary refill of arms and hands.
Palpate and grade the brachial and radial pulses.
(Optional) Perform the Allen test.
Palpate for the epitrochlear nodes.
Evaluate the blood pressure in both arms.
Note the size and symmetry of the legs and feet.
Assess color of legs and feet; evaluate for venous pattern.
Evaluate the toenail beds for color and capillary refill.
Note any edema of the legs. Evaluate for pitting.
Evaluate for any ecchymosis or lesions of the lower extremities.
Palpate the legs for temperature.
Assess the texture and turgor of the skin.
Palpate and grade the femoral, popliteal, dorsalis pedis, and posterior tibial pulses.
Palpate the upper and medial thigh for the superficial inguinal lymph nodes.
(Optional) Auscultate with a Doppler to assess any weak peripheral pulses.
(Optional) Assess the ankle-brachial index (ABI).
(Optional) Perform the color changes test to check for arterial insufficiency.
(Optional) Perform the manual compression test.
(Optional) Perform the Trendelenberg test.

Signature_____ Date _____

Guide for Use in Practice

Technique	Normal Findings	Abnormal Findings
Note size and symmetry of arms and hands as well as muscle atrophy or hypertrophy.	*Arms and hands are symmetrical with full joint movement.*	Muscle atrophy, hypertrophy
Assess color of arms and hands; evaluate for venous pattern.	*Color is pink, symmetrical, and consistent without prominent venous pattern.*	Pallor, erythema
Evaluate the nail beds for color and angle.	*Nail beds are pink. Nail-base angle is 180 degrees without clubbing.*	Decreased capillary refill
Note any edema of the arms and hands. Evaluate for pitting.	*No indentation remains when you remove your fingers.*	Lymphedema
Evaluate for any ecchymoses or lesions of the upper extremities.	*Ecchymoses and lesions are absent.*	Ecchymoses, lesions, bruising, delayed wound healing
Palpate the arms and hands for temperature.	*Arms and hands are warm and equal in temperature.*	Coolness of an extremity
Assess skin texture and turgor.	*Texture is firm, even, and elastic. Turgor is intact, as shown by rapid return of skin after pinching.*	Rough or dry texture and poor turgor
Assess capillary refill.	*Capillary refill is <3 seconds.*	Capillary refill takes 3 seconds or longer
Palpate and grade the brachial and radial pulses.	*Pulse is graded +3/4.*	Pulse is <+3
When indicated, perform the Allen test.	*Color returns within 2–5 seconds, indicating adequate circulation.*	Lack of color return
Palpate for the epitrochlear nodes.	*Normally, the epitrochlear nodes are not palpable. If palpated, note size, consistency, mobility, and tenderness.*	Enlarged nodes
Evaluate the blood pressure in both arms. Document the arm with the higher pressure and take subsequent blood pressures in that arm.	*Adult blood pressure is 100–140 mm Hg systolic and 60–90 mm Hg diastolic.*	Difference >10 mm Hg in both arms
Note size and symmetry of the legs as well as muscle atrophy or hypertrophy.	*Legs are symmetrical with full joint movement.*	Atrophy
Assess color of the legs; evaluate for venous pattern.	*Color is symmetrical and consistent without predominant venous pattern.*	Pallor, erythema, edema, and tenderness; color change to white in the toes; dilated and tortuous veins
Evaluate nail beds for color and capillary refill.	*Nail beds are pink, with capillary refill <3 seconds.*	Delayed capillary refill
Note any edema of the legs. Evaluate for pitting.	*No edema is found.*	Edema from chronic venous insufficiency, DVT, and lymphedema; calf or leg swelling; unilateral pitting edema; localized pain or tenderness
Evaluate for any ecchymosis or lesions of the lower extremities.	*Ecchymosis and lesions are absent.*	Ecchymosis, lesions, gangrene

Palpate the legs for temperature.	*Legs and feet are warm and equal in temperature.*	One extremity cooler than the other; warm, edematous, and tender extremity
Assess the texture and turgor of the skin.	*Texture is firm, even, and elastic. Turgor is intact when skin rapidly returns after pinching.*	Rough or dry texture and poor turgor
Palpate and grade the femoral, popliteal, dorsalis pedis, and posterior tibial pulses.	*Pulses are +3/4.*	Pulse lower than +3
Palpate the upper and medial thigh for the superficial inguinal lymph nodes.	*They may be palpable and up to 1–2 cm, movable, and nontender.*	Nodes >2 cm
Assess the ABI.	*Ankle pressure is slightly higher or equal to the brachial. The result is 1.0 (100%) or greater.*	ABI of 0.90 or less (indicates arterial insufficiency)
Perform the color change test.	*Color returns to the feet and toes within 10 seconds. The superficial veins of the feet fill within 15 seconds.*	Return of color taking longer or persistent dependent rubor
Perform the manual compression test.	*If the valves are competent, a wave transmission is not palpable.*	A transmission wave
Perform the Trendelenberg test.	*The saphenous veins fill from the bottom up while the tourniquet is on.*	Filling from above while the tourniquet is on or rapid retrograde filling when the tourniquet is removed

2. Lactation after childbirth is stimulated by
   A. increased testosterone levels
   B. the baby
   C. pituitary gland dysfunction
   D. prolactin secretion

3. A nurse is providing patient education to a group of prepubescent girls at a local elementary school. What would the nurse be most likely to include in the presentation?
   A. Information about fetal development
   B. Information about dating
   C. Information about the stages of breast development
   D. Information about menopause

4. While studying the breast and axillae, students learn that variations in the color of the skin and nipple relate to
   A. ethnic background
   B. age
   C. number of pregnancies
   D. premenopausal or postmenopausal status

5. Benign conditions of the breast include
   A. ductal carcinoma
   B. fibrocystic changes
   C. Paget's disease
   D. precancerous lesions

6. The American Cancer Society currently recommends that palpation of the breast be done in what pattern?
   A. Circular
   B. Radial
   C. Horizontal
   D. Vertical

7. Each glandular lobe in the breast has lobules with milk-producing cells. What cells in these lobules produce milk?
   A. Montgomery's cells
   B. Lactiferous cells
   C. Milk cells
   D. Acini cells

ALTERNATIVE CASE SCENARIOS

Mrs. Randall, a 66-year-old African–American woman, is receiving home care for the management of stage III breast cancer. She recently had preoperative chemotherapy and a mastectomy; she is currently undergoing radiation treatments. Medications include oxycodone for moderate to severe pain, acetaminophen (Tylenol) for mild to moderate pain, senna (Senokot) as a laxative, and metoclopramide (Reglan) for nausea. Mrs. Randall can get out of bed for meals, but she has not been eating much because of a lack of appetite and fatigue. The nurse performed and documented an assessment of Mrs. Randall yesterday. Temperature was 37°C (98.6°F) orally, pulse 78 beats/min, respirations 24 breaths/min, and blood pressure 138/70 mm Hg.

Review the following alternative situations related to Mrs. Randall. Based on the changes outlined below, consider what other outcomes, information, and problems would affect the overall picture and shape your responses.

Alternative A

Subjective: "I just hate the way that this surgery has made me look. The redness from the radiation is even making it worse. How can I ever show my husband what this looks like?"

Objective: Mrs. Randall refuses to look at her breast and looks away when it is exposed. She has not gone out of the house since surgery because of fear of meeting someone whom she knows.

- Are the psychosocial or physical needs of the patient in this case more important? Provide rationale.

- What issues related to her body image might be important to assess?

- How should the nurse organize and prioritize data collection, based upon Mrs. Randall's multiple problems?

Alternative B

Subjective: "I just feel so useless. Usually I am cooking up a storm, because my family loves my Southern cooking. I've always prided myself on having the neatest and cleanest house on the block and I just can't get up enough energy to clean. All of those things that I used to do I just can't anymore."

Objective: Unable to find strength and energy to perform usual role functions such as shopping, cooking, and cleaning. Appears saddened about the change in her physical capacity. Agrees to referral to chore services to assist temporarily.

- How are the psychosocial or physical needs of the patient in this case related? Provide rationale.

- What will the nurse assess related to the patient's role performance?

- How will the nurse individualize assessment to Mrs. Randall's specific needs, considering her condition, age, and culture?

DOCUMENTATION

Form for Use in Practice

Patient Name _____ Date _____

Date of Birth _____

Initial Survey

Reason for seeking health care: _____

History of present illness

- Location:

- Intensity:

- Duration:

- Description:

- Aggravating factors:

- Alleviating factors:

- Functional impairment:

- Pain goal:

Vital signs: T (route)_____   P (site)_____   R_____   BP (site)_____   SpO$_2$_____

Weight: _____ Height: _____ BMI: _____

General appearance: _____

General level of distress: _____

Level of anxiety: _____

Risk Factors and History:

- Family history of breast cancer:

- Previous diagnosis with breast cancer:

- Previous diagnosis with cysts or benign breast disease, fibroadenoma, or breast abscess:

- Previous breast surgery:

- Recent treatment for breast infection:

- Date of last menstrual period:

- Prescribed medications:

- Natural supplements:

- Over-the-counter medications:

- Smoking/tobacco use:
- Blood cholesterol level:
- Blood glucose level:
- Physical activity:
- Typical diet:
- Alcohol use:
- Recreational drug use:

Common Symptoms:

Symptom	Yes	No	Additional data
Breast pain			
Rash			
Lumps			
Swelling			
Discharge			
Trauma			

Physical Assessment:

Right breast • Inspect • Palpate
Left breast • Inspect • Palpate
Self–breast examination • When taught • Date of last self-examination • How often do you perform BSE
Mammogram • Date of last mammogram • Results

Signature_____ Date _____

Guide for Use in Practice

Technique	Normal Findings	Abnormal Findings
Inspect breast skin appearance:		
• Color and texture	*Skin tone determines actual color. Pale, linear stretch marks (striae) may be evident after pregnancy or if a woman has gained and then lost significant weight.*	Redness (erythema) and heat; hyperpigmentation; unilateral vascular appearance; *peau d'orange* appearance; rash or ulceration
• Size and shape	*Wide variation exists, from small to very large (pendulous).*	Significant size or shape difference between breasts

• Symmetry	*Symmetrical, or a left breast slightly larger than the right breast*	Significant asymmetry
• Contour	*Should be uninterrupted*	Retractions or dimpling
• Nipple and areola characteristics	*Areola round or oval, and pink to dark brown or black. Most nipples are everted, but it may be normal for one or both nipples to be inverted. An extra (supernumerary) nipple along the embryonic nipple line is a common variation.*	Recent nipple changes from everted to inverted or in the angle the nipple points; discharge; cracking or crusting
Reinspect with the patient lifting the arms over head, pressed firmly on the hips, leaning forward from the waist, and then lying supine.	*Findings consistent with those outlined above*	Any change in color, size (especially if unilateral), symmetry, or contour of the breast, or change in nipple characteristics
Inspect the axillae while the patient is sitting.	*No signs of rashes, infection, texture changes, or unusual pigmentation*	Rashes or infection; velvety axillary skin or deep pigmentation; lumps; lesions
Palpate the axillae while the patient is sitting. Feel for the central nodes. Also assess the pectoral, lateral, and subscapular nodes.	*One or more small, soft, nontender nodes*	Firm, hard, enlarged nodes (>1 cm) fixed to underlying tissues or skin; tender, warm, or enlarged nodes
Palpate breast tissue from clavicle to inframammary fold and from midsternum to posterior axillary line. Make sure to examine the tail of Spence. The patient should be supine with her arm raised overhead and a small pillow or towel rolled under the side being examined. The American Cancer Society currently recommends the vertical pattern. Using the finger pads of the first three fingers, palpate in small, concentric circles beginning in the axilla and moving in a straight line down toward the bra line. Apply light, medium, and then deeper pressure at each point. Continue in vertical overlapping lines until the sternal edge is met.	*The breast of a nulliparous woman feels smooth, elastic, and firm. Prior to menstruation, breasts are often engorged secondary to increased progesterone. After pregnancy, breasts feel softer and have less tone. Tissue is consistent with no lumps, discharge, excessive tenderness, pain, or inconsistency.*	Dilated, painful mammary ducts; lump; thickening; inverted nipple
Palpate the nipple.	*Nipple without discharge*	Discharge
Ask the patient to demonstrate self breast examination (SBE).	*Patient performs techniques correctly.*	Patient requires teaching on correct procedure.
For women with previous mastectomy, inspect the scar and axilla. Palpate the scar and chest wall with the pads of two fingers in a circular motion to assess for breast changes. Palpate the axilla and supraclavicular lymph nodes.	*No signs of inflammation, rash, color changes, thickening or irritation, lymphedema, lumps, tenderness, or swelling*	Inflammation, rash, color changes, thickening or irritation, lymphedema, lumps, tenderness, swelling
For male patients, inspect the nipple and areola. Palpate the areola and breast tissue for nodules or masses.	*No swelling, ulceration, drainage, or lumps*	Firm, glandular tissue (gynecomastia); an ulcer or hard, irregular mass

Abdominal Assessment

OBJECTIVE SUMMARY

The gastrointestinal (GI) system is responsible for the ingestion and digestion of food, absorption of nutrients, and elimination of solid waste products from the body. Parts of the GI system also reside in the head, neck, and thoracic regions. Findings need to be evaluated based on the organ systems found in those regions as well. GI symptoms are common and send people of all ages in search of relief. Diagnosis of abdominal diseases depends heavily on accurate and thorough history taking. During the health history, it is essential to delineate the sequence of the patient's symptoms. Additionally, it is important to master the abdominal assessment to provide quality health care.

READING ASSIGNMENT

Read Chapter 22 in Jensen's *Nursing Health Assessment: A Best-Practice Approach*.

VOCABULARY/TERMINOLOGY

- **Accessory digestive organs**: Liver, pancreas, and gall bladder.
- **Alimentary canal:** The tube lined with mucous membrane that stretches from mouth to anus and connects the digestive tract from its beginning to its end.

- **Anorexia nervosa:** Disease in which a patient intentionally limits food intake to the point of starvation as a result of disturbed body image.
- **Ascites:** Accumulation of fluid in the abdomen. It is found in patients with *cirrhosis* or primary or metastatic tumors of the liver.
- **Blumberg's sign:** Assessment technique elicited during abdominal assessment to check for *peritonitis*.
- **Borborygmi:** Sounds made by a growling stomach.
- **Bruit:** Auscultatory sound (swishing) that indicates turbulent blood flow from constriction or dilation of a tortuous vessel.
- **Chemical digestion:** Breakdown of food through a series of metabolic reactions with hydrochloric acid, enzymes, and hormones.
- **Constipation:** Decrease in normal frequency of defecation with hard, dry stool.
- **Diarrhea:** Passage of loose, unformed stools.
- **Dysphagia:** Difficulty swallowing. May result from stress, esophageal stricture, gastroesophageal reflux disease (GERD), or tumor.
- **Friction rub:** Harsh, grating sounds on auscultation; occur in the right upper quadrant (RUQ) and left upper quadrant (LUQ) over the liver and spleen. Caused by tumors or inflammation of the underlying organs.

- **Hepatitis:** Viral infection with inflammation of the liver. Hepatitis A is transmitted by the fecal-oral route, usually within 30 days of exposure. The disease is vaccine-preventable. Hepatitis B is transmitted through contact with bodily secretions of infected people. Hepatitis C is the most commonly diagnosed form of hepatitis in the United States. It is transmitted through contact with the blood of infected people.

- **Hernia:** Part of an internal organ that bulges through a weak area of muscle. Most hernias occur in the abdomen. There are several types: inguinal, umbilical, or along an old incision.

- **Malnutrition:** general term for a medical condition caused by an improper or insufficient diet. It most often refers to undernutrition resulting from inadequate consumption, poor absorption, or excessive loss of nutrients.

- **McBurney's point/sign:** *McBurney's point* is the name given to the point over the right side of the abdomen that is one third of the distance from the ASIS (anterior superior iliac spine) to the umbilicus (the belly button). This point roughly corresponds to the most common location of the base of the appendix where it is attached to the cecum. Deep tenderness at McBurney's point, known as *McBurney's sign*, is a sign of acute appendicitis.

- **Mechanical digestion:** Breakdown of food through chewing, peristalsis, and churning.

- **Obesity:** Weight greater than 20% of ideal.

- **Odynophagia:** Painful swallowing in the mouth or esophagus. It can occur with or without dysphagia.

- **Omentum:** Large fold of peritoneum that hangs down and extends from the stomach to the posterior abdominal wall after associating with the transverse colon.

- **Parietal pain:** Acute pain, results from inflammation of the peritoneum. It is usually severe and localized over the involved structure. Patients describe it as steady, aching, or sharp, especially with movement.

- **Peritoneum:** Serous membrane that covers and holds the organs in place. It contains a parietal layer that lines the walls of the abdomen and a visceral layer that coats the outer surface of the organs.

- **Peritonitis:** Inflammation of the lining of the abdominal cavity; symptoms include fever, nausea, and vomiting.

- **Rebound tenderness:** Tenderness greater when the examiner quickly withdraws the hand from the point of the pain than when pressing slowly on the tender area.

- **Referred pain:** Pain that occurs in distant sites innervated at approximately the same spinal level as the disordered structure.

- **Rovsing's sign:** When the examiner depresses deeply and evenly in the left lower quadrant (LLQ) and quickly withdraws fingers, the patient reports pain in the right lower quadrant (RLQ) during LLQ pressure, suggesting appendicitis.

- **Striae:** Stretch marks.

- **Visceral pain:** Pain that occurs when hollow organs are distended, stretched, or contract forcefully.

STUDY GUIDE

Activity A **FILL IN THE BLANK**

1. Fill in the blank in the following sentences:

   A. The abdomen is a large cavity extending from the _____ of the sternum down to the _____ of the pubic bone.

   B. Accessory organs of the GI system within the abdomen include the _____, _____, and _____.

   C. On average, _____ of food ingested today are eliminated _____ later.

   D. During pregnancy, _____ decreases activity, contributing to constipation.

   E. Elderly people have changes in _____ _____ that may affect their ability _____.

Activity B   LABELING

1. Correctly label the items listed on the box below.

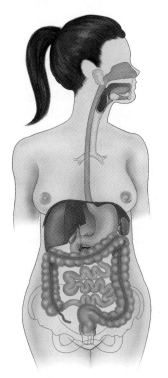

Cecum, Descending colon, Esophagus, Gallbladder, Liver, Pancreas, Rectum, Stomach

Activity C   MATCHING

1. **Match the organ with its function.**

Answer	Organ	Function
	1. Pancreas	**A.** Vestigial structure with no absolute purpose
	2. Stomach	
	3. Ureter	**B.** Muscular duct
	4. Gallbladder	**C.** Inhibits insulin and glucagon secretion
	5. Jejunum	
	6. Liver	**D.** Central of the three divisions of the small intestine
	7. Appendix	
		E. Primary organ of the digestive tract
		F Stores and concentrates bile
		G. Stores fat-soluble vitamins A, D, E, and K; vitamin B_{12}; and copper and iron

2. **Match the health problem with the race or ethnicity most often affected.**

Answer	Health Problem	Race/Ethnicity
	1. Stomach cancer	**A.** Non-Hispanic black women
	2. Inflammatory bowel disease (IBD)	**B.** Asian Americans
		C. Americans of Jewish ancestry
	3. Colon cancer	**D.** Ashkenazi Jews
	4. Obesity	**E.** Native Americans
	5. Thalassemia	**F.** Americans of Greek descent
	6. Steatorrhea	

3. **Match the auscultated sound with its description.**

Answer	Auscultated Sound	Description
	1. Bruit	**A.** Soft-pitched humming noise with a systolic and diastolic component
	2. Venous hum	
	3. Friction rub	**B.** Grating sound that increases with inspiration
		C. Swishing sound

Activity D   SHORT ANSWER

1. Describe the abdomen, including the landmarks and muscles associated with it.

_____

_____

_____

_____

2. Name the genitourinary organs that lie within the abdominal cavity, including their functions.

_____

_____

_____

_____

3. Explain the digestive process from the start to when food is turned into chyme.

_____

_____

_____

_____

4. Explain physiological changes that occur in the abdomen of a pregnant woman.

_____

_____

_____

_____

5. Explain physiological changes that occur in the alimentary canal of the older adult and how they affect the body's ability to process food from ingestion through elimination.

_____

_____

_____

_____

6. Discuss food-borne illnesses. Include whom they affect most and why, as well as suggested *Healthy People* goals and interventions.

_____

_____

_____

_____

7. Briefly discuss immunization recommendations against hepatitis A and B.

_____

_____

_____

_____

Activity D **MULTIPLE CHOICE**

1. The peritoneum is a serous membrane that contains
   A. antibodies
   B. a parietal layer
   C. a visceral ligament
   D. a drying agent

2. During digestion the food that is ingested enters the stomach and is churned into
   A. mastication
   B. thyme
   C. chyme
   D. bolus

3. Nursing students are giving a class presentation on the digestive process. Where would the students say the villi are that absorb nutrients?
   A. Duodenum
   B. Pancreas
   C. Jejunum
   D. Cecum

4. Where in the digestive tract is most of the water absorbed?
   A. Stomach
   B. Duodenum
   C. Ileum
   D. Large intestine

5. A 27-year-old woman comes to the emergency department reporting severe right upper quadrant pain. Her temperature is 101.5°C, BP 120/80 mm Hg, pulse 95 beats/min, and respirations 22 breaths/min. She is 8 months pregnant. What might the nurse suspect the patient has?
   A. Acute appendicitis
   B. Chronic gallbladder disease
   C. Gastroenteritis
   D. Braxton-Hicks contractions

6. Older adults often have trouble with swallowing. What might cause this?
   A. Slowing of peristalsis
   B. Decreased saliva
   C. Decreased stomach acid
   D. Constipation

7. A 17-year-old baseball player is brought to the emergency department by EMS. His temperature is 101.3°C, BP is 80/65 mm Hg, and pulse is 100 beats/min. He says he is dizzy when he stands, feels weak, and has heart palpitations and a dry mouth. He collapsed on the ball field while playing in 100°C+ heat. What might the nurse suspect is wrong with this patient?
   A. Heat stroke
   B. Atrial fibrillation
   C. Dehydration
   D. Gastroenteritis

Abdominal pain			
Dysphagia, odynophagia			
Change in bowel function			
Constipation			
Diarrhea			
Jaundice/icteris			
Urinary/renal symptoms			
Kidney or flank pain			
Ureteral colic			

Physical Assessment:

Inspect the abdomen.
Assess for abdominal distention.
Inspect urine.
Inspect emesis.
Inspect stool.
Auscultate all four abdominal quadrants for bowel sounds.
Auscultate all four quadrants for vascular sounds.
Percuss all four quadrants carefully for tympany or dullness.
Percuss the kidneys.
Test for liver span.
Assess approximate liver size.
Assess bladder size by percussing for bladder distension.
Lightly palpate the abdomen in all four quadrants.
Perform single-handed deep palpation.
Palpate the liver.
Use the hooking technique.
Palpate the spleen.
Palpate the left and right kidneys.
Palpate the abdominal aorta.
Palpate the bladder using deep palpation in the hypogastric area.
Palpate inguinal lymph nodes.
Assess for ascites in the liver.
Elicit the abdominal reflex.

Signature_____ Date _____

Guide for Use in Practice

Technique	Normal Findings	Abnormal Findings
Inspect the abdomen for contour, peristaltic waves, and pulsations. Look at the skin and umbilicus.	*Usual contour, waves*	Scars, striae, veins, umbilicus with a hernia or inflammation
Assess for distention. Inspect for visible aortic pulsations, peristalsis, and respiratory pattern.	*No distention or visible pulsations; normal breathing*	Distention, abnormal contours, peristaltic wave, pulsation of the aorta
Inspect urine.	*Clear and light yellow*	Cloudy or dark urine; sediment or blood
Inspect emesis.	*None*	Vomiting; green, coffee-ground, or bloody emesis is especially concerning.
Inspect stool.	*Soft and light brown*	Foul-smelling, dark, or currant-jelly stool
Auscultate all four abdominal quadrants for bowel sounds.	*5–30 clicks per minute or one sound every 5–15 seconds. If no sounds are audible, listen for up to 5 minutes.*	Hyperactive, decreased, nonexistent, increased, high-pitched, tinkling, or rushing sounds
Auscultate all four quadrants for vascular sounds.		
Listen over the aorta and renal and iliac arteries for bruits.	*No bruits*	Bruits
Near the liver and over the umbilicus listen for venous hums.	*No venous hums*	Venous hums
Auscultate over liver and spleen for friction rubs.	*No friction rubs*	Friction rubs
Percuss all four quadrants carefully for tympany or dullness.	*Dullness over the liver in the RUQ and hollow tympanic notes in the LUQ over the gastric bubble. Over most of the abdomen, tympanic sounds are heard.*	Pain; dullness over organs, masses or fluid
With the patient sitting, percuss the kidneys with the fist at the costovertebral angle posteriorly. Repeat on the other side.	*Slight or no pain with fist percussion*	Significant pain upon blunt percussion
Test for liver span.	*6–12 cm. If liver span in the MCL is >12 cm, measure in the midsternal line. Normal midsternal liver span is 4–8 cm.*	Hepatomegaly and the firm edge of *cirrhosis*
Assess approximate size of the spleen: 1. Percuss from the left midcoastal line (MCL) along the costal margin to the left midaxillary line (MAL). 2. Percuss at the lowest intercostal space at the left MAL. Ask the patient to take a deep breath and hold it; percuss again. 3. Percuss from the third to fourth ICS slightly posterior to the left MAL, and percuss downward until dullness is heard.	*Tympany*	Dullness at the MAL

Assess bladder size by percussing for bladder distension.	*Bladder at or below the symphysis pubis*	Tenderness over the symphysis pubis; bladder rises above symphysis pubis.
Lightly palpate the abdomen in all four quadrants.	*No tenderness*	Involuntary guarding
Perform single-handed deep palpation. Use the tips of your fingers and depress 4–6 cm in a dipping motion in all four quadrants. Bimanual deep palpation is necessary when palpating a large abdomen. Place your non-dominant hand on your dominant hand and depress your hands 4–6 cm.	*Tenderness near the xiphoid process, over the cecum, or over the sigmoid colon*	Mass
Palpate the liver.	*Palpable liver edge against your right hand during inspiration*	Liver palpable below the costal margin
Use the hooking technique.	*Palpable liver edge against your right hand during inspiration*	Liver palpable below the costal margin
Palpate the spleen.	*Spleen not palpable*	Palpable spleen tip
Palpate the left and right kidneys.	*Unable to palpate the kidneys except in slender patients.*	Kidneys palpable
Palpate the abdominal aorta.	*Pulsations palpable; aorta 2 cm*	An enlarged aorta (>3 cm) or one with lateral pulsations
Palpate the bladder using deep palpation in the hypogastric area.	*Bladder neither tender nor palpable*	A bladder that is full or enlarged; a tender bladder
Palpate inguinal lymph nodes.	*Inguinal lymph nodes nontender and slightly palpable*	Nodes palpable or enlarged
Assess for ascites in the liver by assessing for shifting dullness, fluid wave, or both.	*Dullness does not shift; no fluid wave.*	Dullness moves to the most dependent area. The tap causes a fluid wave through the abdomen.
Elicit the abdominal reflex.	*Umbilicus moves toward the stimulus. This reflex may be masked and not determinable in obese patients.*	Absent abdominal reflex

CHAPTER 23

Musculoskeletal Assessment

OBJECTIVE SUMMARY

This chapter discusses the structure and function of the musculoskeletal system. It provides instructions for a comprehensive musculoskeletal assessment, including health history, physical examination (with specific procedures for joint problems), and related laboratory and diagnostic tests. A patient would undergo a complete musculoskeletal examination during the first visit to a health care provider or when a condition that involves all the joints is suspected. More commonly, patients undergo focused assessments on a specific area with injury or pain, such as a shoulder, knee, or elbow.

READING ASSIGNMENT

Read Chapter 23 in Jensen's *Nursing Health Assessment: A Best-Practice Approach*.

VOCABULARY/TERMINOLOGY

- **Abduction:** Movement of a part away from the center of the body.
- **Acromegaly:** Hormonal disorder that develops when the pituitary gland produces too much growth hormone during adulthood. Bones increase in size, including those of the hands, feet, and face.
- **Acromioclavicular (AC) joint:** Joint at the top of the shoulder that is the junction between the acromion and the clavicle.
- **Acromion process:** Anatomical feature on the shoulder blade (scapula), together with the coracoid process extending laterally over the shoulder joint.
- **Adduction:** Movement of a part toward the center of the body.
- **Amphiarthrotic joint:** Slightly moveable joint.
- **Antalgic:** Counteracting or avoiding pain.
- **Apraxic:** Difficulty initiating or continuing walking.
- **Arthralgia:** Pain in the joints.
- **Articulation:** Joint.
- **Ataxia:** Neurological finding of gross lack of coordination of muscle movements.
- **Atrophy:** Wasting or shrinking of the muscle.
- **Ballottement:** Sign that indicates increased fluid in the suprapatellar pouch over the patella at the knee joint.
- **Bouchard's nodes:** Hard, nontender bony growths or gelatinous cysts on the proximal interphalangeal joints. A sign of osteoarthritis.
- **Bursa:** Fluid-filled sac in area of friction to cushion bones or ligaments that might rub against one another.

- **Calcaneus:** Heel bone; largest bone of the human foot.

- **Cancellous bone:** Spongy bone.

- **Cartilage:** Anatomical structure that allows bones to slide over one another, reduces friction, prevents damage, and absorbs shock.

- **Cartilaginous joint:** Slightly moveable joint.

- **Circumduction:** Circular motion that combines flexion, extension, abduction, and adduction.

- **Collateral ligament:** Structure that connects the joint on both sides of the patella to give medial and lateral stability and to prevent dislocation. Felt in the depressions on both sides of the patella.

- **Compact bone:** Bone that forms the shaft and outer layer.

- **Contracture:** Shortening of tendons, fascia, or muscles; may result from injury or prolonged positioning. Once a contracture develops, it is difficult to stretch and may require surgery.

- **Crepitus:** Medical term to describe the grating, crackling, or popping sounds and sensations experienced under the skin and joints.

- **Cruciate (cruciform) ligaments:** Pairs of ligaments arranged like a letter X. They cross within the knee to provide anterior and posterior stability and to control rotation.

- **Diarthrotic joint:** Freely movable joint.

- **Dorsiflexion:** Bending the ankle so that the toes move toward the head.

- **Effusion:** Synovial thickening.

- **Epicondyle:** Rounded projection at the end of a bone, located on or above a condyle, and usually serving as a place of attachment for ligaments and tendons.

- **Eversion:** Sole of the foot is turned away from the other leg.

- **Extension:** Movement of a joint whereby one part of the body is moved away from another. Increases the angle to a straight line or 0 degrees.

- **Fascia:** Flat sheets that line and protect muscle fibers, attach muscle to bone, and provide structure for nerves, blood vessels, and lymphatics.

- **Fibrous joint:** Immovable, such as in the sutures in the skull.

- **Flexion:** Maneuver that decreases the angle between bones or brings bones together.

- **Glenohumeral joint:** Shoulder joint; it involves articulation between the glenoid fossa of the scapula and the head of the humerus.

- **Goniometer:** Scale used for measuring the angle at which a joint can flex or extend.

- **Heberden's nodes:** Hard, nontender bony growths on the distal intraphalangeal joint.

- **Hematopoiesis:** Manufacturing of blood cells.

- **Hyperextension:** Extension beyond the neutral position.

- **Hypertrophy:** Increase in the volume of an organ or tissue due to the enlargement of its component cells.

- **Interphalangeal joint:** Hinge joints of the phalanges of the hand.

- **Intervertebral disc:** Disc that lies between adjacent vertebrae in the spine.

- **Inversion:** Turning of a structure toward the opposite.

- **Kyphosis:** Forward bending of the upper thoracic spine; may accompany osteoporosis, ankylosing spondylosis, and Paget's disease.

- **Ligaments:** Anatomical structure that connects bone to bone to stabilize joints and limit movement.

- **Lordosis:** Increased lumbar curvature.

- **Meniscus:** Cartilage disc between bones to absorb shock and cushion joints.

- **Metatarsophalangeal joint:** Joint between the metatarsal bones of the foot and the proximal bones (proximal phalanges) of the toes.

- **Midcarpal joint:** Articulation between parallel rows of carpal bones. It allows flexion, extension, and some rotation.

- **Monoarticular:** Affecting one joint.

- **Myalgia:** Muscle pain.

- **Myositis:** Inflammation of the muscles.

- **Olecranon process:** Structure centered between the medial and the lateral epicondyles of the humerus.

- **Opposition:** Moving the thumb to touch the little finger.

- **Osteoporosis:** Condition in which bone resorption is faster than deposition. The weakened bone increases risk for fractures, especially in vertebrae, wrist, and hip.

- **Plantar flexion:** Pointing the toes downward toward the ground.

- **Polyarticular:** Pain in several joints.

- **Polydactyly:** Congenital anomaly in which humans have supernumerary fingers or toes.

- **Pronation:** Turning a structure to face downward.

- **Protrusion:** Pushing a structure forward.

- **Radiocarpal joint:** Wrist joint.

- **Retraction:** Returning a structure to neutral position.

- **Scoliometer:** Measuring device that may be used to obtain a measurement of the number of degrees that the spine is deviated in scoliosis.

- **Scoliosis:** Lateral curvature of the spine.

- **Spondylosis:** Spinal degeneration and deformity of the joint(s) of two or more vertebrae. Commonly occurs with aging. Often, there is herniation of the nucleus pulposus of one or more intervertebral discs.

- **Subluxation:** Partial dislocation of a joint.

- **Supination:** Turning a structure to face upward.

- **Synarthrotic joint:** Immovable joint (eg, skull suture). Also called a "fibrous joint."

- **Syndactyly:** Condition where two or more digits are fused together.

- **Synovial joint:** Freely movable joint.

- **Talipes equinovarus:** Club foot.

- **Temporomandibular joint:** Articulation of the mandible and temporal bone.

- **Tendon:** Anatomical structure that connects muscles to bones.

- **Tibiotalar joint:** Ankle.

- **Torticollis:** Lateral deviation of the neck.

- **Valgus:** Part of a limb twisted out from the midline.

- **Varus:** Part of a limb twisted toward the midline.

STUDY GUIDE

Activity A FILL IN THE BLANK

1. Fill in the blank in the following sentences:
   A. There are two types of bones: _____, which forms the shaft and outer layer, and spongy or _____, which makes up the ends and center.
   B. The _____ joint is where the humerus articulates with the _____ of the scapula.
   C. The ankle (_____) is the articulation of the tibia, fibula, and talus.
   D. A person who has had a stroke is at increased risk of _____, or _____, of the shoulder from the weight of the arm and the lack of muscle tone to hold the joint together.

2. Fill in the blanks about scoliosis.
   A. Scoliosis may be _____, caused by a defect in the spine, or _____, caused by habits.
   B. While the patient stands, look for _____of the hips, scapulae, shoulders, and any skin folds or creases.
   C. A _____may be used to obtain a measurement of the number of degrees that the spine is deviated.
   D. During _____ of the spine, feel for any _____ or deformities.

Activity B LISTING

1. List the National Osteoporosis Foundation (NOF) recommended comprehensive approach to prevent osteoporosis:
   A. _____
   B. _____
   C. _____
   D. _____
   E. _____

Activity C MATCHING

1. *Match the connective tissue with its function.*

Answer	Tissue	Function
	1. Cartilage	**A.** Fluid-filled sacs in areas of friction
	2. Tendons	**B.** Connect bone to bone
	3. Bursae	**C.** Connect muscles to bones
	4. Ligaments	**D.** Allow bones to slide over one another

2. *Match the name of the test with what is being tested.*

Answer	Test	What is Being Tested
	1. Phalen's test	**A.** Assesses presence of a flexion contracture of the hip
	2. Ballottement	**B.** Checks for meniscus injury
	3. Bulge test	**C.** Checks for knee injury
	4. McMurray's test	**D.** Evaluates presence of large accumulation of fluid behind the knee
	5. Thomas's test	**E.** Evaluates for carpal tunnel syndrome
	6. Drawer sign	**F.** Differentiates soft tissue swelling from accumulation of excess fluid behind the patella

Activity D SHORT ANSWER

1. Explain the procedure for examining a patient for scoliosis. Include a brief explanation of scoliosis.

_____

_____

_____

_____

2. Explain why it is important for a nurse to ask the patient about any previous musculoskeletal surgeries. Include how it assists the nurse in planning interventions for the patient.

_____

_____

_____

_____

3. Discuss the necessity of assessing the size and shape of the patient's extremities bilaterally.

_____

_____

_____

_____

4. Discuss what is being assessed for during musculoskeletal palpation.

_____

_____

_____

_____

5. Explain the process of palpating the shoulder joint.

_____

_____

_____

_____

6. Name and explain common abnormal findings when inspecting and palpating the hand.

_____

_____

_____

_____

_____

7. Discuss inspection and palpation of the hips.

_____

_____

_____

_____

Activity E MULTIPLE CHOICE

1. A patient presents at the clinic with an enlarged, swollen, hot, and red metatarsophalangeal joint and bursa of the great toe. What diagnosis would the nurse suspect this patient has?
   A. Gouty arthritis
   B. Hallux valgus
   C. Hammertoe
   D. Pes planus

2. A 70-year-old woman has come to the clinic for a bone density test. The results show that she has osteoporosis. What is a medication that might be ordered for this patient?
   A. Testosterone
   B. Thyroid hormone
   C. Raloxifene
   D. Trisphosphonates calcitonin

3. A patient presents at the neurology clinic for an initial visit. The nurse notes that the patient has irregular, uncoordinated movements. How would the nurse note this in the patient's record?
   A. "Patient exhibits spasticity."
   B. "Patient is ataxic."
   C. "Patient is atonic."
   D. "Patient is hypotonic."

4. The nurse is assessing the range of motion (ROM) of a patient's joints. What would the nurse use to assess flexion and extension of a joint if the patient complains of pain on examination?
   A. Calibrater
   B. Scoliometer
   C. Angulator
   D. Goniometer

5. When assessing muscle tone and strength, the nurse would document normal findings as
   A. "extremity muscle strength is 5/5 bilaterally"
   B. "upper and lower extremity muscle strength is 5/5 bilaterally"
   C. "upper and lower extremity muscle strength is 5/5"
   D. "upper extremity muscle strength is 5/5 bilaterally"

6. The nurse is caring for a patient with a diagnosis of degenerative disease of the cervical spine. What might the nurse find on inspection of this patient?
   A. Torticollis
   B. Hypotonicity
   C. Atrophy
   D. Hypertonicity

7. When assessing a patient's foot, how would the nurse document an exaggerated arch height?
   A. "Patient has pes valgus."
   B. "Patient has pes planus."
   C. "Patient has pes cavus."
   D. "Patient has pes varus."

8. When assessing the foot and ankle of a clinic patient, the nurse notes that the patient complains of pain along the Achilles' tendon. What might this patient have?
   A. Strain
   B. Plantar fasciitis
   C. Sprain
   D. Bursitis

ALTERNATIVE CASE SCENARIOS

Mrs. Gladys Runningbird is an 82-year-old Native American who recently fell, requiring hospitalization. Twelve days ago, she was transferred from the hospital to a skilled nursing facility. Today, her temperature is 36.6°C orally, pulse is 82 beats/min, respirations are 18 breaths/min, and blood pressure is 122/64 mm Hg. Current medications include alendrolate sodium (Fosamax) for osteoarthritis. Supplements are a multivitamin, vitamin D, calcium, and magnesium.

Review the following alternative situations related to Mrs. Runningbird. Based on the changes outlined below, *consider what other outcomes, information, and problems would affect the overall picture and shape your responses.*

Alternative A

Subjective: "I was just trying to go to the bathroom."

Objective: Mrs. Runningbird has forgotten to call for the nurse prior to going to the bathroom. The patient subsequently slipped and fell.

She states that she has no pain. She is alert and oriented, and her vital signs are stable.

- What factors place Mrs. Runningbird at risk for falling?

- How will the nurse work with Mrs. Runningbird to reduce the risk of falling?

- What assessments will the nurse make prior to moving Mrs. Runningbird?

Alternative B

Subjective: "I hurt so bad. Could you please give me something for the pain?"

Objective: Mrs. Runningbird has osteoarthritis more prominent in her hips, knees, and feet instead of in her hands. The osteoarthritis is making ambulation and self-care difficult.

- What different assessments would the nurse perform related to the body parts affected?

- What nursing diagnoses might be different for osteoarthritis in the lower body as opposed to in the hand?

- How might nursing interventions differ based on compromise to the lower part of the body?

DOCUMENTATION

Form for Use in Practice

Patient Name _____ Date _____

Date of Birth _____

Initial Survey

Reason for seeking health care: _____

History of present illness

- Location:

- Intensity:

- Duration:

- Description:

- Aggravating factors:

- Alleviating factors:

- Functional impairment:

- Pain goal:

Vital signs: T (route)_____ P (site)_____ R_____ BP (site)_____ SpO_2_____

Weight: _____ Height: _____ BMI: _____

General appearance: _____

General level of distress: _____

Level of anxiety: _____

Risk Factors and History:

- Family history of muscle, joint, or bone problems:

- Previous musculoskeletal trauma or injury:

- Fractures:

- Stroke:

- Polio:

- Infections of the bone or muscles:
- Diabetes:
- Parathyroid problems:
- Daily servings of dairy products:

Medications:

- For women, current and past birth-control methods:
- For postmenopausal women, hormone replacement therapy:
- Calcium and vitamin D supplements:
- Pain or anti-inflammatory medications:
- Muscle relaxants:
- Steroids:

Complementary or Alternative Therapies

- Occupation
- Repetitive motion:
- Lifting or twisting:
- Protective devices:

Hobbies, Lifestyle, and Sports:

- Injury prevention:
- Car seats:
- Helmets:
- Protective gear:
- Smoking history:
- Alcohol use:
- Recreational drug use:

Common Symptoms:

Symptom	Yes	No	Additional data
Pain or discomfort			
Weakness			
Stiffness or limited movement			
Deformity			
Lack of balance and coordination			

Physical Assessment:

• General inspection.
• Assess posture.
• Assess gait and mobility.
• Assess balance.
• Assess coordination.

- Inspect and measure extremities.
- Assess TMJ.
  - Inspection.
  - Palpation.
  - Pain.
  - ROM.
  - Muscle tone and strength.
- Assess cervical spine.
  - Inspection.
  - Palpation.
  - Pain.
  - ROM.
  - Muscle tone and strength.
- Assess shoulders.
  - Inspection.
  - Palpation.
  - Pain.
  - ROM.
  - Muscle tone and strength.
- Assess elbows.
  - Inspection.
  - Palpation.
  - Pain.
  - ROM.
  - Muscle tone and strength.
- Assess wrists and hands.
  - Inspection.
  - Palpation.
  - Pain.
  - ROM.
  - Muscle tone and strength.
- Assess hips.
  - Inspection.
  - Palpation.
  - Pain.
  - ROM.
  - Muscle tone and strength.

• Assess knees.
• Inspection.
• Palpation.
• Pain.
• ROM.
• Muscle tone and strength.
• Assess ankles and feet.
• Inspection.
• Palpation.
• Pain.
• ROM.
• Muscle tone and strength.

Signature_____ Date _____

Guide for Use in Practice

Technique	Normal Findings	Abnormal Findings
Observe posture as the patient stands with feet together. Observe the relation of the head, trunk, pelvis, and extremities. Assess for symmetry in shoulder height, scapulae, and iliac crests. Observe the patient's posture while sitting.	*Posture erect with head midline above the spine. Shoulders equal in height*	Patient leans forward or to the side when standing or sitting; enlarged skull and increased length to the hands, feet, and long bones.
Watch the patient walk across the room while observing from the side and from behind.	*Walking smooth and rhythmic with arms swinging in opposition to legs. Patient rises from sitting with ease.*	Hesitancy, unsteadiness, staggering, reaching for external support, high stepping, foot scraping, inability to raise the foot completely off the floor, persistent toe or heel walking, excessive pointing of toes inward or outward, asymmetry of step height or length, limping, stooping, wavering, shuffling, waddling, excessive swinging of shoulders or pelvis, and slow or rapid speed
Ask the patient to walk on tiptoes, heels, heel-to-toe fashion (tandem walking), and backward. Ask the patient to step to each side, and to sit down and stand.	*Patient performs all correctly.*	Patient cannot perform any of the described maneuvers.
(Optional) Perform the Romberg test.	*Patient is balanced when standing and has a negative Romberg test.*	Patient sways
Ask the patient to rapidly pat the table or thigh, alternating between palm and dorsum of the hand. Assess fine motor coordination of the hand by asking the patient to perform finger to thumb opposition. Assess gross motor coordination in the legs by having the patient run the heel of one foot up the opposite leg from ankle to knee.	*Patient performs rapid alternating movements of the arms and finger-thumb opposition and runs the heel of one foot down the opposite shin.*	Poor coordination

Inspect the extremities.	*No swelling, lacerations, lesions, deformity, atrophy, or asymmetry*	Asymmetry in bone length or muscle size
Assess both extremities at the same time to evaluate for symmetry.	*Symmetry*	Disuse, swelling, edema; discrepancy in leg length of more than 1 cm
Palpate joints for contour and size; palpate muscles for tone. Feel for any bumps, nodules, or deformity. Ask if there is any tenderness during touch.	*No bumps, nodules, deformity, or tenderness*	Limitation of movement, **crepitus** (cracking or popping), and non-verbal and verbal expressions of discomfort or pain
TMJ Inspect the TMJ for symmetry, swelling, and redness.	*Jaw symmetrical bilaterally*	Asymmetrical facial or joint musculature
Palpate the TMJ.	*Muscles are symmetrical, smooth, and nontender.*	Discomfort, swelling, limited movement, and grating or crackling sounds; ear pain or headache; swelling or tenderness
Ask the patient to open the jaw as wide as possible, push the lower jaw forward (protrusion), return the jaw to neutral position (retraction), and move the jaw from side to side 1–2 cm.	*The joint may have an audible or palpable click when opened. The mouth opens with 3–6 cm between the upper and the lower teeth. The jaw moves with ease.*	Difficulty opening the mouth; pain in the TMJ
Ask the patient to repeat the above movements while you provide opposing force.	*Strength of muscles is equal on both sides of the jaw; the patient can perform the movements against resistance. Muscle strength is 5/5, with no pain, spasms, or contractions.*	Decreased muscle strength
Cervical Spine With the patient standing, inspect the cervical spine from all sides. Observing from the side, check for the concave curve of the cervical spine.	*As viewed from behind, the patient holds the head erect, and the cervical spine is in straight alignment. From the side, the neck has a concave curve.*	Lateral tilting of the head and neck; lateral deviation of the neck; hypertrophy of the neck muscles
Stand behind the patient to palpate the cervical spine and neck.	*Paravertebral, sternocleidomastoid, and trapezus muscles are fully developed, symmetrical, and nontender.*	Decreased ROM, pain, and tenderness; neck spasm
Ask the patient to touch the chin to the chest (flexion), look up toward the ceiling (hyperextension), attempt to touch each ear to the shoulder without elevating the shoulder (lateral flexion or abduction), and turn the head to each side as far as possible (rotation).	*Flexion 45 degrees, hyperextension 55 degrees, lateral flexion 40 degrees, and rotation 70 degrees to each side*	Limited hyperextension and flexion; pain, numbness, or tingling
Ask the patient to rotate the neck to the right and left, against the resistance of your hand.	*Muscle strength is sufficient to overcome resistance.*	Weakness or loss of sensation in arms

Shoulder

Compare both shoulders anteriorly and posteriorly for size and contour. Observe the anterior aspect of the joint capsule for abnormal swelling.	*No redness, swelling, deformity, or muscular atrophy. Shoulders smooth and bilaterally symmetric. Right and left shoulders level. Each shoulder an equal distance from the vertebral column*	Deformity, redness, and swelling; unequal shoulder height
Stand in front of the patient and palpate both shoulders, noting any muscular spasm, atrophy, swelling, heat, or tenderness.	*Muscles are fully developed and smooth.*	Tenderness
Ask the person to perform forward flexion, extension, hyperextension, abduction, adduction, circumduction, and internal and external rotation. Cup one hand over the patient's shoulder during ROM to detect any crepitus.	*Movement is fluid. Forward flexion 180 degrees, hyperextension 50 degrees, abduction 180 degrees, adduction 50 degrees, internal rotation 90 degrees, and external rotation 90 degrees*	Limited ROM, pain, crepitation, and asymmetry. Inability to externally rotate the shoulder
Ask the patient to shrug both shoulders, flex forward and upward, and abduct against resistance.	*Full ROM against resistance*	Decreased ability to shrug the shoulders against resistance

Elbow

Inspect size and contour in both the extended and flexed positions. Check the olecranon bursa for swelling.	*Elbows symmetrical with no swelling*	Subluxation, swelling, and redness of the olecranon bursa, effusion, or synovial thickening
Passively flex the elbow to 70 degrees. Palpate the olecranon process and medial and lateral epicondyles of the humerus. Check for synovial thickening, swelling, nodules, or tenderness.	*Elbows smooth with no swelling or tenderness*	Soft, boggy swelling, local heat or redness, subcutaneous nodules at pressure points on the olecranon process or ulnar surface
Ask the patient to bend and straighten the elbow. Have the person pronate and supinate the forearm by laying the forearm and ulnar surface of the hand on a table. Have the patient touch the palm and then the hand dorsum to the table.	*Flexion 150–160 degrees, extension 0 degree; some people cannot extend the elbow fully. Some people can hyperextend the elbow –5 to –10 degrees. Pronation and supination of 90 degrees*	Decreased ROM, pain, or crepitation; redness, swelling, and tenderness of the olecranon process; disabling pain at the lateral epicondyle of the humerus that radiates down the lateral side of the forearm
While supporting the patient's arm, apply resistance just proximal to the patient's wrist, and ask the patient to flex and then extend both elbows.	*Patient can perform full ROM against resistance.*	Decreased strength

Wrist and Hand

Hold the patient's hand in your hands. Use your thumbs to palpate each joint of the wrist and hand for tenderness.	*Joint surfaces smooth without nodules, edema, or tenderness*	Painful finger joints; firm mass over the dorsum of the wrist; edema, redness, and tenderness of the finger and wrist joints

Observe wrist and hand ROM.	*Wrist: flexion (90 degrees), extension (return to 0 degree), hyperextension (70 degrees), and ulnar (55 degrees) and radial (20 degrees) deviation. Meta-carpophylangeal joints: flex-ion (90 degrees), extension (0 degree), and hyperextension (up to 30 degrees). Proximal and distal intraphalangeal joints perform flexion, extension, and abduction. Thumb performs op-position with each fingertip and base of the little finger.*	Decreased or unequal ROM
Perform each motion above against resistance. Ask the patient to grasp your first two fingers tightly while you pull to remove your fingers.	*Muscle strength equal bilaterally and sufficient to overcome resistance*	Weak muscle strength
Hips With the patient standing, inspect the iliac crest, size, and symmetry of the buttocks and number of gluteal folds. Assist the patient to supine with legs straight. Look for swelling, lacerations, lesions, deformity, muscle size, and symmetry. Observe from the anterior and posterior views.	*Hips rounded, even, and symmetrical*	When lying supine, external rota-tion of the lower leg and foot; unequal gluteal folds or unequal height of iliac crests
While the patient is supine, palpate the hip joints, iliac crests, and muscle tone. Feel for bumps, nodules, and deformity. Ask if there is any tenderness with touch. Feel for crepitus when moving the joint.	*Buttocks symmetrical in size. Iliac crests at the same height on both sides*	Asymmetry, discomfort when touched, or crepitus during movement
Observe for full active ROM of each hip.	*Full ROM without discomfort or crepitus*	Straight leg flexion that produces back and leg pain radiating down the leg; when lying down, one leg longer than the other or limited internal rotation
With the patient lying down, apply pressure to the top of the leg while the patient flexes the hip. Apply pressure to the side while the patient abducts the hip.	*Full ROM against resistance*	Asymmetry of strength
Knee Inspect the knee both standing and sitting. Inspect contour, shape, swelling, lacerations, lesions, deformity, muscle size, and symmetry. Look for symmetry in length of long bones.	*Hollows on each side of the patella; knees symmetrical and aligned with thighs and ankles*	Swelling, muscle atrophy, *genu valgus* (knock-knee), *genu varus* (bowlegged), asymmetry in leg muscle size
With the knee flexed, palpate the quadriceps muscle for muscle tone. Palpate downward from 10 cm above the patella; evaluate the patella and each side of the femur and tibia. Palpate the tibiofemoral joints with the leg flexed 90 degrees. Assess the tibial margins and the lateral collateral ligament. Feel for bumps, nodules, or deformity. Ask if there is any tenderness during touch. Feel for crepitus when moving the joint.	*Quadriceps and surrounding tissue firm and nontender. Supra-patellar bursa not palpable. Joint is firm and nontender.*	Pain, swelling, thickening, and heat

Observe for full active ROM of each knee with the patient seated.	*The knee can perform full ROM without discomfort or crepitus.*	Inability to perform full ROM
Ankle and Foot		
Inspect feet with the patient standing and sitting. Look for swelling, lacerations, lesions, deformity, muscle size, and symmetry. Look for toe alignment.	*Feet are of the same color as the rest of the body. They are symmetrical; toes aligned with long axis of leg. No swelling. When the patient stands, weight falls on the middle of the foot.*	Enlarged, swollen, hot, red metatarsophalangeal joint and bursa of the great toe; pain on palpation and ROM; crepitus; hallux valgus (bunion); callus; hammertoe; corn; pes planus; pes varus; pes valgus; pes cavus; plantar fasciitis; talipes equinovarus (club foot)
Palpate for muscle tone, bumps, nodules, or deformity. Holding the heel, palpate the anterior and posterior aspects of the ankle, the Achilles' (calcaneal) tendon, and the metatarsophalangeal joints. Palpate each interphalangeal joint. Ask if there is any tenderness during touch. Feel for crepitus on movement.	*Ankle and foot joints are firm, stable, and nontender.*	Pain or discomfort in the ankle or foot during palpation; pain and tenderness along the Achilles' tendon; small nodules on the tendon; cooler temperature in the ankles and feet than in the rest of the body
Observe for full active ROM of the ankle. Ask the patient to curl the toes and return them to straight (flexion and extension). Ask the patient to keep the soles on the ground and raise the toes upward (hyperextension). Ask the patient to spread the toes wide open, as far apart from each other as possible (abduction) and return the toes to original position (adduction).	*Ankle ROM: dorsiflexion 20 degrees, plantar flexion 45 degrees, inversion 30 degrees, and eversion 20 degrees. Toes flex, extend, hyperextend, and abduct.*	Limited ankle or foot ROM without swelling; inflammation and swelling with limited ROM
Ask the patient to perform dorsiflexion and plantar flexion against the resistance of your hand. Then ask the patient to flex and extend the toes against your resistance.	*Muscle strength is equal bilaterally and able to overcome resistance.*	Asymmetry of strength
Thoracic and Lumbar Spine		
With the patient standing, look at the patient from the side for the normal S pattern (convex thoracic spine and concave lumbar spine). Observe from behind, noting whether the spine is straight. Observe if the scapulae, iliac crests, and gluteal folds are level and symmetrical. Ask the patient to bend forward; reassess that vertebrae are in a straight line and scapulae are equal in height.	*Spine in alignment both standing and sitting*	Kyphosis, lordosis, flattened lumbar curve, listing, scoliosis
Palpate the spinous processes for any bumps, nodules, or deformities. Ask if there is any tenderness. Feel for crepitus when the spine bends.	*Spinous processes in a straight line. Patient denies tenderness. Paravertebral muscles are firm. No crepitus*	Pain on palpation; unequal spinous processes
Observe for full active ROM of the spine.	*Full ROM without crepitus or discomfort*	Limited ROM

Neurological Assessment

All those who perform neurological assessments use some of the same methods and, at times, share the same goals. Generally, physicians assess neurological function primarily to localize pathology and to make a medical diagnosis. Nurses perform neurological assessment mainly to identify actual or potential health problems related to neurological dysfunction, and the patient's response to those problems. Common to all settings and types of neurological assessment is use of an organized approach to maximize the value of information derived from collected data. This approach consists of general patient observation, data-gathering from the health history (often performed simultaneously), and a systematic neurological examination.

READING ASSIGNMENT

Read Chapter 24 in Jensen's *Nursing Health Assessment: A Best-Practice Approach.*

VOCABULARY/TERMINOLOGY

- **Abnormal plantar reflex:** Great toe extends upward and the other toes fan out.

- **Abnormal reflex posturing:** Reflexive movements that are out of the normal range.

- **Adiadochokinesia:** Lack of coordination during rapid alternating movements.

- **Afferent (sensory) stimulation:** Stimulation that travels through the brainstem to the cerebral cortex.

- **Aphasia:** Impaired ability to interpret or use the symbols of language.

- **Ascending tracts:** Tracts of the nervous system that generally carry specific sensory information from the periphery to higher levels of the central nervous system (CNS).

- **Ataxia:** Unsteady, wavering movement with inability to touch the target.

- **Autonomic nervous system:** Division of the nervous system that maintains involuntary functions of cardiac and smooth muscle and glands. It has two components: sympathetic (fight or flight) and parasympathetic (rest and digest).

- **Basal ganglia:** Four paired tracts of gray matter on both sides of the thalamus deep within the brain tissue. They modulate automatic movements, receiving input from the cerebral cortex and sending output to the brainstem and thalamus to facilitate smooth motor function.

- **Brain death:** High cervical cord or extensive medulla damage. The brain is no longer showing electrical activity.

- **Brainstem:** Brain area integral to intact neurological functioning. Both afferent and efferent fibers pass through it from the spinal cord to the cerebrum and cerebellum.

- **Broca's area:** Brain area that regulates verbal expression and writing ability.

- **Brudzinski's sign:** Resistance or pain in the neck and flexion in the hips or knees.

- **Central nervous system (CNS):** Brain and spinal cord.

- **Cerebellum:** Area under the occipital lobe in the posterior part of the brain; coordinates voluntary movement, posture, and muscle tone, and maintains spatial orientation and equilibrium.

- **Clasp-knife spasticity:** Resistance is strongest on initiation of the movement and "gives way" as the examiner slowly continues the movement. Type of hypertonicity noted in patients with Parkinson's disease.

- **Clonus:** Alternating flexion/extension movements (jerking) in response to a continuous muscle stretch.

- **Cogwheel rigidity:** Seen in patients with Parkinson's disease; manifested by a ratchet-like jerking noted in the extremity on passive movement.

- **Corneal reflex:** Blinking in response to corneal stimulation by a cotton wisp.

- **Cranial nerves:** The 12 paired nerves that exit from the brain, not the spinal cord. Some cranial nerves have only a sensory component, some have only a motor component, and others have both.

- **Cushing's response:** Increased intracranial pressure.

- **Dermatome:** Area of skin innervated by the afferent sensory fibers in the dorsal root of a spinal nerve.

- **Descending tracts:** Tracts of the nervous system that carry information related to motor function and muscle movement. They control voluntary movement, carrying impulses from the cortex to the cranial (corticobulbar tract) and peripheral (corticospinal tract) nerves.

- **Diplopia:** Double vision.

- **Dorsal column:** Area that carries information about localized touch (stereognosis), deep pressure, vibration, position sense (proprioception), and movement (kinesthesia).

- **Dysarthria:** Deficits in speech articulation.

- **Dysphagia:** Difficulty swallowing.

- **Expressive aphasia:** Problems with speaking or finding words.

- **Extraocular movements:** Movements of the eye.

- **Extrapyramidal tract:** Tract that originates in the reticular formation and is modulated by the brainstem, basal ganglia, and cerebellum. It travels down and synapses in the ventral root of the spinal cord; however, it does not directly innervate the peripheral motor system. This tract controls gross automatic movements such as reflexes, walking, complex movements, and postural control.

- **Flaccid (atonic):** Absolutely no resistance to movement.

- **Foramen magnum:** Opening at the base of the skull.

- **Frontal lobe:** Brain lobe responsible for complex cognition, language, and voluntary motor function.

- **Hypertonia:** Increased resistance of the muscles to passive stretch.

- **Hypothalamus:** Endocrine organ that controls vital functions of temperature, heart rate, blood pressure, sleep, the anterior and posterior pituitary, the autonomic nervous system, and emotions. It maintains overall autonomic control.

- **Hypotonia:** Muscle tone that seems decreased or "flabby."

- **Kernig's sign:** Resistance to straightening or pain radiating down the posterior leg.

- **Lead-pipe rigidity:** State of stiffness and inflexibility that remains uniform throughout the range of passive movement, associated with diseases of the basal ganglia.

- **Medulla:** Brain area that contains the vital autonomic centers for respiratory, cardiac, and vasomotor function. It works with the pons to regulate smooth breathing rhythm and also controls involuntary functions such as sneezing, swallowing, vomiting, hiccoughing, and coughing.

- **Midbrain:** Area of the brain that contains many motor neurons and relays information to and from the brain through ascending sensory tracts and descending motor pathways.

- **Motor function:** Ability to move (to cause movement).

- **Nuchal rigidity:** Rigidity in the neck.
- **Paresthesia:** Abnormal prickly or tingly sensations.
- **Parietal lobe:** Lobe in the brain positioned above (superior to) the occipital lobe and behind (posterior to) the frontal lobe. Integrates sensory information from different modalities, particularly determining spatial sense and navigation.
- **Peripheral nervous system (PNS):** Part of the nervous system that resides or extends outside the CNS to serve the limbs and organs. Unlike the CNS, the PNS is not protected by bone, leaving it exposed to toxins and mechanical injuries. The peripheral nervous system is divided into the somatic nervous system and the autonomic nervous system.
- **Pons:** Structure on the brain stem, superior to the medulla oblongata, inferior to the midbrain, and rostral to the cerebellum. Its white matter includes tracts that conduct signals from the cerebrum down to the cerebellum and medulla, and tracts that carry the sensory signals up into the thalamus. Contains the ascending and descending neuron tracts and assists the midbrain to relay information. It contains two respiratory centers: one that controls the length of inspiration and expiration, and the other that controls respiratory rate.
- **Pronator drift:** Drifting downward of the hand into pronation, a sign of weakness.
- **Pupillary reaction:** Size (before and after light stimulus) and speed of the pupils' response to light.
- **Receptive aphasia:** Difficulty understanding verbal communication.
- **Reflex arc:** Neural pathway that mediates a reflex action. Involves a receptor-sensing organ, afferent sensory neuron, efferent motor neuron, and effector motor organ.
- **Reticular formation:** Brain area that relays sensory information, excitatory and inhibitory control of spinal motor neurons, and control of vasomotor and respiratory activity. It is responsible for increasing wakefulness, attention, and responsiveness of cortical neurons to sensory stimulation.

- **Rigidity:** Steady, persistent resistance to passive stretch in both flexor and extensor muscle groups.
- **Romberg test:** Neurological test to detect poor balance. The patient stands with feet together and arms at sides. The examiner notes any swaying. The patient is asked to close the eyes during the Romberg for additional testing.
- **Sensation:** Reaction to a stimulus.
- **Sensory function:** Body's ability to feel or react to a tactile sensation.
- **Spasticity:** Muscular hypertonicity; disorder of the CNS in which certain muscles continually receive a message to tighten and contract; characterized by increased resistance to rapid passive stretch, especially in flexor muscle groups in the upper extremities, resulting from hyperexcitability of the stretch reflex.
- **Thalamus:** Endocrine organ directly above the brainstem that serves as the major relay station and gatekeeper for both motor and sensory stimuli to the cerebral cortex.
- **Triple flexion response:** Reflex withdrawal of the lower extremity to plantar stimulus through flexion of ankle, knee, and hip.
- **Wernicke's area:** Area of the brain that integrates understanding of spoken and written words.

STUDY GUIDE

Activity A **FILL IN THE BLANK**

1. Fill in the blanks about the structure and function of the nervous system:

   A. In the voluntary division, fibers that connect the CNS to _____ facilitate _____ in response to stimuli.

   B. The brain is a network of _____ that control and integrate the body's activities.

   C. Cell bodies are on the _____ (gray matter or cerebral cortex), while axons that connect to other parts of the nervous system (white matter or brain tissue) _____ of the brain.

   D. Neurons communicate with one another at _____.

2. Fill in the blanks about the brain:

A. Controls motor function on the opposite side of the body.

_____

B. Receives input on sensory function including temperature, touch, pressure, and pain, also from the opposite side of the body.

_____

C. Is responsible for visual imaging, auditory processing, and language comprehension and expression.

_____

D. Is responsible for complex cognition; language and voluntary motor function.

_____

E. Recognizes the size, shape, and texture of objects.

_____

F. Serves as the primary visual area.

_____

G. Registers auditory input and is responsible for hearing, speech, behavior, and memory.

_____

Activity B **MATCHING**

1. *Match the part of the brain with its function.*

Answer	Part of Brain	Function
	1. Limbic system	**A.** Controls vasomotor and respiratory activity
	2. Basal ganglia	**B.** Is the opening at the base of the skull
	3. Reticular formation	**C.** Mediates survival behaviors
	4. Foramen magnum	**D.** Relays information to and from the brain
	5. Midbrain	**E.** Modulates automatic movements

2. *Match the nursing diagnosis with the appropriate intervention.*

Answer	Diagnosis	Intervention
	1. Unilateral neglect	**A.** Provide environmental cues.
	2. Impaired verbal communication	**B.** Set alarm watches.
	3. Acute confusion	**C.** Provide safe, well-lit, and clutter-free environment.
	4. Impaired memory	**D.** Anticipate patient's needs.
	5. Risk for aspiration	**E.** Reduce environmental stimuli.
	6. Risk for intracranial adaptive capacity	**F.** Request swallowing evaluation by speech therapy.

3. *Match the pathological indication with the common pupillary finding.*

Answer	Pathological Indication	Finding
	1. Denervation of the nerve supply from diabetic neuropathy or alcoholism	**A.** Unequal pupil size-abnormal
	2. Anoxia, sympathetic effects, atropine, tricyclics, amphetamines, or pilocarpine drops for glaucoma treatment	**B.** Horner's syndrome
		C. Argyll Robertson
	3. Third nerve palsy	**D.** Third nerve palsy
	4. Anisocoria related to compression of the optic nerve	**E.** Adie's pupil
	5. Preganglionic, central, or post-ganglionic lesion	**F.** Dilated and fixed pupils
	6. Neurosyphilis, meningitis	

Activity C **SHORT ANSWER**

1. Explain why sensations from the right side of the body are dealt with in the left side of the brain.

_____

_____

_____

_____

2. Discuss the dermatomes and what part of the body they cover.

_____

_____

_____

_____

3. Discuss what reflexes are and make a brief statement about what they do.

_____

_____

_____

_____

4. Explain the abbreviated acute neurological assessment.

_____

_____

_____

_____

5. Explain how it is determined if a patient has a head injury.

_____

_____

_____

_____

6. Discuss the risk factors for stroke, including patient teaching for those patients who are at high risk for having a stroke.

_____

_____

_____

_____

7. Explain a focused neurologic assessment, noting subjects a nurse should include.

_____

_____

_____

_____

Activity D **MULTIPLE CHOICE**

1. By the end of the second year, a child's brain is what percent of its adult size?
   A. 55%
   B. 65%
   C. 75%
   D. 85%

2. As adults age, peripheral nerve function and impulse conduction decrease. What is the result of this decrease?
   A. Decreased proprioception
   B. Decreased cognitive function
   C. Increased need for sleep
   D. Increased absorption of fats

3. A labor and delivery nurse is caring for a 39-year-old patient in labor. The fetus is in a breech presentation. For what is the fetus at increased risk?
   A. Macrocephaly
   B. Autism
   C. Low 10-minute Apgar scores
   D. Trisomy 21

4. A nurse has been asked to provide an educational event for the families of patients of a nursing home. What would the nurse teach during this educational event?
   A. People older than 65 years have the highest rate of traumatic brain injury-related hospitalization and death.
   B. People older than 70 years have the highest rate of traumatic brain injury-related hospitalization and death.
   C. People older than 75 years have the highest rate of traumatic brain injury-related hospitalization and death.
   D. People older than 80 years have the highest rate of traumatic brain injury-related hospitalization and death.

5. While participating in a research class, a nursing student learns that maternal exposure to pesticides is linked to increased incidence of what?
   A. Alimentary canal defects
   B. Cleft palate
   C. Cerebral palsy
   D. Anencephaly

6. The Glasgow Coma Scale is predictive of outcome from a traumatic brain injury when combined with
   A. patient's age and eye-opening response
   B. patient's age and pupillary response
   C. level of consciousness (LOC) and pain response
   D. LOC and pupillary response

7. When providing patient teaching, what can the nurse assess?
   A. Complex cognitive function
   B. Patient's ability to handle money
   C. Patient's ability to perform ADLs
   D. Patient's mental status

8. Nursing students are doing a class presentation on stroke. What is the term they would use for deficits in articulation?
   A. Aphasia
   B. Nystagmus
   C. Dysarthria
   D. Dystonia

ALTERNATIVE CASE SCENARIOS

Mr. Gardner, a 56-year-old African American, has a history of hypertension, smoking, and mild baseline dementia. He was admitted to an acute care unit via the emergency department (ED) following a stroke. He lives alone, has poor hygiene, and is wearing multiple layers of mismatched clothing. He does not remember the last time he took his blood pressure medication. Vital signs are T 36.8°C orally, P 88 beats/min, R 22, and BP 168/92 breaths/min. Mr. Gardner is alert, but appears somewhat fearful and agitated. He asks for cigarettes and is oriented to name only. Speech is comprehensible but slurred.

Review the following alternative situations related to Mr. Gardner. Based on the changes outlined below, *consider what other outcomes, information, and problems would affect the overall picture and shape your responses.*

Alternative A

Subjective: "I feel so sleepy."

Objective: Mr. Gardner lives with his wife of 35 years in a single family home. She brought him to the hospital because he fell from a ladder while cleaning his gutters 2 days ago. He landed on his head and has been sleeping more since. His wife stated that he was difficult to wake up this morning. His vital signs are T 36.8°C orally, P 88 beats/min, R 22 breaths/min, BP 118/66 mm Hg. He is oriented to place and person, but was incorrect about the date by 2 days. PERRLA, hand grasp equal, follows commands when repeated several times. Arouses to loud voice and touch. He was admitted to an acute care unit via the ED after diagnosis with a subdural hematoma and his admission assessment was performed.

- Is Mr. Gardner's condition stable, urgent, or an emergency?
- How will the nurse focus, organize, and prioritize subjective and objective data collection?
- Which nursing diagnosis is the highest priority? What is the rationale?
- How will the nurse implement and evaluate the interventions?

Alternative B

Subjective: "It's the worst headache that I've ever had."

Objective: Mr. Gardner states that his headache pain is a 9 on 1 to 10 scale (with 10 being the highest rating). Tylenol with codeine fails to relieve the pain. Vitals are T 37°C orally, P 60 beats/min, R 16 breaths/min, BP 156/56 mm Hg. Pupils asymmetrical with left 4-2 and right 6-4. Complaining of blurred vision; ptosis present on right. Slight weakness with left arm strength 3+ and left leg strength 4+. Legs symmetrical at 4+. Complaining of nausea; no vomiting. He was admitted to the intensive care unit with a diagnosis of subarachnoid hemorrhage from a cerebral aneurysm.

- Is Mr. Gardner's condition stable, urgent, or an emergency?
- How will the nurse focus, organize, and prioritize subjective and objective data collection?
- Which nursing diagnosis is the highest priority and what is the rationale?
- How will the nurse intervene and evaluate the interventions?

DOCUMENTATION

Form for Use in Practice

Patient Name _____ Date _____

Date of Birth _____

Initial Survey

Reason for seeking health care: _____

History of present illness

- Location:

- Intensity:

- Duration:

- Description:

- Aggravating factors:

- Alleviating factors:

- Functional impairment:

- Pain goal:

Vital signs: T (route)_____   P (site)_____   R_____   BP (site)_____   SpO$_2$_____

Weight: _____ Height: _____ BMI: _____

General appearance: _____

General level of distress: _____

Level of anxiety: _____

Risk Factors and History:

- Date and result of last blood pressure reading:

- Date and result of last cholesterol level:

- History of neurological problem:

- Seizure history:

- History of head injury:

- History of infectious or degenerative diseases:

- Emotional/coping changes:

- Personality changes:

- Alterations in level of independence:

- Loss of role function:

- Depression, apathy, or irritability:

- Change in ability to tolerate stress:

- Diabetes mellitus:

- Carotid artery disease:

- Atrial fibrillation:

- Sickle cell disease:

- Smoking history:
- Diet:
- Activity level:
- Occupation:

Common Symptoms:

Symptom	Yes	No	Additional data
Headache or other pain (see Chapter 14)			
Weakness of single limb or one side of the body			
Generalized weakness			
Involuntary movements or tremors			
Difficulty with balance, coordination, or gait			
Dizziness or vertigo			
Difficulty swallowing			
Change in intellectual abilities			
Difficulty with concentration, memory, attention span			
Difficulties with expression or comprehension of speech/language			
Alteration in touch, taste, or smell			
Loss or blurring of vision in one or both eyes, diplopia (double vision)			
Hearing loss or tinnitus (ringing in the ears)			

Physical Assessment:

Assess LOC.
Evaluate cognitive function.
Assess orientation.
Observe clarity and fluency of speech.
Assess pupil size, shape, and reactivity.
Test accommodation.
Assess gaze for eye contact and drifting.
Observe abnormal movements.
(Optional) Test cranial nerves.
Inspect muscle bulk. Observe and palpate muscle groups. Assess tone.
Assess and grade muscle strength.
Ask the patient to walk down a corridor.

Perform the Romberg test.
Assess finger-to-nose coordination or rapid alternating movements to test upper extremity cerebellar function. Assess lower extremities by the heel-to-shin test.
Assess light-touch sensation.
Assess pain sensation.
(Optional) Test temperature sense.
Ask point localization.
Assess vibration sense.
Assess motion and position sense.
Test for stereognosis.
Test graphesthesia.
Assess point discrimination.
Assess touch sensation.
(Optional) Assess and grade deep tendon reflexes.
(Optional) Test plantar response.
(Optional) Test abdominal reflex.
(Optional) Test crimasteric reflex in men.
(Optional) Test the bulbocavernous reflex in men.
(Optional) Test the anal reflex.
Auscultate over the carotid artery.

Signature_____ Date _____

Guide for Use in Practice

Technique	Normal Findings	Abnormal Findings
Assess LOC. Initial outcome determines extent and method of the rest of the examination.	*Patient alert; opens eyes spontaneously*	Patient stuporous, unresponsive, comatose
If LOC results show that the patient can interact, evaluate cognitive function (many components may have been done during history).		
Assess orientation by directly questioning the patient about person, place, and time.	*Patient is oriented.*	Patient struggles with response.
Observe clarity and fluency of speech. Ask the patient to repeat words or phrases with multiple combinations of consonants and vowels.	*Speech is clear and articulate.*	Deficits in articulation; speech/language deficits
Assess pupil size, shape, and reactivity. Record both initial and response sizes.	PERRL (pupils equal, round, reactive to light)	Nystagmus, unequal pupils, constricted, dilated, palsy
Test accommodation.	*Pupils constrict and converge bilaterally.* PERRLA.	Nystagmus, unequal pupils, constricted, dilated, palsy

Assess gaze for eye contact and drifting.	*Gaze is purposeful and conjugate.*	Dysconjugate gaze
Observe abnormal movements.	*Movements smooth and symmetric*	Abnormal flexion and extension, hemiplegia, quadriplegia, paralysis, tic, myoclonus, fasciculation, dystonia, tremor, chorea, and athetosis
(Optional) Test cranial nerves.	Refer to Table 24–6 of the Jensen text for a description of normal findings for each cranial nerve.	Refer to Table 24–6 of the Jensen text for a description of abnormal findings in each cranial nerve.
Inspect muscle bulk. Observe and palpate muscle groups to check for any wasting (atrophy). To assess tone, determine degree of resistance of muscles to passive stretch.	*The relaxed muscle shows some muscular tension. Good muscle bulk and tone.*	Absolutely no resistance to movement; tone seems decreased or "flabby"; increased resistance of muscles to passive stretch; spasticity; rigidity; cogwheel rigidity
Assess muscle strength. Grade strength on a scale of 0–5+.	*Strength 4–5+*	Motor strength 0–3+
Ask the patient to walk down a corridor.	*Patient walks smoothly without swaying.*	Spastic hemiparesis, scissors gait, Parkinsonian gait, cerebellar ataxia, sensory ataxia, waddling, dystonia, and athetoid gait
Perform the Romberg test.	*Patient maintains position without opening the eyes.*	Moderate swaying with eyes open or closed; pronounced increase in swaying (sometimes with falling) with eyes closed
Assess finger-to-nose coordination or rapid alternating movements to test upper extremity cerebellar function.	*Good coordination of movements*	Ataxia, lack of coordination, tremor, hypotonia, nystagmus
Assess lower extremities by the heel-to-shin test.		
Pull the end of a cotton swab so that it is wispy. Ask the patient to close the eyes. Apply light touch to the skin with the swab.	*Patient correctly identifies light touch.*	Increased touch sensation (hyperesthesia); absent touch sensation (anesthesia); hypesthesia (reduced touch sensation)
Ask the patient to state where he or she feels the sensation.		
Break a tongue blade or cotton swab so that the end is sharp. Ask the patient to close the eyes; lightly touch the patient's skin with the sharp end. Ask the patient to state where he or she feels the sensation.	*Pain sensation intact*	Increased pain sensation (hyperalgesia); absent pain sensation (analgesia); reduced pain sensation (hypalgesia)
(Optional) Test temperature sense.	*Temperature sensation intact*	Abnormal temperature sensation
Ask the patient to close the eyes. Using a finger, gently touch the patient on the hands, lower arms, abdomen, lower legs, and feet. Have the patient identify where he or she feels the sensation.	*Point localization intact*	"Stocking-glove" distribution suggests peripheral nerves; dermatomal distribution suggests isolated nerves or nerve roots; reduced sensation below a certain level is associated with the spinal cord. Crossed face-body pattern suggests the brainstem; hemisensory loss suggests stroke.

Strike a low-pitched tuning fork on the side or heel of the hand to produce vibrations. Ask the patient to close the eyes. Hold the fork at the base; place it over body prominences, beginning at the most distal location. Ask the patient to state where the sensation is felt and when it disappears.	*Vibration sense is intact.*	Vibration sense lost at any point
Ask the patient to close the eyes. Move the distal joints of the patient's fingers and then toes up or down. If the patient cannot identify these movements, test the next most proximal joints.	*Intact motion and position sense*	Involuntary writhing, snakelike movements of a limb (athetosis)
Ask the patient to close the eyes and identify a familiar object (eg, coin) placed in the palm (*stereognosis*).	*Patient correctly identifies the object.*	Inability to identify objects correctly (astereognosis)
Use a blunt object to trace a number (eg, "8") on the patient's palm. Ask the patient to identify which number has been traced (*graphesthesia*).	*Patient correctly identifies the number.*	Compromised cortical sensory function
Ask the patient to close the eyes. Hold the blunt end of two cotton swabs approximately 2 in. apart and move them together until the patient feels them as one point.	*More discrimination distally than centrally*	Lost cortical sensory function
Ask the patient to close the eyes. At the same time, touch a body area on both sides. Ask the patient to state where he or she perceives the touch.	*Sensations are felt on both sides.*	Lost or reduced stimulus on the opposite side of the damaged cortex
(Optional) Assess deep tendon reflexes. Grade on a scale of 0–4, with 0 representing absent and 4 corresponding to significantly hyperactive.	*DTRs are 2+ bilaterally without clonus.*	Clonus
(Optional) Test plantar response by stroking the sole with a blunt instrument.	*The toes flex (a flexor-plantar response).*	Babinski's sign, triple flexion
(Optional) Stroke the upper quadrants of the abdomen with a tongue blade or reflex hammer.	*The umbilicus moves toward each area of stimulation symmetrically.*	Depression or absence of this reflex
(Optional) Stroke the inner thigh of the male patient.	*The testicle and scrotum rise on the stroked side.*	Response is diminished or absent.
(Optional) Apply direct pressure over the bulbocavernous muscle behind the scrotum.	*Muscle contracts and elevates the scrotum.*	Response is diminished or absent.
(Optional) Scratch the tissue at the side of the anus with a blunt instrument.	*The anus puckers*	Response is diminished or absent.
Auscultate over the carotid artery.	*No bruit*	Bruit

Male Genitalia and Rectal Assessment

CHAPTER 25

OBJECTIVE SUMMARY

This chapter provides an overview of normal anatomy and focuses on physical assessment of the male genitalia, which includes the seminal vesicles, scrotum, penis, testicles, prostate gland, and epididymides. While the rectum and anus are terminal structures of the gastrointestinal tract (see Chapter 22), nurses frequently integrate a holistic nursing assessment of these organs into the physical examination of the male genitalia. A basic understanding of pertinent anatomy assists nurses to perform assessments with confidence and knowledge.

READING ASSIGNMENT

Read Chapter 25 in Jensen's *Nursing Health Assessment: A Best-Practice Approach.*

VOCABULARY/TERMINOLOGY

- **Bulbourethral gland:** Also called a *Cowper's gland*; one of two small exocrine glands in the reproductive system of human males. They are homologous to Bartholin's glands in females. They are located on either side of the urethra immediately below the prostate gland and secrete a clear fluid called *pre-ejaculate.*

- **Corpora cavernosa:** A pair of sponge-like regions of erectile tissue; contain most of the blood in the penis during penile erection.

- **Corpus spongiosum:** Mass of spongy tissue surrounding the male urethra within the penis.

- **Cremasteric muscle:** Muscle layer that allows the scrotum to relax or contract.

- **Ejaculatory duct:** One of two structures in the male anatomy, about 2 cm in length, formed by the union of the vas deferens with the duct of the seminal vesicle. Both ejaculatory ducts pass through the prostate and empty into the urethra at the colliculus seminalis. During ejaculation, semen passes through the ducts and exits the body via the penis.

- **Epididymis:** Elongated cordlike structure along the posterior border of the testis; its coiled duct provides for storage, transit, and maturation of spermatozoa and is continuous with the ductus deferens.

- **Foreskin:** In uncircumcised males, loose, hood-like skin that covers the glan.

- **Glan:** Sensitive bulbous structure at the distal end of the penis.

- **Hernia:** Loop of intestine that prolapses through the inguinal wall or canal or abdominal musculature.

- **Penis:** Final excretory organ of urination; with sexual excitement, it becomes firm or erect to allow penetration for intercourse.

- **Prepuce:** In uncircumcised males, loose, hood-like skin that covers the glan; also called *foreskin.*

- **Priapism:** Long and painful erection.

- **Prostate:** Right and left lobes divided by a slight groove known as the *median sulcus*. These two lobes are in close contact with the anterior rectal wall and palpable during digital rectal examination. It produces the greatest volume of ejaculatory fluid.

- **Scrotum:** Pouch covered with darkly pigmented, loose, rugous (wrinkled) skin. A septum divides the scrotum into two sacs, each of which contains a testis, epididymis, spermatic cord, and muscle layer known as the *cremasteric muscle*.

- **Seminal vesicles:** Glands that produce and secrete ejaculation fluid known as *semen*. Small pouches located between the rectum and the posterior bladder wall; the vesicles join the ejaculatory duct at the base of the prostate.

- **Seminiferous tubules:** Inside each testicle is a series of coiled ducts where spermatogenesis occurs.

- **Smegma:** Thin, white, cheesy substance that develops between the foreskin and the glans.

- **Spermatic cord:** Anatomic cord that suspends the testes in the scrotum.

- **Testis:** Male gonad; either of the paired egg-shaped glands normally situated in the scrotum, in which the spermatozoa develop.

- **Urethra:** Located in the middle of the corpus spongiosum, which ends in the cone-shaped glan with its expanded base, or *corona*. A small slit in the distal tip of the glan is the *urethra meatus*. This tube-like structure evacuates urine from the body, and is the exit point for ejaculatory fluid and sperm.

- **Vas deferens:** Structure that transports sperm from the epididymis to the ejaculatory duct.

STUDY GUIDE

Activity A FILL IN THE BLANK

1. Fill in the blanks about the male reproductive tract and the male rectum.

   A. The _____ are located on either side of the urethra immediately below the prostate gland.

   B. The distal end, commonly referred to as the _____ _____, is identifiable during a colonoscopy as having a _____ edge.

C. The anorectal junction is lined with mucous membrane arranged in longitudinal folds called _____, which contain a complex system of veins and arteries commonly referred to as the _____.

D. The lower portion, which is controlled by _____, is sensitive to stimulation.

Activity B MATCHING

1. *Match the part of the male reproductive tract with its function.*

Answer	Part	Function
	1. Epididymis	A. Contains most of the blood in the penis during penile erection
	2. Prepuce	
	3. Corporus cavernosum	
	4. Root	B. Lies deep within the perineum
	5. Corona	C. Connects the efferent ducts from the rear of each testicle to its vas deferens
	6. Seminiferous tubule	
	7. Prostate gland	
		D. Separates the glan from the shaft
		E. Covers the glans in an uncircumcised male
		F. Produces the greatest volume of ejaculatory fluid
		G. Is where spermatogenesis occurs

2. *Match the abnormal condition of the penis with the appropriate description.*

Answer	Abnormal Condition	Description
	1. Genital piercing	A. Inflammation of the glan and prepuce
	2. Epispadias	B. A prepuce that cannot be retracted over the glan
	3. Paraphimosis	
	4. Hypospadias	C. Deviation of the meatus, which makes it difficult to urinate when standing
	5. Phimosis	
	6. Balanitis	D. An exposed lower urinary tract in severe cases

E. Possible infection

F. A retracted prepuce that cannot be placed back over the glan

Activity C LABELING

1. Label the terms listed below on the figure provided:

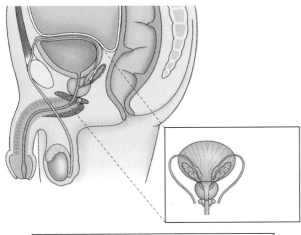

corpus cavernosum, penis, prepuce, prostate, scrotum, seminal vesicle, testes, vas deferens

Activity D SHORT ANSWER

1. Discuss the onset of puberty in the adolescent male and the physiological events that occur.

_____

_____

_____

_____

2. Explain the effects of aging on the reproductive organs of a male.

_____

_____

_____

_____

3. Explain the need for an acute assessment in a male patient presenting with problems of the male reproductive system. Include the causes and the signs and symptoms of these patients' problems.

_____

_____

_____

_____

4. Discuss the need for surgery to treat problems with the male reproductive tract, prostate, and rectum.

_____

_____

_____

_____

5. Explain why nurses may be hesitant to obtain sexual histories from their patients. Discuss why it is important to obtain this information. Include obtaining information concerning sexual dysfunction.

_____

_____

_____

_____

6. Describe the process of performing a testicular self-examination.

_____

_____

_____

_____

Activity E MULTIPLE CHOICE

1. Which of the following cultural groups has the highest incidence of prostate cancer?

A. Caucasian men

B. Native American men

C. African–American men

D. Asian–American men

2. When providing information to a patient about prostate screening, what is one method the nurse would discuss?

A. STE screening

B. PDA screening

C. OTC screening

D. PSA screening

3. A patient with what type of cancer is subject to priapism?

A. Prostate

B. Leukemia

C. Penile

D. Testicular

4. A patient presents at the clinic with scrotal pain. What is the presumptive diagnosis?

A. Testicular torsion

B. Priapism

C. Hydrocele

D. Varicocele

5. An Advanced Practice Nurse is preparing to do a rectal examination on a 77-year-old patient. The patient complains of pain as soon as the examination begins. What might this patient have?

A. Penile atrophy

B. Scrotal enlargement

C. Benign prostatic hyperplasia (BPH)

D. Rectal fissures

6. The nurse is assessing a 2-year-old boy who was admitted with severe stomach pain. When changing this patient, the nurse notes perirectal redness. What might this patient have?

A. Enterobiasis

B. Diarrhea

C. Constipation

D. Anal fissures

7. When assessing for prostate cancer, the PSA is used in combination with what?

A. STE

B. SBE

C. DRE

D. PDA

ALTERNATIVE CASE SCENARIOS

Mr. Gardner, a 50-year-old Caucasian man, was diagnosed with benign prostatic hyperplasia (BPH) 3 years ago. He is visiting the clinic today because he is having increased difficulty with urination. Mr. Gardner has been married to his second wife for 3 months. He has two children from his first marriage and two stepchildren. Mr. Gardner's temperature is 37.0°C, pulse is 84 beats/min, respirations are 16 breaths/min, and blood pressure is 122/68 mm Hg. Current medications include tamsulosin (Flomax) for the prostatic hyperplasia and lovastatin for his elevated lipid

levels. Additional supplements include a multivitamin and fish-oil tablets that he takes to prevent cardiovascular disease.

Review the following alternative situations related to Mr. Gardner. Based on the changes outlined below, *consider what other outcomes, information, and problems would affect the overall picture and shape your responses.*

Alternative A

Subjective: "My bladder feels really full. It hurts more than it usually does."

Objective: Mr. Gardner is unable to void and his bladder scan shows 1,000 mL. Bladder palpable above the pubis.

- Is Mr. Gardner stable, urgent, or an emergency?
- How will the nurse work with Mr. Gardner to promote health and reduce risk for illness?
- How will the nurse focus, organize, and prioritize the subjective and objective data collection?
- Which nursing diagnosis is highest priority and what is the rationale?

Alternative B

Subjective: Mr. Gardner has had surgery for BPH. He is worried about his sexual relationship with his wife.

Objective: Two-week postoperative visit. No hemorrhage, bladder spasms, urinary incontinence, or infection. Urinary catheter removed. Eating high-fiber diet and taking stool softeners. Asking about the return to normal sexual function.

- Is Mr. Gardner stable, urgent, or an emergency?
- How will the nurse work with Mr. Gardner to promote health and reduce risk for illness?
- How will the nurse focus, organize, and prioritize the subjective and objective data collection?
- Which nursing diagnosis is highest priority and what is the rationale?

DOCUMENTATION

Patient Name _____ Date _____

Date of Birth _____

Initial Survey

Reason for seeking health care: _____

History of present illness

- Location:

- Intensity:

- Duration:

- Description:

- Aggravating factors:

- Alleviating factors:

- Functional impairment:

- Pain goal:

Vital signs: T (route)_____ P (site)_____ R_____ BP (site)_____ SpO$_2$_____

Height: _____ Weight: _____ BMI: _____

General appearance: _____

General level of distress: _____

Level of anxiety: _____

Risk Factors and History:

- Family history:

- Testicular cancer:

- Prostate cancer:

- Penile cancer:

- Infertility in siblings:

- Hernia:

- Current or chronic illnesses

	Yes	No	Comments
Diabetes			
Neurologic impairment			
Hypertension			
Respiratory problems (specify)			
Cardiovascular disease			

- Previous surgery on penis, scrotum, or rectum:
- Previous STIs:
- Injury to or other problems with scrotum, penis, or testes:
- Prostate gland problem:
- Cancer:
- Sports and activity:
- Use of protective gear:
- Immunizations against hepatitis A or B
- Self-genital examination:
- Clinical testicular examinations:

Sexual History

- Age at first sexual intercourse:
- By choice?
- Sexual relationships with men, women, or both:
- Type of sex (penile-vaginal, penile-rectal, recipient rectal, oral):
- Frequency of intercourse:
- Sex with multiple partners:
- Number of partners in the last 6 months:
- Use of drugs or alcohol before sexual intercourse:
- Sexual satisfaction:
- Contraceptive use:
- Protective barrier use:
- Pregnancy:

Medications

- Prescriptions:
- Herbal supplements;
- Recreational drugs:
- OTC drugs:

Common Symptoms:

Symptom	Yes	No	Additional data
Pain			
Problems with urination			
Erectile dysfunction			
Penile lesions, discharge			
Scrotal enlargement			

Physical Assessment:

With the patient supine, inspect the groin. Observe genital hair distribution.
Observe the penis for surface characteristics, color, lesions, and discharge. Inspect the posterior side. In the patient with an uncircumcised penis, ask him to retract the prepuce.
Inspect the glan.
Inspect and palpate the shaft.
Inspect and palpate the external urethral meatus. Strip or milk the penis from base toward glan. Note color, consistency, or odor of any discharge.
Inspect the scrotal septum. Inspect the anterior and posterior scrotum for any sores or rashes.
Inspect the sacrococcygeal areas for surface characteristics and tenderness.
With the patient on his side, spread the buttocks and inspect the perineal area.
Inspect the inguinal canal area and femoral area for bulges or masses.

Signature_____ Date _____

Guide for Use in Practice

Technique	Normal Findings	Abnormal Findings
With the patient supine, inspect the groin. Observe genital hair distribution.	*Skin clear, intact, and smooth. Hair diamond shaped or in an escutcheon pattern. Hair appears coarser than at the scalp and has no parasites.*	No hair, patchy growth, distribution in a female or triangular pattern with the base over the pubis; infestations such as pediculosis, scabies, or any parasites; inflammation, lesions, or dermatitis; erosions and pustules; large red, scaly patches that are extremely itchy
Observe the penis for surface characteristics, color, lesions, and discharge. Inspect the posterior side. In the patient with an uncircumcised penis, ask him to retract the prepuce.	*Dorsal vein apparent on the dorsal surface of the penis, which has no edema, lesions, discharge or nodules. In the circumcised patient, the glan and corona are visible, lighter in color than the shaft, and free of smegma. In the uncircumcised penis, the prepuce retracts easily. Smegma may be present around the corona.*	Piercings, phimosis (foreskin cannot retract), paraphimosis (foreskin is retracted and fixed), and *balanitis* (related to diabetes)
Inspect the glan.	*It is glistening pink, smooth in texture, and bulbous.*	*Hypospadias* (urethral meatus on underside) and *epispadias* (meatus on upper side)
Inspect and palpate the shaft.	*Smooth without lesions or pain. Normal variations include ectopic sebaceous glands on the shaft that appear as tiny, whitish-yellow papules.*	Lesions, bleeding, pain on touch, discharge
Inspect and palpate the external urethral meatus. Strip or milk the penis from base toward glan. Note color, consistency, or odor of any discharge.	*It is located centrally on the glan. The orifice is slit-like and millimeters from the tip of the penis. The external urethral meatus has no discharge, stenosis, or warts.*	Yellow, milky-white, or greenish discharge with a foul odor. Urethral meatus on the underside or upper side of penis

Ask the patient to hold the penis out of the way, and inspect the scrotal septum. Inspect the anterior and posterior scrotum for any sores or rashes.	*It is divided into two sacs. Sebaceous cysts or sebaceous glands may be normally noted on the scrotal sac. Anterior and posterior scrotal skin darker in pigmentation with a rugous or wrinkled surface.*	Scrotal lesions, edema, and redness; inconsistencies in size or texture; testicular torsion, epididymitis, variocele, hydrocele, and spermatocele
Inspect the sacrococcygeal areas for surface characteristics and tenderness.	*Skin is clear and smooth with no palpable masses or dimpling.*	A dimple with an inflamed tuft of hair or a tender palpable cyst in the sacrococcygeal area
With the patient on his side, spread the buttocks and inspect the perineal area.	*Skin surrounding the anus is coarse with darker pigmentation. Anal sphincter is closed.*	Warts, loose sphincter, lesions, hemorrhoids, fissures, fistulas, or polyps. Infestations from pinworms or fungal infections
Inspect the inguinal canal area and femoral area for bulges or masses.	*No bulges or masses are found*	Bulges or masses (suggest a hernia)

CHAPTER 26

Female Genitalia and Rectal Assessment

OBJECTIVE SUMMARY

This chapter focuses on genital and rectal assessment of the female patient across the lifespan. By identifying key factors in the process of this assessment, the nurse can explore opportunities for positive communication and accurate information regarding women's health. Nurses can guide female patients in risk reduction and health promotion from the onset of puberty to the menopausal years and beyond.

READING ASSIGNMENT

Read Chapter 26 in Jensen's *Nursing Health Assessment: A Best-Practice Approach.*

VOCABULARY/TERMINOLOGY

- **Ambiguous genitalia:** Congenital anomaly found in newborns in which hyperplasia of the adrenal glands causes excessive androgen production. The clitoris may look like a penis and the fusion of the labia resembles a scrotal sac. This emergent condition requires referral for diagnostic evaluation.

- **Ampulla:** Second portion of the uterine tube. It is an intermediate dilated portion, which curves over the ovary. It is the most common site of human fertilization.

- **Anterior pituitary gland:** Gland that secretes follicle-stimulating hormone (FSH) and lutenizing hormone (LH).

- **Bartholin's glands:** Located at the base of the vestibule, secrete clear mucus into the vaginal introitus during intercourse. They are positioned at 7 and 5 o'clock positions of the posterior vestibule.

- **Cervix:** Posterior portion of the uterus that protrudes into the vagina. The cervix is smooth, rounded, and has a midline opening called the **os.**

- **Clitoris:** Embryologic homologue of the penis; responds in an erectile fashion when stimulated. Nerve fibers in the clitoris respond to touch and produce pleasurable feelings for the female.

- **Dyspareunia:** Pain with intercourse.

- **Fallopian tubes:** Two tubes that transport ova from the ovary to the uterus. They are approximately 12 cm long and 1 mm in diameter and composed of four tissue layers: peritoneal (serous), subserous (adventitial), muscular, and mucous.

- **Fimbria:** One of the three parts of the fallopian tubes. A fringe of tissue around the ostium of the Fallopian tube, in the direction of the ovary.

- **Follicle-stimulating hormone (FSH):** Hormone responsible for growth and maturation of the ovarian follicle and production of testosterone, which maintains spermatogenesis in the male.

- **Frenulum:** Ventral surface of the glans where the labia minora fuse.

- **Gonadotropin-releasing hormone (GnRH):** Tropic peptide hormone responsible for the release of FSH and LH from the anterior pituitary. GnRH is synthesized and released from neurons within the hypothalamus.

- **Hymen:** Fold of mucous membrane that surrounds or partially covers the external vaginal opening. Its name comes from the ancient Greek for "hymenaeus," which means "vaginal flap."

- **Hypothalamus:** Endocrine structure that is of the three main sources for producing the hormones that regulate the female reproductive system.

- **Isthmus:** One of the three parts of the fallopian tubes.

- **Labia majora:** Two folds that extend from mons pubis downward to the perineum.

- **Labia minora:** Two small folds that extend from clitoral hood to the posterior fourchete of the vagina.

- **Lutenizing hormone (LH):** Hormone that functions to lutenize the follicle, which increases production of progesterone by the granulose cells. The lutenizing process ultimately produces the corpus luteum.

- **Menopause:** 12 consecutive months without menses. Cessation of fertility.

- **Metabolic syndrome:** Cluster of increased blood pressure, elevated insulin levels, excess body fat around the waist, and abnormal cholesterol levels that together increase risks for heart disease, stroke, and diabetes.

- **Mons pubis:** Most anterior structure comprised of subcutaneous fatty tissue covered by pubic hair. It is directly over the pubic bone and creates a cushion that protects the bone during intercourse.

- **Ovaries:** Two almond-shaped structures measuring approximately 3 cm by 2 cm. They develop after puberty and reduce in size (atrophy) after menopause. Held in place by ligaments called the infundibulopelvic and ovarian ligaments. They provide ova to be fertilized by sperm and secrete the hormones, estrogen and progesterone.

- **Paraurethral (Skene's) glands:** Glands that produce clear fluid that aids in lubrication during intercourse.

- **Perineum:** Area between the vaginal introitus and the rectum. This is the location where an episiotomy is occasionally done to facilitate difficult childbirth.

- **Posterior fourchette:** Fold of skin that forms the posterior margin of the vulva.

- **Urethral meatus:** Exterior opening of the urethra.

- **Uterus:** Often referred to as the "womb." Organ that holds the endometrial lining and is prepared to accept an implanted ovum. It lies between the bladder and the rectum and is approximately 7 to 8 cm long and 4 to 5 cm at its widest part.

- **Vagina:** Tube of muscular tissue that extends from vaginal introitus to uterus. The three-layer vaginal muscle wall is extremely expandable especially during childbirth. It is lined by glandular mucous membrane, within which are folds called rugae.

- **Vaginal introitus:** Lies posterior to the urethra and is the outer opening of the vagina.

- **Vestibule:** Area that lies between the labia minora and is bound anteriorly by the clitoris and posteriorly by the perineum. Within the vestibule lies the urethra at the upper middle area, with bilateral paraurethral Skene's glands at the 7 and 5 o'clock positions, respectively.

STUDY GUIDE

Activity A **FILL IN THE BLANK**

1. Fill in the blanks about the external female reproductive tract.

   A. Lays directly over the pubic bone and creates a cushion that protects the bone during intercourse _____.

   B. Embryologic homologue of the penis; responds in an erectile fashion when stimulated _____.

   C. Lies posterior to the urethra _____.

   D. The ventral surface of the glans _____.

2. Fill in the blanks about the internal female reproductive system and rectum.

   A. The _____ separates the anterior wall of the vagina from the _____ and _____.

B. The uterine walls consist of an outer layer called the _____, a muscle layer called the _____, and an inner layer called the _____.

C. The fallopian tubes are divided into three parts: _____, _____, and _____.

Activity B **MATCHING**

1. *Match the infection that can occur in the female genitalia with its description.*

Answer	Infection	Description
	1. Pediculosis pubis	**A.** Pain or tenderness in the Bartholin's area
	2. Contact dermatitis	**B.** Usually dysuria, hematuria, or frequently no response to antibiotics given for UTI
	3. Abscess of Bartholin's gland	
	4. Chancre	**C.** Seen with primary syphilis; 1-cm button-like papule at the area of inoculation
	5. Urethral caruncle	
		D. Acute external itching or burning, which may extend to the inner thigh
		E. Mild to severe itching, especially in the mons pubis and perineum

2. *Match the abnormal condition with the appropriate description.*

Answer	Abnormal Condition	Description
	1. Endometrosis	**A.** The affected patient presents with amenorrhea and low pelvic tenderness.
	2. Solid ovarian mass	
	3. Fluctuant ovarian cyst	**B.** Benign (99%) condition of the uterus and uterine walls
	4. Leiomyoma	
	5. Acute salpingitis	**C.** Caused by retrograde menstrual flow into the peritoneal cavity.
	6. Ectopic pregnancy	

D. Another name for pelvic inflammatory disease

E. Most common symptoms are lower quadrant pain, nausea, and referred pain in the neck or shoulder.

F. Benign cystic teratoma

Activity C **LABELING**

1. Label the position of the terms listed below:

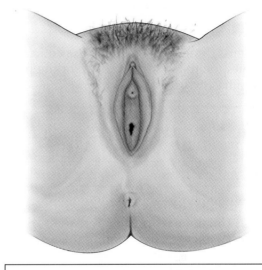

anus, clitoris, hymen, labia majora, labia minora, mons pubis, perineum, urinary meatus, vaginal introitus

Activity D **SHORT ANSWER**

1. Describe the vagina.

_____

_____

_____

_____

2. Discuss the age of onset of puberty in girls, including ethnic variations and physiological changes that occur in adolescent females going through puberty.

_____

_____

_____

_____

3. Explain the definition of menopause and the physiological changes that occur in a woman as she ages.

_____

_____

_____

_____

4. Explain the need for the nurse to obtain data about whether a patient douches and what educational topics this might open up.

_____

_____

_____

_____

5. Discuss dysuria and identify the education topics the nurse should cover for the patient who has dysuria.

_____

_____

_____

_____

6. Discuss the sexually transmitted infection (STI) Chlamydia. Include potential consequences of not treating the infection.

_____

_____

_____

_____

7. Explain osteoporosis and screening for it.

_____

_____

_____

_____

Activity E MULTIPLE CHOICE

1. A 43-year-old woman comes to the ob/gyn clinic for her yearly examination. She tells the nurse that she wants to renew the prescription for her birth-control pills. During the assessment interview, the patient tells the nurse that she smokes ½ pack a day and drinks several drinks a day. What should the nurse include in patient education?
   A. Women who drink should not use hormonal contraceptives.
   B. Women older than 40 years should not use birth-control pills.
   C. The recommended contraceptive for women older than 40 years is tubal ligation.
   D. Women older than 40 years who smoke should not take birth-control pills.

2. The nurse is teaching a health class at the local high school and today will be discussing human papillomavirus (HPV) with a group of 10th-grade female students. What important information should be given to these young women?
   A. The use of condoms prevents the spread of HPV.
   B. Everyone should get the HPV vaccine by the age of 10 years.
   C. Someone with multiple partners has the highest risk of developing HPV.
   D. If you practice "safe sex," you will not get HPV.

3. What is the greatest risk factor for cervical cancer?
   A. HIV
   B. HPV
   C. Genetics
   D. Age

4. A 35-year-old woman visits her family doctor and reports mood swings, swelling of her breasts, acne, bloating, and weight gain every month, starting about 2 weeks prior to her period. What disorder is this patient describing?
   A. Premenstrual syndrome (PMS)
   B. Dysmenorrhea
   C. Premenstrual dysphoric disorder (PMDD)
   D. Ectopic pregnancy

5. A man brings a 29-year-old woman with a history of ovarian cysts to the emergency department. The patient is in severe left-sided pain and tells the nurse that "this is how it feels every time I have had a cyst." She is found to have a ruptured ovarian cyst, and the physician recommends that she be evaluated for what?

   A. Gonorrhea

   B. Tubal pregnancy

   C. Polycystic ovarian syndrome

   D. Premenstrual syndrome

6. The nurse is caring for a 17-year-old girl who is 16 weeks pregnant. The patient's history shows infection with multiple STIs. What should the nurse do?

   A. Give the patient information about contraception.

   B. Verify that the baby's father does not have an STI at the current time.

   C. Ask the patient what she plans to do about her pregnancy.

   D. Verify that prior STIs were treated according to protocol.

7. Research has shown that in vitro fertilization has a higher

   A. risk of fetal loss

   B. risk of STI

   C. rate of single births

   D. rate of fetal congenital abnormalities

8. A 57-year-old woman calls the clinic reporting painful intercourse followed by spotting. She tells the nurse that she hasn't had a period in 2 years. What should the nurse tell her?

   A. "Go to the emergency department to be checked right away."

   B. "You may have an STI."

   C. "These findings are common in postmenopausal women."

   D. "Make an appointment to see the doctor as soon as possible."

ALTERNATIVE CASE SCENARIOS

Teresa Nguyen, a 28-year-old Vietnamese American woman, is being seen in the clinic for the first time with clear vaginal secretions and pelvic pain. Her temperature is 33.8°C orally, pulse 82 beats/min, respirations 16 breaths/min, and blood pressure 102/66 mm Hg. She is taking no medications.

   Review the following alternative situations. Based on the changes outlined below, *consider what other outcomes, information, and problems would affect the overall picture and shape your responses.*

Alternative A

Subjective: Teresa Nguyen is having heavy vaginal discharge that is white and creamy. States that she has had an increase in vaginal itching. Recently placed on oral antibiotics for a strep throat infection.

Objective: T 37°C orally, P 68 beats/min, R 20 breaths/min, BP 118/78 mm Hg. White creamy discharge present on labia.

• How are the nurse's concerns different with this problem?

• What further assessment information will the nurse collect?

• How will the RN and the nurse practitioner collaborate to assess her?

Alternative B

Subjective: Teresa Nguyen states that she has had a sudden onset of severe and sharp midabdominal pain rated 10/10 scale.

Objective: Vital signs are T 37.2°C orally, P 124 beats/min, R 28 breaths/min, BP 88/60 mm Hg. Guarding abdomen, sighing with pain. Appears pale and in acute distress. Abdomen taut and tender. Last menstrual period was 10 weeks ago.

• Is Teresa's condition stable, urgent, or an emergency?

• How will the nurse focus, organize, and prioritize the subjective and objective data collection?

• How will the physical assessment be altered based upon the symptoms?

DOCUMENTATION

Form for Use in Practice

Patient Name _____ Date _____

Date of Birth _____

Initial Survey

Reason for seeking health care: _____

History of present illness

- Location:

- Intensity:

- Duration:

- Description:

- Aggravating factors:

- Alleviating factors:

- Functional impairment:

- Pain goal:

Vital signs: T (route)_____   P (site)_____   R_____   BP (site)_____ SpO_2_____

Weight: _____ Height: _____ BMI: _____

General appearance: _____

General level of distress: _____

Level of anxiety: _____

Risk Factors and History:

Family History

Problem	Yes	No	Details
Diabetes			
Heart disease			
Cancer			
Thyroid problems			
Gynecologic conditions			
Hypertension			
Asthma			
Allergies			
DES use in mother			
Multiple pregnancies			
Congenital anomalies			

Menstrual History

- Age at first menstrual period:
- First day of last menstrual period:
- Character or consistency of flow:
- Tampon use:
- Days of flow during cycle:
- Pads or tampons used per day:
- Cessation of menstrual periods:
- Irregular cycles:
- Absent menses for less than 12 consecutive months:

Obstetrical History

- Previous pregnancy:
- Living children:
- Vaginal or cesarean births:
- Complications before, during, or after pregnancy:
- Miscarriage:
- Elective termination:
- Spontaneous miscarriage:
- Incomplete miscarriage:

Gynecologic History

- Most recent Pap smear results and date:
- Previous Pap abnormalities:
- Previous procedures or surgeries:
- Vaginal infections:
- Use of over-the-counter (OTC) vaginal medications:
- Pelvic infections:
- Use of scented vaginal products:
- Douching:

Immunizations

- HPV:

Sexual History

- Age at first sexual intercourse:
- Type of sex currently engaged in (vaginal, oral, anal):
- Approximate sexual partners:
- Type of sexual partners (male, female, both):
- Current relationships (monogamous?):
- Sexual abuse:

- Pain or bleeding with or after intercourse:
- Urinary burning or infections related to intercourse:

Contraception

- Type used:
- Use of condoms or other barrier methods:
- Problems:

Medications and Supplements

- Prescribed medications:
- OTC medications:
- Antibiotics:
- Herbal therapeutics:
- Vitamins:

Tobacco Use

- Smoking:
- Alcohol:
- Drug use:

Common Symptoms:

Symptom	Yes	No	Additional data
Pelvic pain			
Vaginal discharge, burning, or itching			
Menstrual disorders			
Structural problems			
Hemorrhoids			

Physical Assessment:

Inspect pubic hair.
Inspect the skin, inguinal area, and clitoris.
Inspect the labia majora and vaginal opening.
Inspect the vestibule, urethra, and Skene's glands.
Inspect the perineum.
Assess the urethra and Skene's glands. Palpate the Bartholin's glands.
Locate the cervix. Ask the patient to squeeze the vaginal muscles around your finger. Ask the patient to then bear down slightly.
(APRN) Conduct the speculum examination. Inspect the cervix and vaginal walls.
(APRN) Perform the Pap smear.

| (APRN) Inspect the vaginal wall during insertion and removal of the speculum. |
| (APRN) Perform the bimanual examination. Palpate the cervix for size, shape, and movement. |
| (APRN) Palpate the uterus. |
| (APRN) Palpate the ovaries. |
| (APRN) Perform the rectovaginal examination. |

Guide for Use in Practice

Technique	Normal Findings	Abnormal Findings
Inspect pubic hair for amount and distribution. Look for lice or nits.	*Hair evenly distributed and growing downward. No lice or nits*	Pediculosis pubis (crab lice)
Inspect the skin. Bilaterally observe the inguinal area. Inspect the clitoris, noting the size and shape.	*Clitoris 1–1.5 cm long*	Vulvar or vaginal pain, flu-like symptoms, sores on the vulva or genital region, scattered vesicles along the labia, matching vesicles on the labia, surface ulcerations or crusted lesions, inguinal lymphadenopathy
Inspect the labia majora for size and symmetry. Inspect the vaginal opening.	*No protrusions seen from the vagina. Small inclusion cysts are common and may come and go without notice.*	Vulvar or vaginal itching; vaginal secretions; growths along the vagina or rectum; fleshy pink or grey papilloma or wart-like projections at the vulva, vagina, or anus; lesion; itching; burning; pain; bleeding or watery discharge
Inspect the vestibule. Inspect the urethra for position and patency. Observe the Skene's glands at the 1 o'clock and 11 o'clock positions lateral to the urethra.	*No discharge or redness. Skene's glands small, noninflamed, and occasionally not seen*	Vulvovaginal and rectal puritus, dyspareunia, vulvovaginal edema, erythemia, excoriation, thick white secretions
Inspect the perineum.	*Smooth with no lesions or tears. Healed scars from any episiotomies. Anus intact*	Contact dermatitis, chancres, swelling, lacerations, protrusions
Separate the inner portion of the labia minora. Gently press the index finger forward to assess the urethra and Skene's glands. Palpate the Bartholin's glands on each side.	*No swelling or tenderness noted on either side*	Abscess of Bartholin's gland, urethral caruncle, swelling, tenderness
Locate the cervix. Ask the patient to squeeze the vaginal muscles around your finger to check vaginal tone. Ask the patient to then bear down slightly to assess for pelvic organ prolapse.	*Cervix readily identifiable. No signs of prolapse*	Prolapse
(APRN) Conduct the speculum examination. Inspect the cervix and vaginal walls.	*The cervix of a nulliparous woman has a small round os, while the parous woman has a horizontal or fish-mouth-looking slit. It is smooth, pink, and positioned midline in the vagina. Clear secretions are present.*	Tear of the cervix resulting in an irregular slit; nabothian cyst; polyp; DES syndrome, cervical dysplasia

(APRN) Perform the Pap smear.	*The Pap smear is used to evaluate cells from the cervix for precancerous or cancerous status.*	Collection of cells from the endocervix or cervix may cause some spotting or bleeding; this can occur with a pap or with an STI screening.
(APRN) Inspect the vaginal wall during insertion and removal of the speculum.	*No lesions, bleeding, erythema, or edema*	Thin or thick secretions; foul odor, purulent yellow to green discharge; pain on examination; cervical redness; contact bleeding; pH > 4.5; creamy white to gray secretions
(APRN) Perform the bimanual examination. Palpate the cervix for size, shape, and movement.	*Normal size is approximately 7 × 4 cm (occasionally larger in multigravid women).*	Cystocele, rectocele, uterine prolapse, fibroid, ovarian cyst, solid ovarian mass, bleeding
(APRN) Palpate the uterus.	*Feels pear shaped and smooth and is freely mobile*	Abnormal uterine bleeding and blockage, abdominal pressure, constipation, incontinence, dysmenorrhea, uterine enlargement, mass
(APRN) Palpate the ovaries.	*Ovary is often not felt, especially in older menopausal women. If palpated, it feels like a small almond.*	Pain, tenderness over the ovary, irregular menses, intraperitoneal bleeding; solid ovarian mass
(APRN) Perform the rectovaginal examination.	*Septum feels smooth and intact. Posterior portion of the uterus may be felt and is smooth.*	*Rectocele* (bulging of rectum into the vagina) or *rectovaginal fistula* (opening between vagina and rectum allowing feces to enter the vagina)

Pregnant Women

CHAPTER 27

OBJECTIVE SUMMARY

This chapter describes normal anatomical and physiological changes of pregnancy, as well as expected variations based on age, risk factors, and environment. It considers how cultural variations can affect care during pregnancy. It also explores specific symptoms common to pregnancy and the nurse's role in their identification and management.

READING ASSIGNMENT

Read Chapter 27 in Jensen's *Nursing Health Assessment: A Best-Practice Approach*.

VOCABULARY/TERMINOLOGY

- **Bishop's score:** A prelabor scoring system to assist in predicting whether induction of labor will be required.

- **Braxton-Hicks' contractions:** Contractions that begin in the second trimester and prepare the body for labor. They are usually irregular in frequency and duration, with fewer than five in 1 hour. They are also short (<30 seconds) but may be painful.

- **Chloasma:** (Mask of pregnancy) A blotchy hyperpigmented area on the cheeks, nose, and forehead, common in pregnant women.

- **Diastasis recti:** Separation of the muscles of the abdominal wall.

- **Fundal checks:** Measurements of the height of the fundus of the pregnant woman to assess fetal growth and development.

- **"Growing pains":** Sharp pains in the lower abdomen of the pregnant woman caused by the stretching of ligaments.

- **Hyperemesis gravidarum:** Severe morning sickness, which may cause dehydration and require hospitalization of the pregnant woman.

- **Lightening:** Engagement of the fetal head in the entry to the birth canal. Often an indication of early labor.

- **Linea nigra:** Hyperpigmented line between the symphysis pubis and the top of the uterine fundus of the pregnant woman.

- **Melasma:** (Also known as *chloasma* or *mask of pregnancy*) Tan or dark facial skin discoloration that commonly occurs in pregnant women.

- **Naegele's rule:** Method for calculating the due date of a pregnancy, by which the estimator subtracts 3 months from the first day of the last menstrual period (LMP) and adds 7 days, or about a 40-week pregnancy.

- **Nonstress test:** Test to assess fetal well-being

- **Os:** Cervical opening.

- **Placenta abruption:** Separation of the placenta from the uterine wall before the fetus is delivered. Life-threatening situation for both mother and fetus.

- **Placenta previa:** A placenta that actually covers the os. Cesarean section is necessary or else mother and fetus can die from hemorrhage.

- **Pruritus gravidarum:** A condition characterized by intense itching, which occurs in 1:300 pregnancies, beginning in the third trimester, first on the abdomen, later extending to the entire body surface.

- **Quickening:** Maternal feeling of the fetus kicking and moving (usually at about 20 weeks of pregnancy).

- **Striae gravidarum:** Stretch marks.

- **Teratogens:** Substances or infections that can cause malformations in the embryo or fetus.

STUDY GUIDE

Activity A FILL IN THE BLANK

1. Fill in the blanks about the first and second trimesters of pregnancy.

   A. At 20 weeks' gestation, an ultrasound may reveal the fetal _____.

   B. The fetal survey also indicates _____ and _____ of the placenta.

   C. When the placenta actually _____ the os at the end of the pregnancy, vaginal birth is not possible, and a _____ is planned.

   D. In the 2 weeks leading up to the 20-week mark, the pregnant woman may feel _____ that she confuses with gas.

2. List the tasks of the registered nurse in the outpatient setting when working with pregnant women:

   _____

   _____

   _____

   _____

   _____

   _____

   _____

   _____

Activity B MATCHING

1. *Match the laboratory test performed during pregnancy with its purpose.*

Answer	Laboratory Test	Purpose
	1. Triple- or quad-screen	A. To look for "colonizer"
	2. 50-g glucose challenge	B. To check for presence of syphilis, which crosses the placental barrier to the fetus
	3. GBS	C. To check for rubella, which can cause congenital heart malformations, intrauterine growth restriction, cataracts, and deafness in the fetus
	4. Rubella titer	
	5. VDRL	D. To screen for gestational diabetes at 26–28 weeks
		E. To screen for Down's syndrome and other trisomies, neural tube defects, gastroschisis, and other fetal abnormalities

2. *Match the nursing diagnosis with the appropriate intervention.*

Answer	Nursing Diagnosis	Intervention
	1. Health-seeking behaviors	A. Assess the family's structure, resources, and coping abilities.
	2. Readiness for enhanced parenting	B. Be available to answer questions.
	3. Readiness for enhanced family coping	C. Use nutritional guidelines to plan a diet high in protein, fiber, fruits, and vegetables.
	4. Anxiety	D. Use family-centered care.

Activity C SHORT ANSWER

1. Explain what you would teach a pregnant woman in the third trimester about sleeping.

_____

_____

_____

_____

2. Explain an ectopic pregnancy and how it is treated.

_____

_____

_____

_____

3. Describe the embryo through the first trimester of development.

_____

_____

_____

_____

4. Describe pregnancy during the second trimester; include fetal development, quickening, and the placenta.

_____

_____

_____

_____

5. Discuss pregnancy during the third trimester; include fetal development and activity and key tasks.

_____

_____

_____

_____

6. Explain the fetal survey, including what information it gives the provider.

_____

_____

_____

_____

7. Discuss Naegele's rule.

_____

_____

_____

_____

8. Discuss conditions in pregnancy that require an acute assessment.

_____

_____

_____

_____

Activity D MULTIPLE CHOICE

1. What ethnic group has the best rate for fewest infant deaths from congenital heart defects, maternal deaths, and babies with fetal alcohol syndrome?

A. White non-Hispanic population

B. Hispanic population

C. Asian–American population

D. African–American population

2. What ethnic/cultural groups show high rates of fetal and infant deaths?

A. Alaska Native/Asian American

B. American Indian/Alaska Native

C. White Caucasian/Asian American

D. American Indian/Asian American

3. A pregnant woman should drink at least

A. 1/2 L/day of water

B. 1 L/day of water

C. 1.5 L/day of water

D. 2 L/day of water

4. Feelings of fullness in the breasts of a pregnant woman is due in part to

A. addition of a fat layer and a slowing or growth in alveoli

B. rapid growth of alveoli and decrease in the fat layer

C. rapid growth of alveoli and addition of a fat layer

D. slowing of growth in alveoli and increase in duct system

5. A pregnant patient at her first prenatal visit asks the nurse how much weight she should gain during the first part of her pregnancy. What would the nurse answer for the weight gain during the first trimester?

  A. Less than 7 lb

  B. 7 to 10 lb

  C. 10 lb

  D. 8 to 12 lb

6. A patient at her prenatal visit is found to have 1+ protein in her urine. What might this be indicative of?

  A. Bladder infection

  B. Preeclampsia

  C. Pyelonephritis

  D. Eclampsia

ALTERNATIVE CASE SCENARIOS

Michelle Sherman is visiting the clinic following a positive home pregnancy test. She is a 21-year-old Native American, accompanied by her male partner and their 22-month-old son. Ms. Sherman, 5'4", is concerned because she has not yet lost all the weight she gained during her first pregnancy and is starting this pregnancy at 205 lb. She reports that she quit smoking during her last pregnancy, but resumed smoking a half pack each day after the baby was born to manage the high stress while being a new mother. She thinks her last menstrual period was 6 weeks ago and reports that it was lighter than usual.

Review the following alternative situations related to Michelle. Based on the changes outlined below, *consider what other outcomes, information, and problems would affect the overall picture and shape your responses.*

Alternative A

Subjective: Michelle also states that she is worried because she is spotting on her panty liner.

Objective: Inspection of the panty liner shows a dime-sized spot that is brownish in color.

- Is Michelle stable, urgent, or an emergency?
- How will the nurse work with Michelle to promote health and reduce risk for illness?
- How will the nurse focus, organize, and prioritize the subjective and objective data collection?
- Which nursing diagnosis is highest priority and what is the rationale?

Alternative B

Subjective: Michelle also states that her lower left abdomen is getting more and more painful since this morning.

Objective: Gentle palpation of the place Michelle indicates elicits a grimace and a request that the nurse stop.

- Is this situation stable, urgent, or an emergency?
- How will the nurse work with Michelle to promote health and reduce risk for illness?
- How will the nurse focus, organize, and prioritize the subjective and objective data collection?
- Which nursing diagnosis is highest priority and what is the rationale?

DOCUMENTATION

Form for Use in Practice

Patient Name _____ Date _____

Date of Birth _____

Initial Survey

Reason for seeking health care: _____

History of present illness

- Location:
- Intensity:

- Duration:
- Description:
- Aggravating factors:
- Alleviating factors:
- Functional impairment:
- Pain goal:

Vital signs: T (route)_____ P (site)_____ R_____ BP (site)_____ SpO$_2$_____

Weight: _____ Height: _____ BMI: _____

General appearance: _____

General level of distress: _____

Level of anxiety: _____

Family History

- Diabetes:
- Hypertension:
- Twins/multiple pregnancies:
- Genetic illnesses:

Personal History

- Ethnic group:
- Religious preference:

Pregnancy History

- Previous miscarriages:
- Terminations:
- Previous pregnancies:

Medical Concerns:

Issue	Yes	No	Details
Abnormal Pap smears			
Sexually transmitted infections			
Breast reduction or implants			
Abnormal mammograms			
Fertility problems			
Depression			
Anxiety			
Eating disorder			
Headaches/migraines			
Allergies			
Abuse			

Contraception

- Type:
- Last used:

Other Concerns:

- Support system:
- Tobacco use:
- Alcohol use:
- Drug use:
- Recent immigration:
- Financial concerns:
- Access to care:

Common Symptoms:

Symptom	Yes	No	Additional data
Morning sickness			
Growing pains			
Increased vaginal discharge			
Increased urination			
Breast tenderness or discharge			
Periumbilical pain in the second trimester			
Fetal hiccups			
Braxton-Hicks' contractions			

Physical Assessment:

Take weight, blood pressure, other vital signs, and pain level.
Obtain a urine sample. Test urine for glucose and protein.
Inspect the skin. Look for linea nigra, chloasma, and striae.
Check the fetal heartbeat.
Palpate the fundus to feel the fetal back.
Measure the uterine fundus.
Inspect the breasts.

Signature_____ Date _____

Newborns and Infants

CHAPTER 28

OBJECTIVE SUMMARY

This chapter examines health assessment of newborns and infants. It discusses important past and present health history and pertinent findings of the physical examination. Because infants are preverbal and totally reliant on parents/guardians, the nurse must develop excellent observation skills and involve parents in the assessment and care planning.

READING ASSIGNMENT

Read Chapter 28 in Jensen's *Nursing Health Assessment: A Best-Practice Approach*.

VOCABULARY/TERMINOLOGY

- **Baby bottle tooth decay:** A condition that develops from a child going to bed with a bottle. Sugar sticks to and coats the primary teeth. Bacteria in the mouth break down the sugars to use for food. As this breakdown occurs, the bacteria produce acids that attack the teeth and cause decay.

- **Barlow's sign:** Upon testing, the head of the femur comes out of the acetabulum, confirming a hip dislocation.

- **Brachycephaly:** Abnormal head shape caused by laying the infant on one side without enough "tummy" time while the child is awake.

- **Central cyanosis:** Blueness in the center portions of the torso or of the lips, tongue, or oral mucous membranes; a sign of poor oxygenation.

- **Circumoral cyanosis:** Blueness surrounding the mouth.

- **Craniosynostosis:** Premature closure of the cranial sutures.

- **Craniotabes:** Soft areas on the skull felt along the suture line; normal in infants, particularly those born prematurely.

- **Hydrocephalus:** Enlarged head from increased cerebrospinal fluid.

- **Mongolian spot:** Bluish pigmented area(s) on the lower back or buttocks. Common in infants of Asian, African, or Hispanic descent.

- **Ortolani's maneuver:** Test for hip dislocation. The infant is positioned supine on the examining table. With the baby's legs together, the examiner flexes the knees and hips 90 degrees. Then, with the examiner's middle fingers over the greater trochanters and thumbs on the inner thighs, he or she abducts the baby's hips while applying upward pressure.

- **Plagiocephaly:** Abnormal head shape from consistent positioning on the back or one side to sleep without enough "tummy time" while awake.

- **Pneumatic otoscopy:** Visualization of the movement of the tympanic membrane by the use of an otoscope with an air bulb to puff air into the air.

STUDY GUIDE

Activity A FILL IN THE BLANK

1. Fill in the blanks about the development of an infant.

   A. During the _____ of life, the growth rate is more _____ than at any other time in childhood.

   B. Motor development progresses in predictable patterns: _____, _____, and _____.

   C. The infant learns language through _____, _____, and _____ with the environment.

   D. Nurses assess newborn and infant motor development using standardized screening tools, such as the _____.

2. According to the American Academy of Pediatrics and American Heart Association, the nurse must ask four key assessment questions about the newborn's health:

   - _____
   - _____
   - _____
   - _____

Activity B MATCHING

1. *Match the newborn reflex with how to elicit it.*

Answer	Newborn Reflex	How to Elicit
	1. Moro	A. Turn the head of the supine infant to one side.
	2. Galant	B. Stroke one side of the infant's foot upward from the heel and across the ball of the foot.
	3. Tonic neck	
	4. Babinski	
	5. Stepping	C. Occurs when the infant is startled or feels like he or she is falling.
		D. Hold the infant upright. Allow the soles to touch a flat surface.
		E. Place the newborn in ventral suspension. Stroke the skin on one side of the back.

2. *Match the odor with the disease it indicates*

Answer	Odor	Disease
	1. Mousy odor	A. Ingestion of a chemical such as kerosene, bleach, glue, alcohol
	2. Foul odor of umbilical area	
	3. Noxious mouth odor	B. Retained foreign body
	4. Rotten or offensive odor from the nose or vagina	C. Maple syrup urine disease
	5. Maple syrup odor to the urine	D. Omphalitis
		E. Phenylketonuria

3. *Match the skin condition with its description.*

Answer	Skin Condition	Description
	1. Intertrigo	A. Spots that start out as light brown pigmented lesions and grow and darken as the child grows
	2. Lichen simplex chronicus	
	3. Café-au-lait spots	
	4. Port wine stains	B. Rash resulting from infection with *Candida albicans*
	5. Candidal diaper dermatitis	C. Congenital capillary lesions
		D. Inflammation of the skinfolds resulting from skin-on-skin friction
		E. Discrete patches of eczema (thickened skin with scaling)

Activity C SHORT ANSWER

1. Explain why it is necessary to regularly assess the motor, physical, and language skills of infants.

2. Discuss the expected increase in length and weight of an infant during the first year of life.

3. At the first sign of respiratory distress in an infant or newborn, the nurse must take steps to intervene. Explain why.

4. Discuss the initial visit the parents should have with the primary health care provider before the infant is born.

5. Safe sleep habits for newborns and infants are important areas of teaching to new parents. Explain what the nurse would teach them and why.

6. Explain the need for immunizations and when they should be given.

Activity D MULTIPLE CHOICE

1. Parents bring a 4 month old to the clinic for a checkup. The mother tells the nurse that the infant is exclusively breastfed. Why might this infant need iron supplements?
   A. The mother is Hispanic.
   B. The baby is not eating solid food.
   C. The mother's iron stores are low.
   D. The mother doesn't eat iron-rich food.

2. Baby bottle tooth decay can affect a child's self-image because
   A. it affects the front teeth and is visible
   B. it causes the primary teeth to break off
   C. it leads people to think the child has bad parents
   D. it makes other children think the child's family is too poor for a dentist

3. Motor development of an infant progresses
   A. outer to inner
   B. fine to gross
   C. cephalocaudally
   D. distal to central

4. The staff educator for a pediatric unit is presenting a class to a group of new nurses. Today they are talking about emergent situations in infants. What would the staff educator tell the new nurses is what causes most emergent situations in infants?
   A. Respiratory decompensation
   B. Cardiac problems
   C. Congenital problems
   D. Child abuse

5. The American Academy of Pediatrics recommends that an infant have the first well-child appointment at what age?
   A. 3 to 5 days
   B. 4 to 6 days
   C. 1 week
   D. 2 weeks

6. Teaching for the parents of a newborn would focus most heavily on what?

   A. Growth and development

   B. Parenting

   C. Nutrition

   D. Safety

7. When talking about choking, the nurse would advise the parents to survey the environment

   A. from a sitting position

   B. from the infant's perspective

   C. from a cleanliness perspective

   D. from a squatting position

8. Which toy should never be given to an infant?

   A. Pull toy

   B. Latex balloon

   C. Small drum

   D. Ball

ALTERNATIVE CASE SCENARIOS

Keri Downs, 1 month old, is visiting the clinic today for her well-child checkup and hepatitis B immunization. She was born at term and has had no health problems. Her mother is breastfeeding Keri; they have adjusted well.

Keri is the first child in a two-parent family. The mother is a nurse who plans on returning to work in 2 months; the father is an accountant. Paternal grandparents live in the area and provide child care 1 day a week.

Review the following alternative situations related to Keri. Based on the changes outlined below, *consider what other outcomes, information, and problems would affect the overall picture and shape your responses.*

Alternative A

Keri Downs is a 1-week-old infant girl visiting the clinic today because her mother is worried that she is not breastfeeding well and seems listless. She was born at term and her newborn physical was normal.

Subjective: The mother reports, "Keri doesn't seem at all interested in eating and she doesn't respond to me like she was the first few days. Her cry sounds funny and her skin has an orange-yellow tint."

Objective: Keri is listless with a high-pitched, irritable cry. Abdomen soft, nondistended. T 37°C, P 150 bpm, R 35 breaths/min. Skin is hot to touch and very dry. Sclera, mucous membranes, and skin are dark yellow in color. Fontanels are sunken. Mother states Keri hasn't stooled in all day and diapers have small amounts of dark urine. Changing 2 to 3 diapers per day. Weight 6 lb 12 oz, her birth weight was 7 lb 8 oz, a 10% drop.

- Is Keri's condition stable, urgent, or an emergency?

- How will the nurse work with Keri to promote health and reduce risk for illness?

- How will the nurse focus, organize, and prioritize the subjective and objective data collection?

- Which nursing diagnosis is highest priority and what is the rationale?

Alternative B

Keri Downs is a 3-month-old infant visiting the clinic today because her mother states that it "must be time for her shots." She was born at term and her newborn physical was normal. This is her first clinic visit since birth. Keri seems happy and content. She readily smiles when the mother laughs and plays with her.

Subjective: Mother says that the baby is happy and content. She breastfeeds well every 3 to 4 hours and has been gaining weight as measured by a home scale. Keri calms readily with classical music and she enjoys watching her mobile.

Objective: Keri is alert and interacts by smiling and cooing. Abdomen soft, nondistended. T: 37°C, P 134 bpm, R 32 breaths/min. Skin is warm to touch and supple. Anterior fontanel is flat with a slight pulsing sensation when palpated. Mother reports Keri has 2 to 3 soft yellow stools and 4 to 5 wet diapers per day. She measures in the 50th percentile for weight, length, and head circumference.

- Is Keri's condition stable, urgent, or an emergency?

- How will the nurse work with Keri and her mother to promote health and reduce risk for illness?

- How will the nurse focus, organize, and prioritize the subjective and objective data collection?

- Which nursing diagnosis is highest priority and what is the rationale?

DOCUMENTATION

Form for Use in Practice

Patient Name _____ Date_____

Date of Birth _____

Initial Survey

Reason for seeking health care: _____

History of present illness

- Location:
- Intensity:
- Duration:
- Description:
- Aggravating factors:
- Alleviating factors:
- Functional impairment:
- Pain goal:

Vital signs: T (route)_____　P (site)_____　R_____　BP (site)_____　SpO_2_____

Weight: _____ Length: _____ Head circumference: _____ Chest circumference: _____

General appearance: _____

General level of distress: _____

Family: _____

Residence:_____

Pregnancy/Birth History

- Unusual circumstances or health problems during pregnancy:
- Duration of pregnancy:
- Type of labor and delivery:
- Type of anesthesia used for labor:
- Apgar score:
- Any resuscitation at birth:
- Birth weight:
- Discharge from hospital after birth:
- Time in the NICU:

Since Birth

- Infections:
- Illnesses:
- Injuries:
- Hospitalizations:

- Surgeries:
- Well-child checkups:

Medications and Supplements

- Prescription medications:
- OTC preparations:
- Vitamins:
- Immunizations:

Risk Factors

- Sleep practices:
- Sleep with a bottle:
- Childproofed home:
- Use of car seat:
- CPR training of parents:

Common Symptoms:

Symptom	Yes	No	Additional data
Respiratory complaints and/or distress			
Fever			
Skin disorders			
Gastrointestinal distress			
Crying/irritability			

Physical Assessment:

(For newborns) Take the Apgar score.
(For newborns) Determine gestational age.
Evaluate reflexes.
Begin the general survey.
Notice interactions between infant and parent.
Take temperature.
Assess apical pulse and respiratory rate.
(Optional) Take blood pressure.
Assess for pain.
Weigh the infant. Measure from crown of head to heel. Measure head and chest circumferences.
Ask about urination and bowel movements.
(For bottle-fed infants) Ask how many ounces per feeding and how many feedings per day.
Observe sleep states and behavior.
Assess parent and infant for signs of domestic violence.
Inspect skin, hair, and nails.

Assess head size and shape. Check for symmetry. Palpate fontanels and sutures.
Observe face. Look for symmetry of movement.
Check neck range of motion (ROM).
Inspect and palpate the trachea. Auscultate for any bruits. Palpate clavicles. Palpate lymph nodes.
Look for symmetry and spacing of eyes. Inspect the lids for proper placement. Observe palpebral fissures. Inspect inside lining of lids (palpebral conjunctiva), bulbar conjunctiva, sclera, and cornea.
Assess ocular alignment. Assess pupils for shape, size, and movement. Test their reaction to light.
(Optional, for advanced practice) Use an ophthalmoscope to obtain the red reflex.
Observe for light perception and ability to fix on and follow a target.
Assess ear placement.
(Optional, for advanced practice) Visualize the tympanic membranes and check eardrums.
Inspect the nose. Check patency.
Inspect the lips, mouth, and throat. Defer throat examination to the end, unless the infant cries. The uvula can easily be visualized when the infant is crying.
Observe breathing movements and pattern. Auscultate all lobes of the lungs from the front, back, and under the arms on both sides.
Assess oxygenation.
Palpate the point of maximum impulse (PMI).
Auscultate the heart; inspect and auscultate the neck vessels.
Note character and quality of brachial and femoral pulses.
Observe the nipples.
Inspect the abdomen. Auscultate bowel sounds. Percuss the abdomen.
Palpate the abdomen. Try to locate the kidneys using deep palpation in both upper quadrants.
Palpate for hernias in the umbilical and inguinal regions.
Observe for symmetry of movement and strength of the musculoskeletal system.
Note shape and appearance of the hands, palms, fingers, feet, and toes.
Perform Ortolani's maneuver and elicit Barlow's sign.
Integrate neurological evaluations from previous portions of the examination. Inspect, then palpate along the length of the spine.
(For females) Inspect the genitalia. Gently part the labia and observe the structures of the vestibule. Visualize the vaginal opening.
(For males) Inspect the penis. Note cleanliness and placement of the urethral meatus. Evaluate the scrotum for size, color, and symmetry.
Inspect the anus.
(Optional) Perform the rectal examination.

Signature_____ Date _____

Guide for Use in Practice

Technique	Normal Findings	Abnormal Findings
(For newborns): Take the Apgar score.	*Score of 7–10*	5-minute score <7 (continue to score every 5 minutes until the score is above 7, the newborn is intubated, or the newborn is transferred to the nursery)
(For newborns) Determine gestational age.	*Total New Ballard Score 37–40 weeks*	Prematurity or postmaturity
Evaluate reflexes: rooting, suck, Moro (startle), Galant's (trunk incurvation), stepping, palmar grasp, tonic neck, and Babinski.	*Reflex responses appropriate or extinguished by the expected age*	Diminished reflexes; reflexes continuing past the expected age
Begin the general survey, keeping in mind the age of the infant in months and the correlated expected development.	*Good muscle tone, symmetrical appearance. Respirations unlabored, no signs of acute distress*	Hypotonia, asymmetry, labored breathing
Notice interactions between infant and parent.	*Parent picks up on infant cues. Infant appears alert and engaged in the environment, unless sleeping.*	Infant listless and uninterested in interaction. Parent pays little attention to the infant and does not pick up on cues. Unusual odors. Poor hygiene or inappropriate dress for the weather
For newborns, take axillary temperature. After the first month of life, take either axillary or tympanic temperature.	*97.7°F–98.6°F (36.5°C–37°C)*	Elevated or decreased temperatures
Assess apical pulse and respiratory rate for a full minute each with the infant at rest.	*Pulse for newborn 110–160 bpm, decreasing slightly to 80–140 for infants older than 1 month. Respiratory rate 30–60 breaths/min for newborns and 22–35 for infants older than 1 month*	Tachycardia, bradycardia, tachypnea, bradypnea
Blood pressures are not measured routinely in the infant. If the blood pressures are taken, measure pressures in all four extremities.	*Systolic pressures of 50–70 for newborns and 70–100 for infants older than 1 month*	Difference between upper and lower extremity blood pressures
Assess for pain.	*Infant appears comfortable and not excessively irritable.*	Crying indiscriminately
Weigh the infant using an infant scale that is calibrated regularly. Use the tape measure and carefully measure from crown of head to heel. Measure head and chest circumferences. Plot all measurements on a standardized growth chart.	*Measurements are above the 10th percentile and below the 90th percentile. Compare measurements with previous visits. Infant is gaining height and weight at a steady pace.*	Measurements below the 10th percentile or above the 90th percentile; small head; small chest circumference
Inspect the general condition of the skin, hair, and nails. Ask about urination and bowel movements.	*Soft, supple skin and shiny hair. Infant wets a diaper four to six times per day and has regular bowel movements that are soft and not watery.*	Parental reports of fussing, crying, and not seeming satisfied after feeding. Sallow skin tones with poor turgor, dry brittle hair and nails, losing weight or falling behind on growth charts compared to previous visits, consuming <100 kcal/kg/day

If the infant is bottle feeding, ask the parent how many ounces per feeding and how many feedings per day.	*Infant is consuming approximately 100 kcal/kg/day*	Failure to thrive (weight that falls below the fifth percentile for the child's age)
Determine mental status by observing sleep states and behavior throughout the examination. Observe for developmentally appropriate behavior.	*An alert 1 month old engages with the eyes when face to face with the parent or nurse and responds to the voice by turning toward the sound or tracking with the eyes. An older infant reaches for an object the parent or examiner offers.* *Crying stops with gentle rocking in the arms or while holding the infant against the shoulder. As the infant matures, the infant may smile and interact with the examiner, as long as movements are not sudden or threatening and the voice maintains a calm and reassuring quality.*	Interaction between infant and parent does not seem synergistic; older infant is excessively clingy or does not warm up to the examiner after a period of interaction. Excessive irritability and inconsolable crying. High-pitched cry, or lethargy and listlessness
Assess the parent and infant for signs of domestic violence.	*Parent relaxed, confident demeanor with appropriate affect, good grooming, and appropriate interaction with and concern for the infant. Infant shows appropriate grooming and dress, no injuries, and willingness to engage.*	Bruises, fractures, inappropriate clothing, injuries with no or conflicting explanations, poor hygiene
Inspect skin, hair, and nails.	*Skin soft, not excessively dry, and supple. Snaps quickly back to original shape after gentle pinching. Free of rashes, lesions, bruising, and edema. Hair soft and shiny. Nails soft, of an appropriate length, not growing inward, and securely attached to nail beds, which are pink, unless the child is dark skinned*	Rashes, lesions, bruising, excoriation from scratching, sensitivity to touch, edema, nails lifting off the nail bed, nails dry and brittle, inflammation around nails with nails poking into the skin, poor elasticity and tenting of the skin, pallor or pale mucous membranes, yellow or jaundiced skin tones, periorbital edema, dependent, bruises in varied stages of healing, well-demarcated lesions, or bilateral burns
Assess head size and shape. Check for symmetry. Palpate the anterior and posterior fontanels and sutures. Trace along each suture line with the tips of the fingers to ensure they have not fused prematurely.	*Posterior fontanel palpable until approximately 3 months of age. Anterior fontanel does not close until 9–18 months of age. Anterior fontanel is flat, not sunken or bulging, with the infant at rest and sitting. The fontanel may bulge slightly when the infant is crying. Suture lines are easily palpable. Craniotabes, soft areas on the skull felt along the suture line, are normal in infants, particularly those born prematurely.*	Head flattened from the back or one side; abnormal head shapes; *craniosynostosis* (premature closure of the sutures); bulging fontanels with the infant at rest; sunken fontanels
Observe the infant's face. Look for symmetry of movement.	Symmetrical	Asymmetrical facial movements
Check neck ROM.	*Neck ROM full; head lag and control correlate with expected development*	Persistence of head lag beyond the fourth month; limited neck ROM; webbing on the sides of the neck; enlarged thyroid gland with a bruit

Inspect and palpate the trachea. Auscultate for any bruits. Palpate the clavicles in the newborn. Palpate the preauricular, suboccipital, parotid, submaxillary, submental, anterior and posterior cervical, epitrochlear, and inguinal lymph nodes.	*Trachea midline with no swelling or masses. No bruits. Clavicles smooth with no pain or crepitus. Any palpable lymph nodes are small, mobile, and nontender.*	Deviated trachea; crepitation over the clavicles in a newborn immediately after birth
Look for symmetry and spacing of the eyes. Inspect the lids for proper placement. Observe the general slant of the palpebral fissures. Inspect the inside lining of lids (palpebral conjunctiva), bulbar conjunctiva, sclera, and cornea.	*Eyes parallel and centered in the face. Ptosis absent. Sclera clear and white*	Upward or downward slanting or small palpebral fissures; eyes too close together, too far apart, or asymmetrical; exophthalmos; ptosis
Assess ocular alignment. Assess pupils for shape, size, and movement. Test their reaction to light.	*Some strabismus in the first few months of life. PERRLA*	Strabismus; pupils that are asymmetrical, respond sluggishly, are "blown," or are pinpoint
(Optional, for advanced practice) Use an ophthalmoscope to obtain the red reflex.	*Red reflex present*	If the red reflex cannot be elicited in the newborn, the infant needs a complete eye examination by a specialist. Absence of the red reflex in newborns is associated with *congenital cataracts* and *neuroblastoma*.
Observe for light perception and ability to fix on and follow a target.	*By 3 months can follow objects*	Inability to fix or follow
Assess ear placement.	*Ears symmetrical. Top of pinna lies just above an imaginary line from the inner canthus of the eye through the outer canthus and continuing past the ear.*	Ears that fall below the imaginary line; one ear significantly smaller than the other; extra ridges and pits
(Optional, for advanced practice) Use the pneumatic otoscope to visualize the tympanic membranes and to check the eardrums if otitis media is suspected.	*Tympanic membrane convex, intact, and translucent; visualization of the short process of the malleus. Cone of light visible in anterior inferior quadrant*	Otitis media; perforated eardrum; tympanosclerosis
Inspect the nose. Check patency. Inspect the lips, mouth, and throat. Defer throat examination to the end, unless the infant cries. The uvula can easily be visualized when the infant is crying.	*Nose midline of the face with symmetrical nares. Philtrum below the nose fully formed (ie, not flat); nasolabial folds symmetrical. Nares patent bilaterally. Lips symmetrical and fully formed. Tongue of normal size and does not get in the way of feeding. Mucous membranes moist and pink*	Nasal flaring; flattened nasal bridge; macroglossia (enlarged tongue); flat philtrum and thin upper lip; deviated uvula or a uvula with a cleft; red, inflamed tonsils
Observe breathing movements and pattern. Auscultate all lobes of the lungs from the front, back, and under the arms on both sides.	*Thorax symmetrical. Chest expansion equal bilaterally. No signs of distress or use of accessory muscles. Breath sounds equal bilaterally and typically louder and more bronchial than in adults. Inspiration slightly longer than expiration*	Asymmetrical chest wall, expanded anterior-posterior diameter (pigeon breast) or funnel shape (depressed sternum); retractions anywhere on the chest wall; wheezes, crackles, and/or grunting; absent or diminished breath sounds
Assess oxygenation.	*Pink nail beds with crisp capillary refill time (<3 seconds), pink mucous membranes and tongue*	*Central cyanosis* (blueness in the center portions of the torso or of the lips, tongue, or oral mucous membranes); very pale infant

Palpate the PMI. Auscultate the heart; inspect and auscultate the neck vessels.	*PMI may be difficult to palpate. Heart rhythm regular with a single S_1 and a split S_2. Some murmurs are nonpathologic—typically they are soft and nonspecific in character. Neck vessels nondistended without bruits*	Tachycardia at rest, persistent bradycardia, clubbing, single S_2, ejection clicks, loud and harsh murmurs, central cyanosis, oxygen saturation lower than 90%, disparate readings between upper and lower extremities
Note the character and quality of the brachial and femoral pulses. Compare left to right and upper with lower.	*All pulses equal; pulse rate matches apical heart rate.*	Weak, thready pulses; bounding pulses; palpable pulses in the upper extremities in correlation with diminished pulses
Observe the nipples.	*Areolae full; nipple bud well formed; normal for both male and female newborns to have swollen breasts that may even leak a watery fluid*	Supernumerary (extra) nipples
Inspect the abdomen. Auscultate bowel sounds. Percuss the abdomen.	*Abdomen cylindrical, protrudes slightly, moves in synchrony with diaphragm. Superficial veins visible in fair-skinned infants. Umbilical area clean without discharge, bulging areas, or scarring. Sounds heard in all four quadrants; may be softer immediately after the infant has eaten; dullness noted in the right upper quadrant; tympany over an air-filled stomach and bowel*	Dull sound when percussing above the symphysis pubis; abdominal distention; masses; palpable kidneys; loud, grumbling sounds; bowel sounds heard in the chest
Palpate the abdomen. Try to locate the kidneys using deep palpation in both upper quadrants. Be sure to palpate for hernias in the umbilical and inguinal regions.	*Abdomen soft, without rigidity, tenderness, or masses. Lower liver margins can be palpated from 1 to 2 cm below the right costal margin. Tip of spleen may be palpable in the left upper quadrant. Kidneys cannot be palpated; no hernias*	Abdomen distended and firm
Observe for symmetry of movement and strength of the musculoskeletal system. Note shape and appearance of the hands, palms, fingers, feet, and toes.	*Ankles have full ROM; feet return to neutral without assistance and are flat before the infant begins walking.*	Asymmetrical movements; crepitus with joint movement or any limitation of movement; club foot; talipes valgus
Perform Ortolani's maneuver and elicit Barlow's sign to check for signs of hip dislocation.	*No clicking or clunking sounds are heard. Head of femur remains in the acetabulum.*	Positive Ortolani's and Barlow's maneuvers; asymmetrical thigh and gluteal folds
Integrate neurological evaluations from previous portions of the examination. Inspect, then palpate along the length of the spine.	*No protrusions, lesions, or other unusual findings. No dimples or tufts of hair*	Persistence of newborn reflexes past the time they normally disappear; involuntary movements; abnormal posturing; failure to blink when a bright light is shined in the eyes; absence of a blink upon production of a loud noise; dimpling or tufts of hair on the spine
Inspect the female genitalia. Gently part the labia and observe the structures of the vestibule. Visualize the vaginal opening.	*Labia majora cover the vestibule. The newborn girl may have an enlarged clitoris and labia, and the parent may have noticed a few drops of blood in the diaper. Genital area is clean and free of foul odors.*	Redness, swelling, bleeding (after 1 month of age), torn tissue, a hymen that completely covers the vagina, labial adhesions/fusion, lesions, foul-smelling discharge

Inspect the penis. Note cleanliness and placement of the urethral meatus. Evaluate the scrotum for size, color, and symmetry.	*Urethral meatus at the top of the glans penis and midline. Testes descended bilaterally; area free of edema, masses, and lesions*	*Meatal stenosis*, malpositioned meatus; undescended testes
Inspect the anus. Use the little finger of a gloved hand to palpate it. Rectal examination is not done routinely unless there is evidence of irritation, bleeding, or other symptoms.	*Anus well formed with no redness or bleeding. Muscle contracts with light pressure to the area.*	Redness, bleeding, other signs of irritation; small white worms

Children and Adolescents

This chapter explores health assessment for children and adolescents. It highlights significant past and present health history along with related physical examination findings most pertinent for children and adolescents. These patients live with caregivers who have legal health care decision-making capacity for them. Therefore, caring for children and adolescents requires the nurse to involve both the parent/guardian and child/adolescent in assessment, diagnosis, planning, intervention, and evaluation. Health assessment of the child or adolescent also includes assessing community support, environmental exposures, and potential opportunities for health promotion.

READING ASSIGNMENT

Read Chapter 29 in Jensen's *Nursing Health Assessment: A Best-Practice Approach*.

VOCABULARY/TERMINOLOGY

- **Coarctation of the aorta:** A congenital defect in which the aorta is narrowed after leaving the heart.

- **Cognitive development:** Development related to information processing, conceptual resources, perceptual skill, language learning, and other aspects of brain development.

- **Cryptorchidism:** Undescended testicle; a testicle that has not moved into its proper position in the bag of skin hanging behind the penis (scrotum) prior to the birth of a baby boy.

- **Denver Developmental Screening Test II:** One of several standardized developmental screening tests used in the examination of the child and required for Early and Periodic Screening and Developmental Testing. Considered the gold standard.

- **Head circumference:** Measurement of the circumference of the head at the largest point on the brow above the eyebrows.

- **Hypospadias:** Urethral meatus located on the ventral aspect of the penis anywhere along the urethral groove.

- **Immunization schedule:** Schedule developed by the Centers for Disease Control and Prevention (CDC) for giving immunizations.

- **Innocent heart murmur:** Heart murmur with no accompanying signs or symptoms of heart disease. Common in children.

- **Motor development:** Development of abilities that emerge in the same order and at approximately the same age. Includes skills related to movement, gross coordination, and fine coordination.

- **Psychosocial development:** Progression of psychosocial growth from infancy through adulthood. Erikson's psychosocial theory is considered the gold standard.

- **Pulmonary flow murmur:** Murmur resulting from increased pulmonary flow; the sound is louder with the patient supine and is accentuated by exercise, fever, and excitement.

- **Speech development:** Development of the verbal means of communicating, which includes articulation, fluency, and voice. Development of use of the voice and physical elements of speaking to articulate the spoken language.

- **Standardized growth charts:** Charts developed by the CDC to track the growth and weight of a child as it grows.

- **Still's murmur:** A vibratory functional murmur, which is louder with the patient in the supine position.

- **Tanner's staging:** Scale that defines physical measurements based on external primary and secondary sex characteristics (ie, size of the breasts, genitalia, and development of pubic hair).

- **Venous hum:** Benign medical condition in which 20% of blood flow travels to the brain and back to the heart. Because of the large amount, the blood can move quite fast, causing vein walls to vibrate and leading to an audible humming noise.

- **Wilms' tumor:** Rare kidney cancer that primarily affects children. Also known as nephroblastoma, it is the most common malignant tumor of the kidneys in children.

STUDY GUIDE

Activity A   FILL IN THE BLANK

1. Fill in the blanks about structure and function in children.

   A. Although children grow and develop at variable rates, they do both at _____ according to previously established normal ranges.

   B. For children older than _____, health care providers calculate and plot body mass index on the appropriate BMI chart.

   C. Evaluation of the child's initiation and continuance of sounds, as well as _____, is critical throughout the early years.

2. Fill in the blanks about the acute assessment of children and adolescents.

   A. Children who present in physiological distress compensate with increased _____ and _____ rates.

   B. Transfer to a _____ is indicated for children in distress.

   C. The additional work of breathing is evidenced in a distressed child by _____, _____, or abdominal breathing.

Activity B   MATCHING

1. *Match the nursing diagnosis with the appropriate intervention.*

Answer	Nursing Diagnosis	Intervention
	1. Disturbed sensory perception	A. Assess the influence of cultural norms, values, and beliefs on the parent's perceptions of development.
	2. Readiness for enhanced family processes	
	3. Delayed growth and development	B. Discuss benefits and barriers to staying healthy.
	4. Health-seeking behaviors	C. Encourage attendance at community groups and classes.
		D. Speak in lower tones if possible.

2. *Match the audiologic test with the age group for whom it is used.*

Answer	Audiologic Test	Age Group
	1. Play audiometry	A. 9 months to 2.5 years
	2. Evoked Otoacoustic emissions (OAEs)	
	3. Conditioned Oriented Response (COR) or Visual Reinforcement Audiometry (VRA)	B. Birth to 9 months
		C. 2.5–4 years
	4. Automated Auditory Brainstem Response (ABR)	D. 4 years to adolescence
	5. Conventional audiometry	E. All ages

Activity C SHORT ANSWER

1. Explain the circumstances that require transfer of a child to a tertiary care center.

_____

_____

_____

_____

2. Discuss the circumstances wherein a child younger than 18 years can legally sign for medical care.

_____

_____

_____

_____

3. Explain how the perinatal environment and exposures can affect the child's present health.

_____

_____

_____

_____

4. Explain the criteria for screening a child for tuberculosis (TB).

_____

_____

_____

_____

5. Discuss why the nurse should ask an adolescent whether he or she engages in oral sex or is otherwise sexually active.

_____

_____

_____

_____

6. What can a nurse do for a patient who has not received the full roster of immunizations?

_____

_____

_____

7. Explain the need for infant/child car seats. Include weight/height recommendations and age recommendations.

_____

_____

_____

_____

Activity D MULTIPLE CHOICE

1. What is the best of the following signs that a home has been modified to optimize child safety?

A. Bars are on the outside of all the windows.

B. Storm doors have safety locks.

C. Open windows have well-maintained screens.

D. The yard is surrounded by a 6-ft high fence.

2. A pediatric nurse is giving a talk to the local PTA. What would the nurse explain to these parents is important to protect their children from fire?

A. Fire escape plan from the home

B. Teaching children about how to start a fire

C. Teaching young children how to work the stove

D. Teaching children how to lay a fire when camping

3. Outdoor safety for children includes

A. wearing a helmet while in a stroller

B. wearing sunscreen

C. wearing knee pads on a tricycle

D. wearing knee pads on a bicycle

4. The use of alcohol and drugs in adolescence is often a means of what?

A. Bending to peer pressure

B. Satisfying addictive cravings

C. Hiding from one's self

D. Self-medicating for other problems

5. A child 2 years of age or older should have a maximum of how much sodium daily?

A. 1,000 mg

B. 1,600 mg

C. 2,000 mg

D. 2,400 mg

6. A woman brings her 7-year-old daughter to the clinic. The mother says the child has been complaining of abdominal pain for the past few days and has stayed home from school. The nurse notes the child walks only on tiptoes. What would the nurse suspect is wrong with the child?

   A. Kidney infection

   B. Bladder infection

   C. Appendicitis

   D. Peritonitis

7. It is difficult to assess the location of pain in a child because generally children cannot

   A. describe their pain

   B. isolate their pain

   C. feel their pain

   D. acknowledge their pain

8. A woman who speaks primarily Spanish at home brings her 3 year old to the clinic for a yearly visit. The mother reports concern that her child's language skills are not progressing as expected. The health care provider may have a difficult time assessing this child's language capabilities if

   A. the child is not bilingual

   B. the mother does not speak English

   C. the provider is not bilingual

   D. the provider does not use a translator

ALTERNATIVE CASE SCENARIOS

Simon Chavez, a 4-year-old Hispanic boy, presents to the school-based health center for a preschool physical examination. Simon lives with his 20-year-old mother who stays home all day with him and his newborn sister. Simon's 21-year-old father is a delivery truck driver for a local grocery distributor; he leaves for work at 7 AM and returns most evenings by 5:30 PM, when he assists with care of the children.

Simon has not been in a structured preschool or day care environment. This fall will be his first exposure to care and formalized instruction outside the home. He seems excited about his new opportunity and is willing to discuss the new school with the nurse. Simon has never been hospitalized, but he has been treated in the emergency department twice for coughing and wheezing. He also has had frequent ear infections; the last one was 3 weeks ago. He has never had surgery. He has no known allergies; his only medication is a daily multivitamin with iron.

Review the following alternative situations related to Simon. Based on the changes outlined below, *consider what other outcomes, information, and problems would affect the overall picture and shape your responses.*

Alternative A

Simon has been coughing for 3 days. He has had a temperature off and on for the past 4 days and now he feels very warm.

- Is Simon's condition stable, urgent, or an emergency?

- How will the nurse work with Simon to promote health and reduce risk for illness?

- How will the nurse focus, organize, and prioritize the subjective and objective data collection?

- What nursing diagnosis is highest priority and what is the rationale?

Alternative B

All the background information about Simon remains the same, but he arrives at the emergency department with his mother, who is carrying Simon and screaming, "He is not breathing!"

- Is Simon's condition stable, urgent, or an emergency?

- How will the nurse work with Simon to promote health and reduce risk for illness?

- How will the nurse focus, organize, and prioritize the subjective and objective data collection?

- Which nursing diagnosis is highest priority and what is the rationale?

DOCUMENTATION

Form for Use in Practice

Patient Name _____ Date _____

Date of Birth _____

Initial Survey

Reason for seeking health care:_____

History of present illness

- Location:
- Intensity:
- Duration:
- Description:
- Aggravating factors:
- Alleviating factors:
- Functional impairment:
- Pain goal:

Vital signs: T (route)_____ P (site)_____ R_____ BP (site)_____ SpO_2_____

Weight: _____ Height: _____ BMI: _____

General appearance: _____

General level of distress: _____

Level of anxiety: _____

Family History

Condition	Yes	No	Details/Comments
Diabetes			
Hypertension			
Heart disease			
Elevated cholesterol level			
Asthma			
Allergies			
Cancer			
Liver, kidney, or GI problems			
Arthritis			
Learning problems			
Death before age 50 years			

- Maternal health:

- Paternal health:
- Sibling health:

Prenatal/Natal History

- Maternal health:
- Medications:
- Exposure to toxic substances, alcohol, or illicit drugs:
- Birth history:
- Birth weight:
- Birth date/due date:
- Labor and birth experience:
- Apgar scores at 1 and 5 minutes

Postnatal History

- Departure from hospital:
- Difficulties once home:
- Jaundice (if positive, list details of treatment):

Developmental History

- Age at sitting:
- Age at standing:
- Age at walking:
- Age at first word:
- Age at toilet trained for day and night:

Personal History

- Previous hospitalizations:
- Surgeries:
- Current prescription medications:
- Current over-the-counter medications:

Risk Factors

- Lead-risk screening:

Question	Yes	No	Comments
Does your child live in or regularly visit a house or child-care facility built before 1950?			
Does your child live in or regularly visit a house or child-care facility built before 1978 that is being or has recently (within the last 6 months) been renovated or remodeled?			
Does your child have a brother, sister, or playmate who has or had lead poisoning?			

- Tuberculosis screening:

Question	Yes	No	Comments
Is the child infected with HIV?			
Is the child in close contact with people known or suspected to have TB?			
Is the child in close contact with people known to be alcohol dependent or intravenous drug users or to reside in a long-term care facility, correctional or mental institution, nursing home/facility, or other long-term residential facility?			
Is the child foreign-born and from a country with high TB prevalence?			
Is the child from a medically underserved low-income population, including a high-risk racial or ethnic minority population (eg, African American, Hispanic, Native American)?			
Is the child/adolescent alcoholic dependent, an intravenous drug user, or a resident of a long-term-care facility, correctional or mental institution, nursing home/facility, or other long-term residential facility?			

- Immunizations:
- Use of car seat:
- Storage of hazardous substances:
- Home safety:
- Guns in the home:
- Fire escape plan:
- Pools:
- Swimming ability:
- Helmet use:
- Sunscreen:
- (Older child/adolescent) Use of drugs, alcohol, or tobacco:
- Typical diet:
- Threats at school:
- Thoughts of hurting self or others:
- (Adolescents) Sexual activity:

Common Symptoms:

Symptom	Yes	No	Additional data
Abdominal pain			
Headache			
Leg pain			

Physical Assessment:

Take height, weight, heart and respiratory rates, temperature, and blood pressure.
Plot height and weight on appropriate growth charts; calculate BMI.
Observe the child's demeanor, attentiveness, affect, and speech.
Observe for range of motion (ROM) and musculoskeletal symmetry and coordination.
Inspect and palpate the skin, hair, and nails.
Inspect the head and neck; observe neck ROM. Palpate the head and neck. Palpate the fontanels of the head on children up to 2 years old.
Inspect the eyes.
Assess distance vision.
(Optional) Screen for color blindness in patients 4–8 years old.
Inspect the ears.
(Optional, for APRN) Visualize the tympanic membrane with an otoscope. Use the pneumatic bulb to test for movement.
Palpate the pinna for tenderness and nodules.
Screen for hearing acuity in infants and young children.
Inspect the nose, mouth, and throat. Note the number of deciduous and permanent teeth.
Inspect the thorax and lungs. Palpate the thorax. Percuss the thorax and lungs. Auscultate the thorax and lungs. Percuss the lungs if pneumonia is suspected.
Inspect for visible pulses on the thorax. Palpate and auscultate the point of maximal intensity (PMI).
Percuss the heart if heart enlargement is suspected. Auscultate the heart in all six designated areas on the chest and in the back. Assess with the child in two positions: lying and/or sitting and/or standing. Observe the jugular venous pulsations.
Inspect the peripheral vascular system. Palpate peripheral pulses. Assess blood pressure in each extremity.
Inspect the breasts.
Inspect, palpate, and percuss the abdomen.
Inspect the muscles and joints. Evaluate for scoliosis. Observe ROM in all joints. Palpate muscles and joints.
Assess orientation. Observe for symmetry. Test deep tendon reflexes and evaluate for equality. Ensure active movement and full strength in all extremities.
Assess developmental progress for age.
Inspect the genitalia.
Note if the male is circumcised or uncircumcised with the urethra midline at the end of the glans. Palpate the male scrotum.
Inspect the anus and rectum.

Signature_____ Date _____

Guide for Use in Practice

Technique	Normal Findings	Abnormal Findings
Take height, weight, heart and respiratory rates, temperature, and blood pressure. Plot height and weight on appropriate growth charts; calculate BMI. Routine blood pressures with cuff and sphygmomanometer begin at 3 years of age if newborn blood pressure was recorded in the nursery as within normal limits in all extremities.	*Charts for blood pressure norms are found on the National Heart, Lung and Blood Institute's Website.*	Any blood pressure over the 90th percentile
Observe the child's demeanor. Look for signs of distress, discomfort, or anxiety. Note attentiveness and affect. Listen for speech difficulties.	*A 4 year old is generally talkative and engaged in the visit, and can answer simple questions about self and concerns. By 2 years, the child uses two-word sentences; by 3 years, a child should speak in more complicated sentences with speech that is understandable 75% or more of the time.*	Flat affect, no eye contact, and clinging to the caregiver
Observe for ROM and musculoskeletal symmetry and coordination.	*ROM full with 4–5+/5 strength symmetrically*	Asymmetry of movement and lack of coordination
Inspect and palpate the skin, hair, and nails.	*Skin smooth and dry. Hair smooth and evenly distributed. Nails smooth and without clubbing*	Absence or overgrowth of nails; dimpling, ripples, or discoloration in nails; unusual moles or hyper-pigmented areas; acne; rash; papules, nodules, cysts
Inspect the head and neck; observe neck ROM. Palpate the head and neck. Look for nodules or pain. Palpate the fontanels of the head on children up to 2 years old.	*Head and neck symmetrical with full neck ROM. Anterior and posterior cervical nodes may be palpable but not enlarged, and also are nontender. No nodule or tenderness noted on the head. Anterior fontanel closed by 18 months, posterior fontanel by 6 months*	Limited neck ROM; tender swollen lymph nodes of the neck and posterior head; lymph nodes that are large, nonmovable, or tender
Inspect the eyes.	*PERRL (A). EOMs at 180 degrees. Corneal light reflexes equal. No deviation during cover and alternate cover tests. Fundoscopic examination reveals a distinct disk with no vessel nicking.*	Unequal and nonreactive pupils; unequal EOMs or CLR; deviation with the cover test
Assess distance vision using a screening test based on developmental stage	*Toddlers: 20/200 bilaterally* *3 years: 20/40 bilaterally* *4 years: 20/30 or better bilaterally* *5–6 years: visual acuity approximate that of adults (20/20 in both eyes).*	Distance vision outside expected parameters for age
Screen for color blindness in patients 4–8 years old.	*Color recognition*	Inability to recognize one or more colors
Inspect the ears.	*Formed pinna, the top of which touches an imaginary straight line through both pupils*	Ear deformities; low-set ears

(Optional, for APRN) Visualize the tympanic membrane with an otoscope. Once visualized, use the pneumatic bulb to test for movement of the tympanic membrane.	*Tympanic membrane gray, nonerythematous with the light reflex and landmarks visualized*	Tympanic membrane erythematous or yellow, drainage in the canal, limited mobility
Palpate the pinna for tenderness and nodules.	*Tympanic membrane mobile; no tenderness or nodules on pinna*	Tenderness with manipulation of the pinna; swollen, erythematous turbinates; pale swollen turbinates
Screen for hearing acuity in infants and young children.	*Child responds to audio cues.*	Lack of Moro reflex, inability to localize sound, lack of understandable language by 24 months
Inspect the nose, mouth, and throat. Note the number of deciduous and permanent teeth.	*Nose midline; nares patent; turbinates pink with unrestricted air passage. Tonsils present and between +1 and +4. No caries. No erythema or exudate*	Dental caries; erythema and exudate
Inspect the thorax and lungs. Palpate the thorax. Percuss the thorax and lungs. Auscultate the thorax and lungs. Percuss the lungs if pneumonia is suspected.	*No increased work of breathing or retractions. No tenderness along intercostal spaces. Lungs resonant. Breath sounds clear in all lobes. No crackles, gurgles, or wheezes*	Pain along ribs; respiratory distress
Inspect for visible pulses on the thorax. Palpate and auscultate the PMI.	*PMI at the MCL in infancy, moving slightly laterally to the fourth ICS just to the left of MCL in children younger than 7 years and then to the fifth ICS in children older than 7 years. No bounding PMI*	Visible PMI
Percuss the heart if heart enlargement is suspected. Auscultate the heart in all six designated areas on the chest and in the back. Assess with the child in two positions: lying and/or sitting and/or standing. Observe the jugular venous pulsations.	*Closure of tricuspid and mitral valves (S1) and the pulmonic and aortic (S2) valves is clear, crisp, and single. No murmurs, rubs, or gallops. Neck vessels not distended or flat*	Murmur
Inspect the peripheral vascular system. Palpate peripheral pulses. Assess blood pressure in each extremity.	*Color pink in all extremities and mucous membranes. Pulses equal in all extremities; no differences between upper-extremity and lower-extremity pulse. If there are slight differences, they are <10 mm Hg.*	Cyanosis; unequal pulses between upper and lower extremities
Inspect the breasts.	*Breast development progresses according to those established in the Tanner Stages (see Chapter 26 of Jensen).*	Onset of pubertal changes before 8 years in girls
Inspect the abdomen. A protuberate abdomen is a common finding in toddlers. Palpate the abdomen. Percuss the abdomen. Percussion can assist in determining the size of the liver.	*No masses, tenderness, or distension. Tympany throughout. Liver at lower right costal margin*	Distension, tenderness, ascities; abdominal masses

Inspect the muscles and joints. Evaluation of scoliosis begins when the child can stand, but it is a focused part of the examination just prior to, and during, puberty. Observe ROM in all joints. Palpate muscles and joints.	*Spine straight. No joint tenderness. ROM full and symmetrical*	Limited ROM in any joint. Joint tenderness with palpation. Scoliosis
Assess orientation. Observe for symmetry. Test deep tendon reflexes and evaluate for equality. Ensure active movement and full strength in all extremities.	*Older children oriented to time and place. Movements symmetrical; DTRs 2+. Strength 4–5+*	Asymmetry of gait, facial features, or movement
Assess developmental progress for age. The Denver Developmental Screening Test is used for children 1 month to 6 years. For children older than 6 years, academic performance is noted.	*Scores within norms for age*	Confusion, unusual behaviors, delayed development progress, and poor academic performance
Inspect the genitalia. Refer to Chapters 25 and 26 of Jensen for sexual maturity and Tanner staging.	*Genitalia show no signs of erythema, discharge, or irritation.*	Onset of pubertal changes before 8 years in girls and 9 years in boys; infections, trauma, labial adhesions for girls; undescended testicles for boys
Note if the male is circumcised or uncircumcised with the urethra midline at the end of the glans. Palpate the male scrotum.	*Testes in the scrotal sac and smooth; no nodules noted*	Hypospadias; testicular nodules; hydrocele, varicocele, spermatocele
Inspect the anus and rectum.	*Skin on anus and rectum without irritation, erythema, or fissures*	Rectal irritation or fissures

Older Adults

OBJECTIVE SUMMARY

This chapter begins with a review of physiologic changes associated with aging and then moves to a discussion of best practices for conducting an interview with an older adult. It includes some common assessment tools used to identify risk for specific geriatric symptoms. The chapter then discusses such tools in the context of physical examination findings. In that section, the normal aging process is separated from findings that represent abnormal changes commonly found in older adults.

READING ASSIGNMENT

Read Chapter 30 in Jensen's *Nursing Health Assessment: A Best-Practice Approach*.

VOCABULARY/TERMINOLOGY

- **Actinic keratoses:** Skin lesions that appear as rough, scaly patches on the face, lips, ears, back of hands, forearms, scalp and neck. Cause is frequent or intense exposure to ultraviolet rays, typically from the sun.

- **Aortic aneurysm:** Weakened and bulging area in the aorta, the major blood vessel that feeds blood to the body.

- **Cellulitis:** Common, potentially serious bacterial skin infection; appears as a swollen, red area of the skin that feels hot and tender; may spread rapidly.

- **Dyspigmentation:** Disorder of pigmentation of the skin or hair.

- **Ectropian:** An eyelid (typically the lower lid) that turns out, leaving the inner eyelid surface exposed and prone to irritation.

- **Entropian:** An eyelid that turns inward so that eyelashes and skin rub against the eye surface, causing irritation and discomfort.

- **Geriatric:** Relating to senior citizens/older adults; relating to the diagnosis, treatment, and prevention of illness in this age group.

- **Herpes zoster:** Commonly known as shingles, viral disease characterized by a painful skin rash with blisters in a limited area on one side of the body.

- **Incontinence:** Loss of bladder or bowel control.

- **Mastectomy:** Surgery to remove all breast tissue from a breast as a way to treat or prevent breast cancer.

- **Parkinson's disease:** Degenerative disorder of the central nervous system that often impairs the sufferer's motor skills, speech, and other functions.

- **Photoaging:** Lifelong cumulative exposure to the sun.

- **Pressure ulcers:** Areas of damaged skin and tissue that develop when sustained pressure cuts off circulation to vulnerable parts of the body.

- **Solar lentigines:** Circumscribed area of a small blemish.
- **Stasis dermatitis:** Skin changes in the leg resulting from "stasis" or blood pooling as a result of insufficient venous return; also called *varicose eczema*.
- **Urinary retention:** Inability to urinate; a common complication of benign prostatic hypertrophy (also known as benign prostatic hyperplasia or BPH).

STUDY GUIDE

Activity A FILL IN THE BLANK

1. Fill in the blanks about structure and function in older adults.

A. Epithelium renews itself every _____ instead of every _____ as in children and adults.

B. Decreased _____ of cells leads to a 50% reduction in rate of wound healing.

C. The number of _____ and sebaceous glands decreases as a result of atrophy, and vascularity and _____ of the skin layer are diminished.

D. It is important to note the difference between normal aging processes and the lifelong cumulative exposure to sun, called _____.

2.

A. Tear production decreases, which leads to _____ .

B. The _____ becomes less elastic, larger, and denser with age and can become progressively yellowed and _____ .

C. Slowed pupillary responses lead to a difficulty in _____ to changes in light, difficulty with night driving, and problems with _____.

D. Increased _____ deposits may be found at the periphery of the cornea around the _____.

Activity B MATCHING

1. *Match the nursing diagnosis with the appropriate intervention.*

Answer	Nursing Diagnosis	Intervention
	1. Imbalanced nutrition, less than body requirements	A. Ambulate with walker three times a day (tid).
	2. Disturbed sensory perception: visual or auditory	B. Assess for depression.
	3. Adult failure to thrive	C. Note laboratory tests such as total protein, albumin, and prealbumin.
	4. Constipation	D. Provide adequate lighting.

2. *For each organ or function, identify whether a change is a part of normal aging.*

Y = Yes, N = No   Organ or Function

1. Thyroid function
2. Inner ear
3. Olfactory receptor neurons
4. Respiratory muscle strength
5. Gastric secretions

Activity C SHORT ANSWER

1. Explain changes in the kidney as a person ages.

_____

_____

_____

_____

2. Discuss natural changes in the musculoskeletal system as a person ages.

_____

_____

_____

_____

3. Discuss current thoughts regarding brain atrophy in the older adult.

_____

_____

_____

_____

4. Significant changes in the endocrine system affect the body as a person ages. Explain these changes.

_____

_____

_____

_____

5. What conditions are considered to require an acute assessment in older adults and why?

_____

_____

_____

_____

6. Discuss the need to set up the environment prior to interviewing an older adult. Explain what the nurse needs to do.

_____

_____

_____

_____

7. Explain the process of interviewing an older adult who is acutely ill.

_____

_____

_____

_____

8. Discuss cultural considerations for older adults.

_____

_____

_____

_____

Activity D   MULTIPLE CHOICE

1. Common conditions or problems that accompany aging are often called
   A. conditions of aging
   B. geriatric symptoms
   C. symptoms of aging
   D. geriatric syndromes

2. What familial condition is it important to assess for in older adults?
   A. Kidney disease
   B. Mental illness
   C. Liver disease
   D. Neurological disease

3. The most commonly used instrument for assessing older adults' nutritional risk is
   A. DETERMINE instrument
   B. CONCERN instrument
   C. EATING instrument
   D. ASCERTAIN instrument

4. How do many older adults define their health?
   A. Ability to work
   B. Ability to function independently
   C. Ability to perform activities related to their hobbies
   D. Ability to maintain their homes and their yards

5. The Morse Fall Scale was developed for whom?
   A. Homebound elders
   B. Independent elders
   C. Hospitalized elders
   D. Nursing home elders

6. A son brings his 80-year-old father into the clinic. The son is concerned because he feels as if his father is growing weak, losing interest in things he used to care about, and no longer coming to dinner on Sundays. The son mentions that his mother died 8 months ago and his father now lives alone. The nurse would know that the father is at risk for what?
   A. Dementia
   B. Depression
   C. Malnutrition
   D. Decreased mobility

ALTERNATIVE CASE SCENARIOS

Mr. Ralph Monroe is a 76-year-old man with a history of Parkinson's disease. He has lived in a nursing home for the past 3 months because of functional limitations. He complains of "terrible constipation" and asks "What causes this?" His daily medications include Sinemet 25/250 four times before meals for Parkinson's, vitamin E 400 IU for prevention of heart disease, calcium 600 mg with vitamin D 800 IU for bone health, and Zestril 5 mg for his blood pressure.

Review the following alternative situations related to Mr. Monroe. Based on the changes outlined below, *consider what other outcomes, information, and problems would affect the overall picture and shape your responses.*

Alternative A

While reviewing Mr. Monroe's chart, the nurse finds that the patient has not had a bowel movement for 7 days.

Subjective: "I just don't have an appetite anymore."

Objective: Alert; conversation with slow, soft speech; dry oral mucosa, fissured tongue; occasional high-pitched bowl sounds on auscultation; distended abdomen, with lumpy mass in left lower quadrant (LLQ); large amount of hard, dry stool in rectal vault.

- Is Mr. Monroe's case stable, urgent, or an emergency?
- How will the nurse work with Mr. Monroe to promote health and reduce risk for illness?
- How will the nurse focus, organize, and prioritize the subjective and objective data collection?
- Which nursing diagnosis is highest priority and what is the rationale?

Alternative B

While reviewing Mr. Monroe's chart, the nurse finds that the patient has not had a bowel movement for 7 days.

Subjective: The staff reports indicate that it was very difficult to waken Mr. Monroe this morning; he slept through breakfast. During the interview, Mr. Monroe does not answer any questions.

Objective: Resident drowsy, difficult to arouse, mumbled answers; dry oral mucosa; fissured tongue; occasional high-pitched bowl sounds on auscultation. Winces with pain response upon abdominal palpation; distended abdomen, with lumpy mass in LLQ; large amount of hard, dry stool in rectal vault. Poor skin turgor.

- Is Mr. Monroe's case stable, urgent, or an emergency?
- How will the nurse work with Mr. Monroe to promote health and reduce risk for illness?
- How will the nurse focus, organize, and prioritize the subjective and objective data collection?
- Which nursing diagnosis is highest priority and what is the rationale?

DOCUMENTATION

Form for Use in Practice

Patient Name _____ Date _____

Date of Birth _____

Initial Survey

Reason for seeking health care: _____

History of present illness

- Location:
- Intensity:
- Duration:
- Description:

- Aggravating factors:
- Alleviating factors:
- Functional impairment:
- Pain goal:

Vital signs: T (route)_____ P (site)_____ R_____ BP (site)_____ SpO$_2$_____

Weight: _____ Height: _____ BMI: _____

General appearance: _____

General level of distress: _____

Level of anxiety: _____

Risk factors and history:
Nutrition—consider using the DETERMINE Nutrition Checklist

Mobility Level and Functional Abilities
Consider using the Katz Index of ADL
Or, if the patient is returning to the community, consider using the Lawton IADL

Risk for Falls
Previous falls:
Dizziness:

Medications/Polypharmacy

Current medications:

Doses:

Schedules:

Purpose of medications:

Vitamins or minerals:

Shared medications:

Adherence to prescriptions:

Side effects:

Skin Breakdown
Consider using the Braden or Norton scale to assess risk for skin breakdown.

Common Symptoms:

Symptom	Yes	No	Additional data
Incontinence			
Sleep deprivation			
Pain			
Cognitive changes			
Depression			
Elder abuse			

Physical Assessment:

Observe normal changes that occur with aging. Assess for any decreasing abilities to function and care for self. Note any changes in mental status.
Measure height and weight. Calculate BMI.
Assess temperature.
Assess apical pulse for 1 minute.
Assess respirations.
Assess pulse oximetry.
Inspect the skin, hair, and nails. Examine carefully for breakdown.
Inspect the head and neck.
Palpate the skull and hair.
Palpate the sternocleidomastoid and trapezius muscles.
Palpate the thyroid.
Inspect the eyes. Test vision, pupillary reflex, and extraocular movements.
(Optional) Perform the ophthalmoscopic examination.
Inspect the ear for any lesions or changes to the auricle.
(Optional) Perform the otoscopic examination.
Inspect the nose, mouth, and throat. Test nasal patency. Make note of the color and moisture of the mucosal membranes of the nose and oral cavity.
Inspect the chest. Palpate the chest wall to test for tactile fremitus. Percuss the lungs. Auscultate breath sounds.
Auscultate heart sounds. Observe neck vessels.
Palpate peripheral pulses.
Palpate breasts.
Inspect, auscultate, palpate, and percuss the abdomen. Perform the rectal examination.
Perform focused assessments of the bones, muscles, and joints. Test the patient's ability to stand from a seated position, walk a short distance, and turn around.
Test cranial nerves.
Test balance and coordination.
Test sensation.
Test reflexes and muscle strength.
Inspect genitals.
Evaluate laboratory data.

Signature_____ Date _____

Guide for Use in Practice

Technique	Normal Findings	Abnormal Findings
Observe normal changes that occur with aging. Assess for any decreasing abilities to function and care for self. Note any changes in mental status.	*Sharper body contours; more angular facial features; posture with general flexion; gait with a wider base of support; steps shorter and uneven; use of arms to aid balance*	Poor hygiene; inappropriate dress; inappropriate affect, inattentiveness, impaired memory, inability to perform ADLs; changes in mental status
Measure height and weight. Calculate BMI.	*BMI of 25–29 (slightly higher than recommended for younger adults)*	BMI above 29 or below 24
Assess temperature.	*36°C–36.8°C (96.9°F–98.3°F).*	Temperatures within normal range for a younger adult
Assess apical pulse for 1 minute.	*60–100 bpm. Pulse rate takes longer to rise to meet sudden increases in demand and longer to return to resting. Resting heart rate lower than for younger adults*	Variation in rhythm
Assess respirations.	*Decreased vital capacity and inspiratory volume; respiratory rate of 16–24 breaths/min*	Respiratory rates >24
Assess pulse oximetry.	*Oxygen saturation >92%*	<92%
Inspect the skin, hair, and nails. Examine skin carefully for breakdown, especially in the perineal area of older adults who are incontinent, and in any area that is at risk for pressure ulcers.	*Increased wrinkling; coarse skin in sun-exposed areas; thinned scalp hair; skin less elastic and dry; thinning of the epidermal layer, more pronounced in the eighth and ninth decades; nail beds with ridges; thickened toenails*	Bruising in various stages of healing; pressure ulcers; patchy white scaly areas on the scalp; very thick yellow overgrown toenails; stasis dermatitis; cellulitis; herpes zoster (shingles)
Inspect the head and neck. Palpate the skull and hair. Palpate the sternocleidomastoid and trapezius muscles. Palpate the thyroid.	*Appearance symmetrical. Facial expression appropriate to situation. Skull smooth with no pain or mass. Hair thin and gray. No pain, enlargement, or masses in thyroid*	Downward gaze with little eye contact; swelling, masses, or tumors; flat affect or facial tension; sunken facial hollows; extremely thick structures; goiter; clicking or crepitus in the temporal mandibular joint; limitations in movement in the neck
Inspect the eyes. Test vision, pupillary reflex, and extraocular movements. (Optional) Perform the ophthalmoscopic examination.	*Senile ptosis; dry eyes that appear irritated and red; decrease in corneal reflex; difficulty focusing properly or presbyopia; difficulty with glare and accommodating to changes in light; smaller pupil size and a slower or sluggish pupillary accommodation; reduced upward gaze; grayish yellow ring surrounding the iris, called arcus senilus; visual fields slightly diminished with confrontation but should not show unilateral differences. Retinal margins may be less distinct; drusen (yellow spots) on the macula*	Ectropian, a turning of the lid outward, or entropian, a turning of the lid inward; reduced visual fields, especially unilaterally; loss of vision
Inspect the ear for any lesions or changes to the auricle.	*No pain, masses, or lesions*	Ulcerated lesions on the auricle

(Optional) Perform the otoscopic examination	*Gray tympanic membrane or ear canal narrowed or occluded with wax. Conductive hearing loss and lateralization of hearing to the ear occluded with wax on the Weber's test, or BC > AC ear occluded with wax on the Rinne's test.*	Loss of hearing
Inspect the nose, mouth, and throat. Test nasal patency. Make note of the color and moisture of the mucosal membranes of the nose and oral cavity.	*Deviation of the nasal septum. Pink to pinkish red and moist mucous membranes. Tongue pinkish red, moist, with no fissures. Slightly dry oral mucosa. Varicosities under the tongue. Intact gag reflex, although possibly mildly diminished*	Vasomotor rhinitis; pale mucosal membranes; malodorous breath; poor dental condition, fractured teeth, or untreated dental caries; bright red tongue; overgrowth of white patchy plaque on the tongue; absent or markedly diminished gag reflex
Inspect the chest. Palpate the chest wall to test for tactile fremitus. Percuss the lungs. Auscultate breath sounds.	*Increased anterior-posterior diameter related to rigidity of the chest wall. Chest wall free of pain, swelling, or masses. Tactile fremitus not increased; percussion resonant. Normal breath sounds. Harsh rhonchi are sometimes found. Some scattered rales at the bases of the lungs*	Increased fremitus or dullness with percussion, especially at the lung bases; hyper-resonance on examination; lung sounds at the bases
Auscultate heart sounds. Observe neck vessels.	*Pulse rates in the 50–60 range; regular heart rate and rhythm with no murmurs, rubs, or gallops; as older adults reach their 80s and 90s, murmurs are common, especially grade 2 systolic murmurs. No jugular venous distention*	Pulses >100; loud (grade 3 or greater) or harsh holosystolic murmurs; loud murmurs heard radiating from the apex to around the side of the chest wall; lower extremity edema, abdominal distension, or other signs of fluid retention; jugular venous distention; arrythmias, especially atrial fibrillation; abdominal aortic pulsations over a wide area
Palpate peripheral pulses.	*Pulses 2–3 on a 4-point scale and symmetrical*	Absent peripheral pulses
Palpate breasts.	*No masses or nodules*	Mastectomy scars
Inspect, auscultate, palpate, and percuss the abdomen. Perform the rectal examination.	*Mass of stool in the LLQ. Flaccid or soft, distended abdomen. Slow but audible bowel sounds. External hemorrhoids*	Asymmetry or masses; abdominal ascites; painful, fiery red, or inflamed hemorrhoids; fecal incontinence or involuntary passage of stool
Obtain height. Perform focused assessments of the bones, muscles, and joints. Test the patient's ability to stand from a seated position, walk a short distance, and turn around.	*Loss of height of up to 6 in by 80 years. Reduced flexion and hyperextension of the neck; kyphosis of the spine; generalized decrease in strength; mildly decreased ROM; enlarged joints, especially at the knees and in the hands; able to change positions and move smoothly, without balance problems, stumbling, or assistance.*	Limited abduction of the shoulder; pain on palpation of the spine after a fall; large nodules in the distal interphalangeal joints; enlargements of the proximal interphalangeal joints; contractures of the hips and knees
Test cranial nerves.	*Decreased upward gaze.*	Blank or blunted affect

Test balance and coordination.	*Slowing of psychomotor finger-nose testing, or finger-to-finger testing. Slightly impaired heel-to-toe walking. Smooth gait with steps that may be wide based*	Difficulty initiating gait; a small, short, stepped gait that gradually becomes normal; a wide-based gait with a heel-to-toe foot slap to the floor; gait in which the leg does not swing through smoothly, catches on the floor, drags, or stops next to the other foot
Test sensation.	*Slightly diminished peripheral sensation and proprioceptive (position) sense*	Unilateral abnormal findings
Test reflexes and muscle strength.	*Reflexes normally diminish with aging; muscle strength against resistance may be slightly diminished.*	Tremors; diminished grip strength; unilateral loss of strength against resistance; severely diminished or absent sensation or proprioception
Inspect genitals.	*Thinning of genital hair, vaginal skin, and testicular or penile atrophy is common.*	Distended lower abdomen with resonant-to-dull percussion of fluid. Underwear smelling of urine, staining of urine, or leaking urine
Evaluate laboratory data.	*Decreased lean muscle and bone mass, increased fat mass, and vasomotor symptoms*	Fatigue, depression, anemia, erectile dysfunction, decreased libido, and decline in immune function

CHAPTER 31

Head-to-Toe Assessment of the Adult

OBJECTIVE SUMMARY

This chapter outlines a comprehensive head-to-toe assessment by a registered nurse. Although the chapter describes some typical assessments, it is important to keep in mind that adaptations are wide ranging, depending on the patient's status, clinical setting, and standards of practice.

READING ASSIGNMENT

Read Chapter 31 in Jensen's *Nursing Health Assessment: A Best-Practice Approach.*

STUDY GUIDE

Activity A   FILL IN THE BLANK

1. Fill in the blanks about clinical indications for an acute assessment.

   A. Skin color is _____ or _____.

   B. Breathing is _____.

   C. Posture is _____.

   D. Facial expression is _____.

   E. Overall appearance indicates _____.

Activity B   SEQUENCING

1. Place the activities of the nurse in the correct order:

   A. Reorganize data.

   B. Collect objective and physical assessment data.

   C. Analyze assessment data.

   D. Collect data related to history and risk factors.

Activity C   MATCHING

1. *Match the nursing diagnosis with the appropriate intervention.*

Answer	Nursing Diagnosis	Intervention
	1. Fatigue	**A.** Ensure adequate hydration.
	2. Diarrhea	
	3. Acute pain	**B.** Identify additional resources available.
	4. Ineffective coping	**C.** Use massage.
		D. Collaborate with provider to treat underlying cause.

2. *Identify whether each of the following pieces of equipment is needed in a comprehensive physical examination.*

Y = Yes, N = No   **Equipment**

      1. Hemoccult testing cards and solution

      2. 3/4″ Huber needle

      3. KOH

      4. H_2O_2

      5. Lubricant

Activity D **SHORT ANSWER**

1. Explain the primary prevention services that nurses offer as part of their professional responsibilities.

_____

_____

_____

_____

2. Discuss how a nurse approaches data about past health history. Include what a nurse does when areas are inconsistent or unclear.

_____

_____

_____

_____

3. List and explain the most important areas for patient teaching during a routine head-to-toe assessment.

_____

_____

_____

_____

4. Explain what questions, other than the review of systems, are important for the nurse to ask the patient.

_____

_____

_____

_____

5. Discuss the nurse's responses to patient questions about abnormal findings during the physical assessment.

_____

_____

_____

_____

6. Explain the differences in the assessment of the hospitalized patient as opposed to the clinic patient.

_____

_____

_____

_____

7. Discuss the need for a screening assessment on hospitalized patients.

_____

_____

_____

_____

Activity E **MULTIPLE CHOICE**

1. When conducting a complete head-to-toe assessment on an adult patient, the nurse needs adaptations for what?

A. Patient problems

B. Cultural background

C. Symptoms of aging

D. Psychosocial problems

2. A common diagnostic test is a serum sodium level. Abnormal findings with this test are most likely the results of what in the body?

A. Too much or too little chloride

B. Too much or too little iron

C. Too much or too little potassium

D. Too much or too little water

3. When doing a complete assessment on a patient, the nurse must analyze findings to do what?

A. Begin giving ordered medication.

B. Initiate a plan of care.

C. Determine the need for referrals.

D. Synthesize needed care.

4. A 27-year-old patient tells the nurse that she is being abused by her spouse. What is one action the nurse might take?

   A. Make a referral to the social worker.

   B. Make a referral to the chaplain.

   C. Report the abuse to the charge nurse.

   D. Report the abuse to the state department of social services.

5. A 54-year-old man is found to be anemic. Which of the following nursing diagnoses are most likely to be recorded in his plan of care?

   A. Decreased activity level

   B. Altered nutrition

   C. Fatigue

   D. Depression

6. When a nurse enters the room of a hospitalized patient, the infusion pump is alarming. The patient is restless, moaning, crying, and exhibiting guarding behavior. An uneaten meal is sitting on the over-bed table; several family members are arguing loudly. What would be a priority?

   A. Turning the alarm off on the infusion pump

   B. Talking with family members

   C. Assessing nutrition

   D. Assessing for pain

7. When obtaining subjective data from a new patient, the nurse focuses on

   A. evaluating risk factors

   B. looking at the family history

   C. assessing the patient's use of alcohol

   D. assessing the patient's coping ability

8. When discussing health assessment, the nursing instructor would tell the students that potential or actual problems are identified to focus on areas requiring what?

   A. Psychosocial evaluation and treatment

   B. Focused assessment

   C. Nutritional assessment

   D. Health teaching

ALTERNATIVE CASE SCENARIOS

Dorothy Jane Suleri, 44 years old, is admitted with diarrhea, obesity, ulcerative colitis, abdominal pain, rosacea, fatigue, and anemia. Her current problem is bleeding related to the colitis, for which she uses prescribed medications. She has had three bloody stools today. She is married with two children, 15 and 13 years old.

Review the following alternative situations related to Ms. Suleri. Based on the changes outlined as follows, consider what other outcomes, information, and problems would affect the overall picture and shape your responses.

Alternative A

Ms. Suleri has a history of ulcerative colitis. She is in remission and has one soft brown stool daily. She has no other symptoms from the colitis. She is on an anti-inflammatory diet, exercises regularly, and has a high-stress job. This is her first visit to the nurse practitioner.

- Is Mrs. Suleri's condition stable, urgent, or an emergency?

- How will the nurse focus, organize, and prioritize subjective and objective data collection?

- What teaching and health promotion needs are identified?

- How will the nurse plan interventions relating to the *Healthy People* goals and U.S. Preventive Services Task Force (USPSTF) recommendations?

Alternative B

Ms. Suleri has a history of ulcerative colitis and pneumonia. She is being discharged from the hospital with the pneumonia resolved and will be seeing the nurse practitioner for follow up in 1 week. At the 1-week appointment:

- How will the nurse focus, organize, and prioritize subjective and objective data collection?

- What teaching and health promotion needs are identified?

- How will the nurse plan interventions relating to the *Healthy People* goals and USPSTF recommendations?

DOCUMENTATION

Form for Use in Practice

Patient Name _____ Date _____

Date of Birth _____

Initial Survey

Reason for seeking health care: _____

History of present illness

- Location:
- Intensity:
- Duration:
- Description:
- Aggravating factors:
- Alleviating factors:
- Functional impairment:
- Pain goal:

Vital signs: T (route)_____   P (site)_____   R_____   BP (site)_____ SpO_2_____

Weight: _____ Height: _____ BMI: _____

General appearance: _____

General level of distress: _____

Level of anxiety: _____

Past Health History

- Allergies:
- Past illnesses:
- Medications:
- Family history:
- Childhood illnesses and immunizations:
- Most recent screening assessments:
- Mental health and psychiatric history:

Review of Systems

- Nutrition:
- Integumentary:
- Head and neck:
- Eyes:
- Ears:
- Nose, mouth, throat:
- Respiratory:
- Cardiovascular:

- Peripheral vascular:
- Breasts:
- Abdominal/gastrointestinal:
- Abdominal/genitourinary:
- Musculoskeletal:
- Neurological:
- Genitalia:
- Endocrine:
- Mental health:

Functional Health Status

- Activities of daily living:
- Growth and development:

Physical Assessment:

Obtain vital signs.
Inspect overall skin color.
Evaluate breathing effort.
Observe appearance.
Assess mood.
Observe nutritional status.
Evaluate personal hygiene.
Assess posture.
Observe for physical deformities.
Perform safety check.
Inspect skin with each corresponding body area.
Palpate skin for moisture, temperature, texture, turgor, and edema.
Evaluate facial structures.
Observe facial expression.
Inspect hair, scalp. Palpate cranium, temporal artery, and temporomandibular joint (TMJ).
Assess cranial nerve V, motor strength and light touch, three facial branches.
Assess cranial nerves V and VII.
Inspect lids, lashes, and brows.
Inspect mouth, lips, buccal mucosa, gums, teeth, hard/soft palates, uvula, tonsils, pharynx, tongue, and floor of mouth (APRN may use light from otoscope).
Grade tonsils.
Note mobility of uvula.
Assess cranial nerve XII; look for symmetry of the tongue when extended.
(Optional) Assess near and distant vision.

For both eyes, inspect conjunctiva and sclera.
For both eyes, inspect cornea, iris, and anterior chamber. Assess cranial nerves III, IV, VI, and extraocular movements (EOMs). Assess visual fields, peripheral vision.
(Optional) Darken room. Obtain light. Assess cranial nerve II.
(Optional, APRN) Perform ophthalmoscope examination.
Turn on lights. For both ears, inspect ear alignment. Palpate auricles, lobes, and traguses.
(Optional, APRN) Change to otoscope head. Perform otoscope examination of canals and tympanic membranes.
Assess cranial nerve VIII (hearing).
(Optional) Obtain tuning fork. Perform Rinne test (on mastoid) if the patient has hearing loss.
(Optional) Perform Weber's test (at midline of skull) if the patient has hearing loss.
Inspect external nose.
Assess nostril patency.
(Optional, APRN) Perform otoscopic examination of mucosa, turbinates, and septum.
Palpate frontal and maxillary sinuses.
Inspect symmetry and flexion, extension, lateral bending, rotation, range of motion (ROM), and strength of upper extremities.
Palpate tracheal position midline.
Palpate carotid pulse.
Inspect jugular veins.
Palpate lymph nodes of upper body.
Assess mental status and level of consciousness.
Assess orientation.
Assess ability to follow commands.
Evaluate short- and long-term memory.
Assess speech.
Assess hearing.
Evaluate circulation, movement, and sensation (CMS). Assess hands and joints. Evaluate nails on upper extremities.
Perform hand grasp for ROM and muscle strength.
(Optional) Perform finger-to-nose test. Test rapid alternating movements. Test stereognosis. Test graphesthesia.
Assess breathing effort, rate, rhythm, and pattern; position to breathe.
Inspect chest shape and skin. If the patient is on an examination table, move to the front of the patient. Inspect costovertebral angle, configuration, and pulsations.
Auscultate breath sounds.
Assess for cough; inspect sputum.
Inspect precordium.

Assess heart rate, rhythm, murmurs, and extra sounds.
Auscultate heart with bell at apex and left sternal border with the patient lying down. Auscultate heart with diaphragm in aortic, pulmonic, left sternal border, tricuspid, and mitral locations with the patient on left side.
Palpate chest for fremitus, thrill, heaves, and point of maximal impulse.
Percuss anterior chest from apex to base and sides.
Auscultate carotid artery.
Inspect the breasts. Palpate breasts and nipple for discharge.
Palpate axillary nodes.
Inspect abdomen.
Auscultate bowel sounds.
Auscultate aorta, renal, and femoral arteries with bell.
Percuss abdomen in all quadrants and for gastric bubble.
Percuss liver margin at right midclavicular line (MCL).
Percuss spleen.
Palpate for abdominal tenderness, distention in all quadrants. Palpate liver, spleen, and kidneys.
Palpate aorta, femoral pulses, and inguinal lymph nodes or hernias.
Evaluate swallowing, chewing, aspiration risk, special diet.
Ask about nausea, vomiting, constipation, diarrhea.
Inspect stool; record last bowel movement. Ask about passing flatus.
Inspect urine color, character, and amount with voiding.
Inspect leg skin and toenails for symmetry, edema, veins, and lesions.
Palpate dorsalis pedis pulses bilaterally. Palpate popliteal pulses and posterior tibial pulses.
Assess capillary refill on both feet.
Inspect and palpate edema on ankles, shins.
Palpate lower extremities for tenderness and temperature.
Palpate lower extremities and joints from hips to toes.
Observe ROM of joints.
Test muscle strength on feet, observe for symmetry. Test muscle strength in hips, knees, and ankles.
Test sensation.
Obtain reflex hammer. Perform deep tendon reflexes—patellar, Achilles, and Babinski.
Move behind the patient. Palpate thyroid.
Inspect skin, symmetry, configuration, and observe respirations.
Palpate spine and scapulae.
Assess tactile fremitus.
Percuss posterior chest from apex to base to sides.

Test flank tenderness (kidney).
Auscultate breath sounds.
Inspect lower back, buttocks (redness, symmetry). Inspect spine.
Evaluate fall risk: history of falling, secondary diagnosis, ambulatory aid, IV therapy, gait, and mental status.
Perform heel-to-shin test for coordination. Have the patient stand. Note muscle strength and coordination when moving.
Observe spinal alignment, hip level, gluteal and knee folds. Assess spine flexion, extension, lateral bending, and rotation.
Ask the patient to walk on heels and then toes, and then to stand on one foot and then the other.
Evaluate risk for skin breakdown.
Assess intravenous, drainage, catheter, suction.
(Males) Palpate the scrotum for tenderness, lumps, and masses. Assess for inguinal hernia.
(Females) Inspect perineal and perianal areas.
(Females, APRN) Insert speculum. Inspect cervix and vaginal walls. Obtain specimens. Remove speculum.
(Females, APRN) Perform bimanual examination of cervix, uterus, and adnexa.
(Males and Females, APRN) Inspect perianal area. With lubricated finger, palpate rectal wall (and prostate in male). Obtain stool sample for occult blood.

Signature_____ Date _____

Guide for Use in Practice

Technique	Normal Findings	Abnormal Findings
Obtain temperature.	*35.8°C–37.3°C.*	Hypothermia, hyperthermia.
Obtain pulse.	*60–100 bpm.*	Tachycardia, bradycardia, irregular rate. If irregular, take apical pulse.
Obtain respirations.	*12–20/min.*	Bradypnea, tachypnea, hyperventilation, Cheyne-Stokes, apnea.
Obtain blood pressure.	*Systolic 100–120/diastolic 60–80 mm Hg.*	Hypertension, hypotension, auscultatory gap.
Obtain oxygen saturation level.	*92%–100%.*	<92%.
Inspect overall skin color.	*Pink.*	Pallor, jaundice, flushing, cyanosis (central versus peripheral), erythema, ruddy, mottled.
Evaluate breathing effort.	*No dyspnea.*	Dyspnea, head of bed elevated, tripod position.
Observe appearance.	*Appears stated age.*	Appears older than stated age.
Assess mood.	*Calm, pleasant, and cooperative. Appropriate affect.*	Flat or inappropriate affect, depression, elation, euphoria, anxiety, irritable, labile.
Observe nutritional status.	*Appears well nourished.*	Appears poorly nourished, overweight, or obese.

Evaluate personal hygiene.	*Good personal hygiene.*	Poor personal hygiene.
Assess posture.	*Posture erect.*	Slouching, bent to one side.
Observe for physical deformities.	*No obvious physical deformities.*	Obvious physical deformity.
Perform safety check.	*Call bell within reach; bedside stand positioned; ID band correct; IVs, medications, tubes, and drains intact.*	Unsafe environment; medications or IVs not verified.
Inspect skin with each corresponding body area. Inspect color; check for rashes and lesions.	*Skin pink, no cyanosis. No telangiectasia, erythema, or papules.*	Changes in skin pigmentation. Lesions or rashes. Infections (eg, cellulitis). Infestations (scabies, lice, and fleas).
Palpate for moisture, temperature, texture, turgor, and edema.	*Skin warm, slightly dry, and intact. Good turgor on upper extremities; no edema, lesions, or tenderness.*	Growths or tumors; wounds or incisions.
Evaluate facial structures.	*Symmetrical structures without edema, deformities, or lesions. Patent nares.*	Asymmetry, edema, deformities, ptosis, lesions. Absence of "sniff," deviated septum, polyps, drainage.
Observe facial expression.	*Appropriate to situation.*	Anxious, facial grimace; facial droop, asymmetry.
Inspect hair, scalp. Palpate cranium, temporal artery, and TMJ.	*Straight hair with normal distribution. Hair supple and thick. Scalp pink and smooth without pests, flaking, lesions, or tenderness. Normocephalic, head midline. Temporal artery 2–3+ bilaterally, nontender. TMJ moves freely, without crepitus or tenderness.*	Facial asymmetry; enlarged bones or tissues; puffy "moon" face; increased facial hair in females; periorbital edema.
Assess cranial nerve V, motor strength and light touch, three facial branches.	*Strong contraction of muscles and senses light touch on forehead, cheek, and chin.*	Decreased or dulled sensation, weakness, or asymmetric movements.
Assess cranial nerves V and VII.	*Facial movements are strong and symmetrical.*	A weak blink from facial weakness.
Inspect eye lids, lashes, and brows.	*No ptosis, lid lag, discharge, or crusting. Even lash distribution. Brows with hair loss on outer third.*	Depressed or absent corneal response.
Inspect mouth with light and tongue blade. Inspect inside lips, buccal mucosa, gums, teeth, hard/soft palates, uvula, tonsils, pharynx, tongue, and floor of mouth (APRN may use light from otoscope).	*Lips, mucosa, gums, palates are pink and smooth. Floor of mouth intact, moist, smooth. Pharynx pink, intact. Tongue pink and rough. No lesions or tenderness. Teeth white, intact with good occlusion.*	Lesions, sponginess, or edema; bleeding gums; missing or discolored teeth; malocclusion; inflammation or tenderness of ducts.
Grade tonsils.	*Tonsils 0–2+. Pink with no discharge or lesions.*	Swollen glands or tonsils (grades 3+ to 4+).
Note mobility of uvula when the patient says "ahh."	*Uvula midline and rises symmetrically.*	Uvula asymmetrical or enlarged.
Assess cranial nerve XII; look for symmetry of the tongue when extended.	*Tongue at midline and extends symmetrically.*	A tongue that deviates to one side.
Assess near and distant vision if appropriate.	*Reads newsprint accurately. Snellen test 20/20.*	<20/20 corrected. Vision blurred. Note use of glasses, contact lenses, or assistive devices.
For both eyes, inspect conjunctiva and sclera.	*Pink, moist conjunctiva; white sclera.*	Sclera yellow with *jaundice.* Conjunctiva pink with *inflammation.*

For both eyes, inspect cornea, iris, and anterior chamber. Assess cranial nerves III, IV, VI, and EOMs. Assess visual fields, peripheral vision.	*Cornea and lens are clear. EOMs intact, no nystagmus. Visual fields equal to examiner's.*	Narrow angle; cloudiness of the lens.
Darken room. Obtain light. Assess cranial nerve II.	*Pupils equal, round, and reactive to light and accommodation (PERRLA L 6–4, R 6–4).*	Asymmetry, pinpoint, or "blown" pupils; describe measure of pupil and response to light.
(APRN) Perform ophthalmoscope examination: check red reflex, disc, vessels, and macula.	*Red reflex symmetric. Discs cream-colored with sharp margins. Retina pink. No hemorrhages or exudates; no arteriolar narrowing. Macula yellow.*	Lack of red reflex; white pupil reflex; blood directly observed in the eye.
Turn on lights. For both ears, inspect alignment; palpate auricle, lobe, and tragus.	*Ears aligned properly. Ears without lesions, crusting, masses, or tenderness.*	Microtia, macrotia, edema, cartilage pseudomonas infection, carcinoma on auricle, cyst, and frostbite.
(APRN) Change to otoscope head. Perform otoscope examination of canals and tympanic membranes.	*Canals with small amount of moist yellow cerumen. Tympanic membranes intact, gray, and translucent; light reflex and body landmarks present.*	Redness, external swelling, and discharge; obstructed canal.
Assess cranial nerve VIII (hearing).	*Whispered words heard bilaterally.*	Unable to repeat whispered words.
Obtain tuning fork. Perform Rinne's test (on mastoid) if the patient has hearing loss.	*Air conduction > bone conduction.*	Bone conduction longer or the same as air conduction.
Perform Weber's test (at midline of skull) if the patient has hearing loss.	*No lateralization.*	Unilateral identification of the sound.
Inspect external nose.	*Midline, no flaring or crusting.*	Asymmetry, swelling, or bruising.
Assess nostril patency.	*Patent bilaterally.*	Unable to sniff; deviated septum; obstructed nares.
Perform otoscopic examination of mucosa, turbinates, and septum.	*Nasal mucosa pink, intact; no polyps. No drainage. Turbinates and septum intact and symmetrical.*	Infection, inflammation of nasal mucosa.
Palpate frontal and maxillary sinuses.	*No frontal or maxillary sinus tenderness.*	Redness and swelling over the sinuses.
Inspect symmetry.	*Neck symmetrical, moves freely without crepitus.*	Neck asymmetrical or with crepitus.
Test flexion, extension, lateral bending, rotation, ROM, and strength.	*Full ROM, strength 4–5+ bilaterally.*	Reduced neck ROM (<4+).
Palpate tracheal position midline.	*Trachea at midline.*	Deviated trachea.
Palpate carotid pulse.	*Carotid pulse 2–3+ bilaterally.*	Reduced carotid pulses.
Inspect jugular veins.	*No jugular venous distention.*	Flat or distended jugular veins.
Palpate preauricular, postauricular, occipital, and posterior cervical chains. Palpate tonsillar, submandibular, submental, and anterior cervical chains. Palpate supraclavicular nodes.	*Not palpable or tender.*	Lymph nodes are not freely movable or are tender.

Assess mental status and level of consciousness.	*Patient alert. Eyes open spontaneously.*	Agitated, asleep, lethargic, obtunded, restless, stuporous. Use coma scale if reduced (eye opening, verbal, motor). Does not respond to stimuli or pain; decorticate rigidity, decerebrate rigidity, or no response to pain.
Assess orientation.	*Oriented × 3.*	A&O X 2 (person and place). A & O X 1 (person), disoriented X 3.
Assess ability to follow commands.	*Follows directions.*	Unable to follow commands.
Evaluate short- and long-term memory.	*Immediate, recent, and distant memory intact.*	Immediate, recent, or distant memory impaired; describe specific details.
Assess speech.	*Speech clear.*	Speech difficult to understand.
Assess hearing.	*Hears voices and responds appropriately.*	Difficulty understanding spoken words. Hard of hearing. Note hearing aids or assistive devices.
Evaluate CMS. Assess hands and joints. Evaluate nails on upper extremities.	*Nails smooth without clubbing. Joints without swelling or deformity. CMS intact.*	Decreased CMS, including color, temperature; capillary refill >3 seconds, pulses, decreased movement, decreased sensation and paresthesia. Nails breakable, cracking, inflamed, jagged, bitten, and clubbing.
Perform hand grasp for ROM and muscle strength.	*4–5+ muscle strength symmetrical.*	Decreased ROM, swelling, or nodules in joints. Muscle strength asymmetrical or 0–3+
(Optional) Perform finger-to-nose test. Test rapid alternating movements. Test stereognosis. Test graphesthesia.	*Finger-to-nose and rapid alternating movements smooth and intact. Patient identifies key or other object. Patient identifies the number 8 or another number.*	Ataxia; lack of coordination (adiadochokinesia); inability to identify objects correctly (*astereognosis*).
Assess breathing effort, rate, rhythm, and pattern; position to breathe.	*Breathes easily, with symmetrical expansion and contraction.*	Dyspnea, orthopnea, paroxysmal nocturnal dyspnea. Rhythm irregular, sitting straight upright or using tripod position to breathe.
Inspect chest shape and skin. If the patient is on an examination table, move to the front of the patient. Inspect costovertebral angle, configuration, and pulsations.	*A:P to transverse ratio 1:2 symmetrical. Skin intact. No pulsations visible. No dyspnea, retractions, or accessory muscle use.*	Barrel chest, funnel chest, pigeon chest, thoracic kyphoscoliosis.
Auscultate breath sounds.	*Bronchovesicular sounds midline, vesicular in lung periphery. Lung sounds clear.*	Diminished or absent breath sounds, bronchial or bronchovesicular sounds in lung periphery. Adventitious sounds (crackles, gurgles, wheezes, stridor, pleural rub).
Assess for cough, inspect sputum.	*No cough or sputum.*	Cough (brassy, harsh, loose, productive); sputum.
Inspect precordium.	*PMI may be visible or absent.*	PMI lateral to MCL; heaves or thrills.

Assess heart rate, rhythm, murmurs, and extra sounds.	*Heart rate and rhythm regular. No gallops, murmurs, or rubs.*	Tachycardia, bradycardia, irregular rhythm, murmurs (systolic versus diastolic), extra sounds (S3, S4, friction rub).
Auscultate heart with bell at apex and left sternal border with the patient lying down. Auscultate heart with diaphragm in aortic, pulmonic, left sternal border, tricuspid, and mitral locations with the patient on left side.	*Heart rate and rhythm regular; no murmurs, gallops, or rubs.*	Irregular rhythm; murmurs, rubs, or gallops.
Palpate chest for fremitus, thrill, heaves, and point of maximal impulse.	*Tactile fremitus symmetrical; no thrill, heave, or lift. Cardiac impulse nonpalpable.*	Asymmetrical fremitus; thrills, heaves, and lifts.
Percuss anterior chest from apex to base and sides.	*Lung fields resonant with dullness over heart area.*	Dull lung percussion.
Auscultate carotid artery.	*No bruit.*	Bruits.
Inspect the breasts. Have the patient raise arms overhead, press hands together, and lean forward Palpate breasts and nipples for discharge.	*No retraction or dimpling; symmetrical movement. No lesions or masses; no discharge. Nontender.*	Retraction, dimpling, or discharge. Mass or lump.
Palpate axillary nodes.	*Axillary nodes not palpable, nontender.*	Positive nodes, especially if immovable or tender.
Inspect abdomen.	*Abdomen symmetrical, rounded, or flat. Smooth, intact skin without lesions or rashes. Peristalsis and pulsations evident in thin patients. Flat, round umbilicus.*	Scars, striae, ecchymosis, lesions, prominent dilated veins, rashes, marked pulsation. Red, everted, enlarged, or tender umbilicus.
Auscultate bowel sounds.	*Bowel sounds present all quadrants.*	Hypoactive, hyperactive, or absent bowel sounds.
Auscultate aorta, renal, and femoral arteries with bell.	*No bruit.*	Venous hum, friction rub, or bruits.
Percuss abdomen in all quadrants and for gastric bubble.	*Dullness throughout.*	Abdomen tympanic in all quadrants. Gastric bubble percussed 6th L ICS at MCL.
Percuss liver margin at right MCL.	*Liver border below ribs.*	Liver border above ribs at R MCL.
Percuss spleen.	*Spleen not palpable.*	Spleen percussed in 10th L ICS posterior to midaxillary line.
Palpate abdominal tenderness, distention in all quadrants. Palpate liver, spleen, and kidneys.	*Abdomen nontender, soft. Liver lower border less than one finger below costal border at right MCL. Spleen and kidneys nonpalpable.*	Large masses, hard, tenderness with guarding or rigidity, rebound tenderness. Liver palpable more than one finger below costal border at right MCL.
Palpate aorta, femoral pulses, and inguinal lymph nodes or hernias.	*Aorta palpable, smooth. Femoral pulses 2–3+. No inguinal nodes or hernias.*	Enlarged aorta (>3 cm) or one with lateral pulsations that are palpable.

Evaluate swallowing, chewing, aspiration risk, special diet.	*Eats >75% of meal without difficulty.*	Dysphagia, impaired chewing, impaired swallowing, medically prescribed diet, tube feedings, significant weight gain/loss.
Ask about nausea, vomiting, constipation, diarrhea.	*No nausea, vomiting, constipation, or diarrhea.*	Nausea, vomiting, constipation, or diarrhea. Describe characteristics of emesis (eg, coffee grounds, blood).
Inspect stool; record last bowel movement. Ask about passing flatus.	*Last bowel movement normal for patient, soft, and brown. Passing flatus.*	Dark stool; stool with bright red blood coating it.
Inspect urine color, character, and amount with voiding.	*Urine clear, yellow, and >30 mL/hr.*	Urine dark, bloody, red, with sediment, cloudy, or <30 mL/hr.
Inspect skin and nails for symmetry, edema, veins, and lesions.	*Toenails white and smooth. Skin intact, slightly pale, and symmetrical, without edema, varicose veins, or lesions.*	Areas of pressure on heels. Lesions, ulcers, varicosities, edema. Mottled, ruddy, reddened, or flaky skin. Indurations with infection or inflammation.
Palpate dorsalis pedis pulses bilaterally. Palpate popliteal pulses and posterior tibial pulses.	*Pulses 2–3+.*	Diminished or absent pulses. Bounding (4+) pulses.
Assess capillary refill on both feet.	*Brisk capillary refill <3 seconds.*	Capillary refill >3 seconds
Inspect and palpate for edema on ankles, shins.	*No edema.*	1+ barely perceptible (2 mm) 2+ moderate (4 mm) 3+ moderate (6 mm) 4+ severe (>8 mm).
Palpate lower extremities for tenderness and temperature.	*Feet warm, no tenderness.*	Tenderness to palpation, feet cool or cold.
Palpate lower extremities and joints from hips to toes.	*No tenderness or swelling.*	Tenderness; swelling.
Observe ROM of joints.	*Full joint ROM.*	Limited or reduced ROM.
Test muscle strength on feet, observe for symmetry. Test muscle strength in hips, knees, and ankles.	*Strength 4–5+.*	Strength 0–3+
Test sensation.	*Appropriately identifies when touched.*	Loss of sensation.
Obtain reflex hammer. Perform deep tendon reflexes—patellar, Achilles, and Babinski.	*Patellar, Achilles DTRs 2+; Babinski negative.*	Reflexes 3–4+ (brisker than normal); 1+–0 (diminished or absent). Positive Babinski.
Move behind the patient. Palpate thyroid.	*Thyroid borders palpable, no enlargement, nodules, or masses noted.*	Thyroid enlargement or masses.
Inspect skin, symmetry, configuration, and observe respirations.	*Chest symmetrical, oval, without barrel chest. AP:transverse ratio = 1:2. Respirations 20 without dyspnea.*	AP ratio approximates 1:1, giving the chest a round appearance.
Palpate spine and scapulae.	*Spine straight, without scoliosis, kyphosis, or lordosis. Scapulae symmetrical.*	Skeletal scoliosis and kyphosis. Asymmetry and paradoxical respirations.
Assess tactile fremitus.	*Tactile fremitus symmetrical.*	Increased tactile fremitus over an area.

Percuss posterior chest from apex to base to sides.	*Lung fields resonant.*	Dullness; hyper-resonance.
Test flank tenderness (kidney).	*No tenderness to indirect percussion*	Kidney tenderness.
Auscultate breath sounds.	*Breath sounds clear.*	Coarse breath sounds; crackles, gurgles (ronchii), and wheezing.
Inspect lower back, buttocks (redness, symmetry). Inspect spine.	*No redness, breakdown. Spine straight, skin intact.*	Any redness, especially over pressure areas; scoliosis, lordosis, and kyphosis.
Evaluate fall risk: history of falling, secondary diagnosis, ambulatory aid, IV therapy, gait, and mental status.	*Scores at low risk on fall scale.*	Hesitancy, unsteadiness, staggering, reaching for external support, high stepping, foot scraping, inability to raise the foot completely off the floor, persistent toe or heel walking, excessive pointing of toes inward or outward, asymmetry of step height or length, limping, stooping, wavering, shuffling, waddling, excessive swinging of shoulders or pelvis, and slow or rapid speed.
Perform heel-to-shin test for coordination. Have the patient stand. Note muscle strength and coordination when moving.	*Smooth, coordinated movement. Moves easily in the environment.*	Poor coordination.
Observe spinal alignment, hip level, gluteal and knee folds. Assess spine flexion, extension, lateral bending, and rotation.	*Spine straight, posture erect. Full ROM in spine.*	*Scoliosis* or low back pain.
Ask the patient to walk on heels and then toes, and then to stand on one foot and then the other.	*Good balance and coordination*	Problems with balance or coordination.
Evaluate risk for skin breakdown.	*Scores at low risk for skin breakdown.*	High scores.
Assess intravenous, drainage, catheter, suction.	*Wound healing, drains intact, catheter draining well, suction on. IV site clean, dry, intact without erythema or tenderness.*	Pressure ulcers; wound drainage that is sanguineous (bloody), serosanguineous (mixed), fibrinous (sticky yellow), or purulent (pus). Signs or symptoms of infection.
(Males) Palpate the scrotum for tenderness, lumps, and masses. Assess for inguinal hernia.	*No redness or discharge; skin intact. No tenderness, lumps, or masses. No hernia.*	No hair, patchy growth, distribution in a female or triangular pattern with base over the pubis; infestations; inflammation, lesions, or dermatitis; crusty, multiple, red, round erosions and pustules; large red, scaly patches that are extremely itchy.
(Females) Inspect perineal and perianal areas.	*No redness or tenderness, skin intact.*	Vulvar or vaginal pain, flu-like symptoms, sores on vulva or genital region, scattered vesicles along the labia, matching vesicles on the labia reflecting "kissing" lesions, surface ulcerations or crusted lesions, inguinal lymphadenopathy.

(Females, APRN) Insert speculum. Inspect cervix and vaginal walls. Obtain specimens. Remove speculum.	*Vaginal walls pink, no lesions. Cervix pink, round, no discharge. No infections, Pap test negative.*	Cervical discharge, lesions, polyps; positive Pap results.
(Females, APRN) Perform bimanual examination of cervix, uterus, and adnexa.	*No pain when moving the cervix, uterus midline; no enlargement, masses, or tenderness. Adnexa and ovaries smooth, no masses or tenderness.*	Pain when moving the cervix; enlargement, masses or tenderness. Rough adnexa and ovaries, masses or tenderness.
(Males and Females, APRN) Inspect perianal area. With lubricated finger, palpate rectal wall (and prostate in male). Obtain stool sample for occult blood.	*No redness or tenderness; skin intact. No hemorrhoids, fissures, lesions, masses, or tenderness. Rectal wall intact. Male: prostate smooth and round. Stool soft and brown.*	Thrombosed hemorrhoids, rectal fissures, hard stool.

STUDY GUIDE ANSWER KEY

CHAPTER 1: THE NURSE'S ROLE IN HEALTH ASSESSMENT

Activity A

1. A. advocacy; B. scholarship and research;
   C. provider of care; D. advanced practice nurse
2. A. Making judgments; B. Gathering information;
   C. Analyzing; D. Synthesizing

Activity B

1. 1 = A; 2 = B; 3 = C
2. 1 = B; 2 = D; 3 = E; 4 = C; 5 = A
3. 1 = E; 2 = D; 3 = A; 4 = B; 5 = C

Activity C

1. Four broad goals are within nursing: (1) to promote health (state of optimal functioning or well-being with physical, social, and mental components); (2) to prevent illness; (3) to treat human responses to health or illness; and (4) to advocate for individuals, families, communities, and populations.
2. The roles in these areas are primarily as providers of direct and indirect care.
3. Evaluation of care is the judgment of the effectiveness of nursing care in meeting the patient's goals and outcomes based upon the patient's responses to the interventions.
4. Critical thinking in nursing entails purposeful, outcome-directed (results-oriented) thinking; is driven by patient, family, and community needs; is based on the nursing process, evidence-based thinking, and the scientific method; requires specific knowledge, skills, and experience; is guided by professional standards and codes of ethics; is constantly re-evaluating, self-correcting, and striving to improve.
5. Cultural competence refers to the complex combination of knowledge, attitudes, and skills that a health care provider uses to deliver care that considers the total context of the patient's situation across cultural boundaries.
6. A comprehensive assessment of a child focuses on cognitive and emotional development in addition to physical growth.
7. The role of the nurse is to facilitate this achievement through health promotion and teaching.

Activity D

1. B
2. C
3. D
4. C
5. A
6. D
7. B

CHAPTER 2: THE INTERVIEW AND THERAPEUTIC DIALOGUE

Activity A

1. A. restatement; B. encouraging elaboration (facilitation); C. active listening
2. A. false reassurance; B. overusing technical language; C. sympathy; D. interruptions

Activity B

1. 1 = A, 2 = C, 3 = B
2. 1 = D, 2 = F, 3 = E, 4 = C, 5 = G, 6 = B, 7 = A
3. 1 = B, 2 = A, 3 = E, 4 = D, 5 = C

Activity C

1. Physical appearance; facial expression; posture and positioning in relation to the patient; gestures; eye contact; voice; and use of touch are all important components of nonverbal communication. Nurses do not assume that touch is culturally acceptable, but ask permission to touch patients first. Nurses ensure that their dress and appearance are professional. Facial expressions are relaxed, caring, and interested. Nurses use gestures intentionally to illustrate points, especially for patients who cannot communicate verbally. To facilitate eye contact, nurses are at eye level with patients. They sit in chairs at eye level with patients who are in bed during interviews. For patients seated on examination tables, nurses are near eye level when standing.
2. Answers will vary based on students' unique experiences.

3. *False reassurance* minimizes uncomfortable feelings and the amount of distressing information that the nurse has to handle. Examples are, "It won't hurt." or "Don't worry. It will be all right." *Sympathy* is feeling what a patient feels from the viewpoint of the nurse. *Giving unwanted advice* is nontherapeutic, because the advice is usually from the nurse's perspective, not the patient's. *Leading or biased questions* carry judgment and encourage patients to respond in the most acceptable way. They also cause patients to feel guilty or inferior because of unhealthy behaviors. *Changing the subject* may happen when a situation is uncomfortable for a nurse because of personal experiences or coping mechanisms. The nurse also might change the subject unconsciously when feeling rushed or stressed. In such cases, she or he may not take time to use active listening. Other communication problems include *distractions, using too many technical terms or providing too much information, talking too much,* and *interrupting.*

4. Nonprofessional involvement occurs when the nurse crosses the boundaries of the professional relationship and establishes social, personal, or economic ties with patients.

5. (1) The *pre-interaction phase* occurs before the nurse meets with the patient. The nurse collects data from the medical record, including the previous history of medical illnesses or surgeries, current medication list, and problem list. She or he uses this information to conduct an interview, already knowing about some past problems and responses to treatments. (2) In the *beginning phase,* the nurse introduces herself or himself by name and states the purpose of the interview. The nurse shakes hands if that seems comfortable for a patient and is appropriate for the setting. To relax the patient, the beginning phase may continue with some neutral discussion. (3) During the *working phase,* the nurse collects data by asking specific closed-ended and open-ended questions. The nurse also charts the patient's history and health problems. The goal is to achieve a balance between listening and documenting. (4) With the *closing phase,* the nurse ends the interview by summarizing and stating the two to three most important patterns or problems. The nurse also asks if the patient would like to mention or needs anything else. The nurse thanks the patient and any family members for taking time to provide information.

6. In intercultural communication, the sender of an intended message belongs to one culture, while the receiver is from another. Cultural differences may exist related to group or ethnicity, region, age, degree of acculturation into Western society, or a combination of these factors. Nonverbal differences in eye contact, facial expression, gestures, posture, timing, touch, and space needs are all culturally influenced. Language differences between patients and the nurse can compound cultural differences and prevent the nurse from understanding the perspectives of patients. Voice volume, vocal tone, inflections, pronunciation, and accents also influence meaning. More than simple language translation, the cultural meanings of health, illness, and treatment are important factors to consider.

7. Communication etiquette refers to the code of conduct and good manners that show respect for others. Such etiquette varies between and within cultures. The nurse must assess the degree to which each patient identifies with cultural norms. Additionally, many patients identify with multiple cultures. The nurse should avoid assuming that patients follow cultural beliefs and assess the degree to which each individual perceives those beliefs. The nurse can bridge cultural differences by being sensitive to variations and using caring communication techniques.

Activity D

1. C
2. C
3. A
4. C
5. D
6. B
7. A
8. D

CHAPTER 3: THE HEALTH HISTORY

Activity A

1. A. history of present illness; B. demographic data; C. symptoms; D. signs
2. A. Onset; B. Location; C. Duration; D. Character; E. Associated/aggravating factors; F. Relieving factors; G. Timing; H. Severity

Activity B

1. 1 = B, 2 = A, 3 = C
2. 1 = D, 2 = G, 3 = F, 4 = E, 5 = B, 6 = A, 7 = C
3. 1 = E, 2 = A, 3 = D, 4 = C, 5 = B.

Activity C

1. A complete family history includes use of a genogram to illustrate family patterns.
2. Nurses assess activities of daily living by asking about feeding, bathing, toileting, dressing, grooming, mobility, home maintenance, shopping, and cooking.
3. The functional health assessment includes health perception, nutrition, elimination, activity, sleep, cognition, self-perception, roles, sexuality, coping, and values.
4. A complete review of systems assesses the history of all body systems including nutrition/hydration, skin/hair/nails, head/neck, eyes/ears, heart, peripheral vascular, breasts, abdominal, musculoskeletal,

neurological, genitalia, rectum, and endocrine/hematological.

5. The history of present illness includes assessment of location, intensity, duration, description, aggravating and alleviating factors, functional impairment, and pain goal.

6. Nurses collect primary data from patients themselves. They collect secondary data from other sources such as the chart or family.

7. A focused assessment is more narrow and specific to the presenting problem; a comprehensive assessment covers all body systems for screening and health promotion.

Activity D

1. A
2. B
3. C
4. D
5. A
6. B
7. C
8. D

CHAPTER 4: TECHNIQUES OF PHYSICAL EXAMINATION AND EQUIPMENT

Activity A

1. A. auscultation; B. percussion; C. palpation; D. inspection
2. A. Organisms are on a patient's skin or immediate environment. B. Organisms are transferred from the patient to the nurse's hands. C. Organisms survive on the nurse's hands for at least several minutes. D. The nurse omits or performs inadequate or inappropriate hand hygiene. E. The nurse's contaminated hands come into direct contact with another patient or environment in direct contact with the patient.

Activity B

1. 1 = C; 2 = A; 3 = D; 4 = E; 5 = B
2. 1 = A; 2 = B; 3 = C

Activity C

1. People with symptoms of a respiratory infection are asked to cover their mouths/noses when coughing or sneezing.
2. The best preventive action is to avoid contact with latex when possible. Health care facilities can establish latex-free zones for patients and staff. Nurses should take care to avoid carrying any latex substances into such zones, including stethoscopes, urinary catheters, and vials with rubber stoppers. To avoid increasing exposure to latex and, subsequently, allergy rates, institutions are

encouraged to substitute powder-free, low-allergen gloves and latex-free gloves for latex gloves when possible.

3. To minimize the adverse effects of hand hygiene, nurses can select less irritating products purchased by institutions and use skin moisturizers after washing hands.

4. Patient-to-patient transmission of pathogens requires five sequential steps: Organisms are present on a patient's skin or immediate environment; Organisms are transferred from the patient to the nurse's hands; Organisms survive on the nurse's hands for at least several minutes; The nurse omits or performs inadequate or inappropriate hand hygiene; The nurse's contaminated hands come into direct contact with another patient or environment in direct contact with the patient.

5. Auscultation is use of the stethoscope to hear movements of air or fluid over the lungs and abdomen. Percussion is tapping motions with the hands to produce sounds that indicate solid or air-filled spaces over the lungs and other areas. Palpation is use of the hands to feel the firmness of body parts, such as the abdomen. Inspection means observation of the patient for general appearance and any specific details related to the body system, region, or condition under examination.

6. The intention of standard precautions is to prevent disease transmission during contact with non-intact skin, mucous membranes, body substances, and blood-borne contacts (eg, needle-stick injury). Because many patients are unaware of being infected, standard precautions serve to help ensure that providers treat all patients equally.

Activity D

1. B
2. C
3. C
4. D
5. C
6. B
7. A

CHAPTER 5: DOCUMENTATION AND INTERDISCIPLINARY COMMUNICATION

Activity A

1. A. charting by exception (CBE); B. PIE note; C. SOAP note; D. narrative notes
2. A. Vital signs; B. Intake and output; C. Routine assessments; D. Diabetic record

Activity B

1. 1 = D; 2 = A; 3 = C; 4 = E; 5 = B
2. 1 = B; 2 = C; 3 = D; 4 = A

Activity C

1. In addition to being a legal document, the medical record is used for communication among health team members, care planning, quality assurance, financial reimbursement, education, and research.
2. Computerized medical records allow several health team members to view the patient record simultaneously. For those with special clearance, they enable the off-site viewing of the electronic record to note changes in patient condition or to order necessary laboratory tests, diagnostic studies, or medications. Computerization ensures that all entries are legible and time dated. It enables the graphing of trends in vital signs or assessment data. It minimizes compliance issues, because programs will not let nurses enter data until they have completed all required fields. This ensures a more complete assessment. Some programs create plans of care from entered assessment data.
3. One such tool, the Risk Assessment Report, provides risk scores on sepsis, pressure ulcers, falls, abnormal laboratory reports, and other criteria of interest.
4. Health care providers who violate HIPPA may face fines of up to $250,000 or jail time (HIPPA, 1996). Employees have been terminated for breaching HIPPA laws concerning confidentiality.
5. As nurses are learning health assessment techniques, they also should focus on learning the language, labeling the findings, and identifying abbreviations.
6. During rounds, nurses present assessment data on nursing issues such as mobility, fluid balance, pain management, and emotional or family issues.

Activity D

1. D
2. B
3. D
4. C
5. C
6. C
7. B

CHAPTER 6: GENERAL SURVEY AND VITAL SIGNS ASSESSMENT

Activity A

1. A. amplitude; B. elasticity; C. pulse deficit; D. rhythm
2. A. Exercise; B. Anxiety/pain; C. Smoking; D. Positioning

Activity B

1. 1 = A, 2 = C, 3 = B
2. 1 = D, 2 = E, 3 = A, 4 = G, 5 = B, 6 = H, 7 = F, 8 = I, 9 = C
3. 1 = C, 2 = D, 3 = E, 4 = A, 5 = B

Activity C

1. Indicators of an acute situation include extreme anxiety, acute distress, pallor, cyanosis, and a change in mental status.
2. Anthropometric measurements are the various measurements of the human body, including height and weight.
3. The oral route cannot be used to measure temperature in patients who are unconscious, orally intubated, or confused, or with those who have a history of seizures. Oral temperatures are also contraindicated in cases of postoperative oral surgery or oral trauma. Oral thermometers are not recommended for children younger than 6 years.
4. Compare a thigh BP with an arm BP if the arm BP is extremely high, particularly in young adults and adolescents, to assess for coarctation of the aorta. Position the patient prone if possible. Place a large cuff around the lower third of the thigh, centered over the popliteal artery. Proceed as directed for the brachial artery. The thigh SBP is 10 to 40 mm Hg higher than the arm SBP, while the DBPs are approximately the same in both sites.
5. Teach patients to consistently weigh themselves at the same time of day and wearing clothing of similar weight.
6. Patients undergoing surgery and those with decreased ventilation should be taught coughing and deep-breathing exercises.
7. The JNC VII published the following recommendations to help maintain controlled BP:

   - If you are more than 10% above ideal body weight, lose weight.
   - Limit alcohol to no more than 1 ounce of ethanol per day.
   - Exercise regularly.
   - Limit sodium intake to less than 100 mmol/L/day.
   - Quit smoking.
   - Reduce dietary saturated fat and cholesterol.

Activity D

1. C
2. A
3. D
4. D
5. B
6. A
7. C
8. B

CHAPTER 7: PAIN ASSESSMENT

Activity A

1. A. somatic pain; B. cutaneous pain; C. chronic pain; D. referred pain
2. A. Vocalizations; B. Facial grimacing; C. Bracing; D. Rubbing painful areas; E. Restlessness; F. Gestures

Activity B

1. 1 = C, 2 = D, 3 = A, 4 = B
2. 1 = H, 2 = E, 3 = A, 4 = G, 5 = C, 6 = D, 7 = B, 8 = F

Activity C

1. There are four steps in nociception: (1) transduction, in which noxious stimuli create enough of an energy potential to cause a nerve impulse perceived by nociceptors (free nerve endings); (2) transmission, in which the neuronal signal moves from the periphery to the spinal cord and up to the brain; (3) perception, in which the impulses being transmitted to the higher areas of the brain are identified as pain; and (4) modulation, in which inhibitory and facilitating input from the brain modulates or influences the sensory transmission at the level of the spinal cord.

2. Many older patients have chronic illnesses such as osteoarthritis or diabetes that cause pain. Although pain is prevalent in older patients, some of them see pain as just part of natural aging. They may be reluctant to report pain, because they want their providers to consider them "good patients," or they may fear that complaints of pain may lead to costly tests or expensive medications that they cannot afford. The older person may hide expressions of pain and be stoic. Although experiencing pain, their outward reaction to it may hide their discomfort.

3. These patients have an altered physiologic response to the pain stimulus, and the repeated use of opioids causes their bodies to become more sensitive to pain. This sensitivity is called opioid hyperalgeisa and can occur as soon as 1 month after opioid use begins. Not only are patients with opioid tolerance more sensitive to pain, they face a high level of bias from health care providers. Because these patients are more sensitive to pain, they often report high levels of pain with little relief from usual doses of opioids. They are often labeled as drug seeking. Many health care providers fear that they will induce addiction in patients by providing them with opioids. Many patients with opioid dependence mistrust the health care system. These attitudes by patients and health care providers can lead to undertreated pain.

4. Re-assessing pain is similar to reassessing a patient taking blood pressure medication or a patient with diabetes who needs regular blood glucose level testing. For patients taking pain medication, re-assessment provides a reliable measure of the drug's efficacy. It allows the nurse to see if pain intensity has decreased since administration—much as blood pressure should be lower once a patient takes blood pressure medication. Most hospitals have a standard time frame for re-assessment, such as 1 hour for oral medication and 30 minutes for pain medication given intravenously. They base these time frames on the time it takes a pain medication to provide a noticeable decrease in pain intensity.

5. Prejudices and bias related to educational, family, or cultural values can affect how nurses perceive the patient's self report of pain.

6. Conditions such as fibromyalgia, irritable bowel syndrome, migraines, and temporomandibular joint pain are more prevalent in women than in men.

7. Patients who have had surgery or a crush-type of injury are at high risk for developing CRPS. Nurses should be aware that when a patient with such an injury continues to complain of high levels of pain and begins to experience a subsequent loss of function, temperature sensitivity, swelling, or other skin changes (eg, hair loss in the affected area), the patient may be developing CRPS.

8. The best practice is to consistently use a scale specific to the patient's age. Pain scales have been developed that are specific to infants and children. Infants in pain may exhibit brow bulge, eye squeeze, nasolabial fold, open lips, stretched mouth, lip purse, taut tongue, chin quiver, and tongue protrusion. The difficulty with these behavioral measures is that they do not discriminate between pain behaviors and reactions from other sources of discomfort, such as hunger. The nurse should assume that if a condition or procedure is painful for an adult, it also is painful for an infant or child. Infants and children may exhibit physiological responses to pain including increased heart rate, respiratory rate, blood pressure, palmar sweating, cortisone levels, oxygen, vagal tone, and endorphin levels. Because the preverbal infant cannot self report pain, the nurse relies on these physiological and behavioral indicators.

Activity D

1. A
2. B
3. A
4. D
5. C
6. A
7. C

CHAPTER 8: NUTRITION ASSESSMENT

Activity A

1. A. healthy eating habits; B. variety; C. 300 to 500 cal/day; D. whole foods
2. A. Garlic; B. Ginger; C. Ginko; D. Grapefruit

Activity B

1. 1 = G; 2 = D; 3 = A; 4 = F; 5 = B; 6 = E; 7 = C
2. 1 = G; 2 = C; 3 = F; 4 = B; 5 = A; 6 = D; 7 = E

Activity C

1. Too high or too low potassium level may cause potentially fatal cardiac dysrhythmias.
2. Nurses should strive to make meal times as enjoyable as possible by encouraging both independent eating and family involvement. It is also advisable to adhere to food preferences as much as possible and to maintain adequate hydration. Other recommendations for maintaining adequate nutrition among long-term care residents include providing clean, comfortable, pleasant surroundings; offering water; providing small, frequent meals; and minimizing distractions during meals.
3. Nurses can help coordinate potential financial resources for patients and their families with limited income.
4. Folate is a B vitamin essential to metabolism and cell synthesis. Dietary sources include leafy greens, lentils, seeds, liver, orange juice, grains, cereals, and breads fortified with folic acid. Groups at risk for folate deficiency include patients with alcoholism, older adults, those who follow "fad" diets, and people of low socio-economic status. Adequate maternal intake of folate before conception and in the first trimester of pregnancy reduces incidence of neural tube defects (eg, spina bifida). The U.S. Public Health Service recommends that all women of childbearing age and capable of pregnancy consume 400 micrograms of synthetic folic acid daily from either foods or supplements.
5. The recommended adequate intake (AI) of water varies depending on gender, age, air temperature, activity level, and state of health.
6. Amidst a growing body of evidence showing the link between herbicide and pesticide use in agriculture and certain cancers, many people are seeking organic food sources. Further, the public has also questioned the use of antibiotics and hormones in raising cattle, pork, and poultry. Increased production of genetically modified foods had contributed to a move toward consuming organically grown foods from plant sources.
7. A psychosocial component of a comprehensive nutritional assessment is important to elicit the patient's feelings about food. Questions to be asked include: Does stress affect your eating or drinking habits? If so, please describe. And Does smoking affect your appetite? If so, describe. Remember that some patients gain weight with stress, while others lose weight and smoking impairs both senses of smell and taste.
8. Common symptoms of malnutrition include sudden or gradual changes in body weight; change in eating habits; changes in skin, hair, or nails; and decreased energy level. Questions you might ask when assessing the patient include
   - What is your present height and weight?
   - How do these compare with 5 years ago?
   - Have there been any changes in your weight over the past year? If so, please describe.
   - How do you feel about your present weight?
   - Have you experienced a change in a regular diet pattern (number, size, and contents of meals)?
   - Have you noticed any changes in your hair, nails, and skin? If so, describe.
   - Would you say that you heal well? Poorly? Other?
   - Do you have any difficulty tolerating hot or cold weather? How much energy would you say that you have?
   - Has your energy level changed recently, say during the past year? If so, describe.

Activity D

1. D
2. A
3. A
4. D
5. B
6. A
7. C
8. D

CHAPTER 9: ASSESSMENT OF DEVELOPMENTAL STAGES

Activity A

1. A. trust vs. mistrust; B. autonomy vs. shame and doubt; C. initiative vs. guilt; D. industry vs. inferiority; E. identity vs. role confusion; F. intimacy vs. isolation; G. generativity vs. stagnation; H. ego integrity vs. despair
2. A. expected pattern; B. variable rates; C. height and weight; D. motor, language, psychosocial, and cognitive development

Activity B

1. 1 = E, 2 = F, 3 = D, 4 = B, 5 = A, 6 = C
2. 1 = B, 2 = C, 3 = A

Activity C

1. Language development consists of two parts. *Receptive language* is the understanding of spoken or written words and sentences, and *productive language* is the individual's use of spoken or written words. Receptive language leads productive language, and throughout the life span receptive vocabulary tends to be larger than productive vocabulary.
2. Healthy children are much more likely to grow into healthy adults, and they need a great deal of support to make healthy and safe choices. Parents also need a great deal of support so that they can choose the healthiest possible lifestyles for themselves and their children.
3. Infant - 1½ times birth length and triple birth weight by age 1 year; Toddler - ½ adult height and quadruple birth weight by age 2 years; Preschooler - 2½ to 3 inches and 5 to 7 lbs/year.

4. Adolescent: Girls: Growth spurt of 2.5 to 5 inches and 8 to 10 lbs. Boys: Growth spurt 3 to 6 inches and 12 to 14 lbs.

5. Sensory memory is retention of a sensory image for a very brief time; there is a slight to no decrease with aging. Short-term memory is memory for things the person is presently and actively thinking about. There is a slight to no decrease with aging. Working memory means active processing of information while it is held in short-term memory. It can decrease somewhat with aging. Episodic long-term memory is recollection of past events and personally relevant information. It decreases with aging, but this finding may be caused by slower processing speed. Semantic long-term memory is retrieval of facts, vocabulary, and general knowledge, and it decreases minimally with aging.

6. Uri Bronfenbrenner proposed a frequently cited systems model of development, which describes the individual's development in interaction with the immediate environment. In this approach, development is continuous, important at all ages, and an active rather than a passive process.

7. In Erikson's view, the older adult with ego integrity has come to terms with life choices and recognizes that the life lived was the only possible one, and that it had dignity, which the person is ready to defend against physical or economic threats.

8. Young adults are more likely to use post-formal thought than are adolescents. They deal directly with such realities as local and national politics, occupational issues, and relationships. They have had enough experience to understand that an approach to a work problem needs to differ from an approach to a romantic problem. Many young adults are skeptical of the notions of a single truth and one final answer. Sometimes thinking cannot simply be abstract, but has to be realistic and practical.

Activity D

1. B
2. D
3. A
4. C
5. B
6. C
7. A
8. D

CHAPTER 10: MENTAL HEALTH ASSESSMENT

Activity A

1. A. observation; B. clinical setting; C. culture; D. investigate an area
2. (In any order): Support systems, Housing, Literacy, Health care accessibility

Activity B

1. 1 = A; 2 = D; 3 = B; 4 = E; 5 = C; 6 = G; 7 = F
2. 1 = F; 2 = G; 3 = E; 4 = A; 5 = B; 6 = D; 7 = C

Activity C

1. The patient would exhibit a slow, shuffling gait; mask-like facial expression; tremors; pill-rolling movements of the hands; a stooping posture; and rigidity.

2. An acute mental health assessment includes questions about harm to self or others. Acute situations include a risk for injury with psychotic states, depression, dementia, and delirium.

3. The art of nursing lies in the ability to communicate and accurately assess the patient, listening for not only what is said, but also what is unsaid. The nurse must be comfortable asking questions about psychosis, suicide, history of abuse, and sexuality. If the nurse is uncomfortable, the patient will sense it and be reluctant to respond. The nurse may even avoid asking relevant questions because of emotions they evoke within himself or herself. It is important to practice asking these types of questions during the laboratory and clinical experience to increase skill and comfort level. The science lies in the knowledge base that the nurse incorporates in the examination, including the accurate labeling of findings and the precise use of reliable and valid tools that screen for mental health issues.

4. Data for the objective assessment are usually organized by **A** (appearance), **B** (behavior), **C** (cognitive function), and **T** (thought process), plus the mini mental status examination.

5. Poor hygiene may be from paranoia of water, homelessness, severe depression, or incapacitation as a result of mental illness. Risk of lice increases with poor grooming. Excessive fastidiousness may accompany obsessive-compulsive disorder (OCD). One-sided neglect may result from stroke, brain trauma, or physical injury. An unkempt state might indicate depression or psychosis.

6. Attention span indicates current level of cognitive functioning. Can the patient follow the conversation? Is the patient easily distractible?

7. **Dementia** is more common in older adults. It is usually a gradual process over months to years. Remote memory and intellect are impaired, with impoverished thoughts. The patient retains alertness and attention. **Confusion** is characterized by a lack of clear and orderly thought and behavior. It can be acute and situational, quickly resolving, or chronic and long lasting. It is usually a finding with dementia and delirium; it sometimes accompanies depression. **Delirium** generally has an underlying medical cause that, once treated, results in the delirium resolving. Onset is acute over a few hours, lasting hours to weeks. Recent and remote memory is impaired. Attention fluctuates. Thoughts are

disorganized, with clouding of consciousness and disorganized perception. Delirium does not usually present with mood components. **Depression** has a slow onset. Its main feature is a disturbance of mood, usually with sadness or numbness of feeling. Memory and concentration may be impaired. Attention is intact.

Activity D

1. A
2. B
3. C
4. C
5. D
6. A
7. D
8. C

CHAPTER 11: ASSESSMENT OF SOCIAL, CULTURAL, AND SPIRITUAL HEALTH

Activity A

1. A. biomedical model; B. social assessment; C. social assessment of the individual; D. primary building blocks; E. social assessment of the community; F. eudaimonistic model of health; G. Gordon's functional health model; H. complementary and alternative medicine model; I. Roy's adaptation model
2. (In any order) Gaining knowledge, Comparing culture care needs, Identifying similarities and differences, and Generating a holistic picture

Activity B

1. 1 = B; 2 = D; 3 = A; 4 = C
2. 1 = C; 2 = D; 3 = G; 4 = F; 5 = E; 6 = A; 7 = B

Activity C

1. Spirituality emphasizes a notion of a path to achieve better understanding and connectedness with nature, inner harmony, other people, or an improved relationship with the divine. Spirituality is also considered an integral part of one's religion or self-directed path modeled after several different religions. In all cases spirituality is concerned with matters of the soul rather than the world of senses and material things. Similar to social and cultural assessments, spiritual assessment involves understanding the relationship between spirituality and health.
2. The traditional biomedical model continues to serve as the philosophical basis for Western medical care. In recent years, however, a trend in the biomedical community has emerged to consider the social, cultural and spiritual aspects of health during decision-making about treatment regimens.

3. Nightingale described the nurse's duty as putting the patient in the best condition for nature (God) to act upon him or her. She maintained that healing can occur only in an environment equipped with proper ventilation, adequate temperature, pure air and water, efficient drainage, cleanliness, light, and diminished noise. These environmental features are as important to health and healing today as they were to Nightingale in the 19th century. Evidence is also growing that care that embraces the patient's biopsychosocial and spiritual dimensions is important to health, because it puts the patient's life context and perceived needs first and offers healing for both body and spirit. This holistic approach to care results in more favorable outcomes than conventional treatments alone.
4. Roy refers to health as the patient's ability to adapt, compensate, manage, and adjust to physiologic–physical health-related setbacks. The adaptation model holds that a person is a set of parts connected to function as a whole. The goal of nursing care is to assist the patient to attain an optimal level of *physical health*: also described as physiological processes involved in the proper functioning of a living organism; *self-concept*: mental health; *role function*: ability to adequately perform in roles occupied in society; and *interdependence*: satisfying interpersonal relationships.
5. Gordon identified 11 categories of **functional health patterns,** which she refers to as behaviors that occur sequentially across time: (1) health perception–health management; (2) nutrition-metabolic; (3) elimination; (4) activity-exercise; (5) sleep-rest; (6) cognitive-perceptual; (7) self perception-self concept; (8) role-relationship; (9) sexuality-reproductive; (10) coping-stress tolerance; (11) value-belief. From the functional health perspective, an optimal healing environment would sustain life to a level expected for and desired by the patient, using various treatment modalities.
6. Social assessment refers to identifying the social context influencing the patterns of health and illness for individuals, communities, and societies. Basic variables of social assessment include gender, age, ethnicity, race, marital status, occupational class, shelter, employment status, and education level. It is important to understand how these variables interact with the broader sociocultural environment. Knowledge obtained from social assessment helps nurses understand and address issues of equity and social justice related to health. It also helps providers to create new ways to improve patients' access to resources.
7. Social assessment of the individual is intended primarily to inform nurses about the patient's physical and mental health as related to the patient's existing resources, constraints, and demands.

Resources might include education, income, housing, and support systems; constraints might be unemployment, single-parent family, minority status, unsafe neighborhood, and lack of social support; demands might involve struggling to live on a fixed income or caring for aging parents. At the community level, the scope of social assessment is broader and more complex. Community social assessment involves gathering data to identify community resources, constraints, and high-priority health concerns.

8. Data generated from the assessment are grouped into three categories: primary, secondary, and potential building blocks. Formal institutions in the area, such as local businesses, schools, libraries, parks, police, and fire stations, constitute the primary building blocks. Secondary building blocks include agencies designed to serve the community that have outside overarching corporations that manage and operate these agencies. An example is a community's small primary care clinic that belongs to, and shares the values and mission of, a national corporate health care system. Potential building blocks are programs and services designed by an individual or agency outside the community to improve some aspect of community well-being. An example is a federally funded participatory action research study aimed at improving the cardiovascular health of a given community with an increased incidence of heart disease.

Activity D

1. B
2. D
3. C
4. A
5. C
6. A

CHAPTER 12: ASSESSMENT OF HUMAN VIOLENCE

Activity A

1. A. child maltreatment; B. family violence; C. elder abuse; D. sibling violence; E. school violence; F. bullying; G. intimate partner violence; H. violence against adults with disabilities; I. hate crimes
2. (In any order) School clinics, WIC clinics, Immunization clinics, Nursing homes

Activity B

1. 1 = D; 2 = A; 3 = B; 4 = E; 5 = C
2. 1 = F; 2 = B; 3 = G; 4 = H; 5 = A; 6 = I; 7 = C; 8 = D; 9 = J; 10 = E

Activity C

1. Common psychological red flags are mood and behavior changes from normal for the specific patient. Depression and anxiety can manifest as a flat, quiet, and sullen affect (emotional dullness), withdrawal, or irritability and impulsive anger (see Chap. 10), which can further manifest as acting-out behaviors (eg, impulsive aggression toward others, risky and dangerous behaviors). Some violence victims use substances such as alcohol, marijuana, methamphetamines, cocaine, and narcotics to feel better while simultaneously numbing feelings of anxiety, low self-worth, sadness, and fear. Nevertheless, a link between human violence and mental health problems is usually hidden, and health care providers may overlook opportunities for healing interventions frequently.

2. Assessment findings are similar and different among violence survivors. Differences in how each person experiences and is affected by violence depend on type and severity and the lived experiences of a person in her or his family, community, and society. Age, ethnicity, socioeconomic status, education, sexual orientation, religion, urban or rural living, culture, and relationships can be highly influential on outcomes. Thus, it is very important not to make assumptions but to use open-ended questions such as, "How are you coping?" and "What has your experience been?"

3. Documentation is an important aspect of violence assessment. Close listening and keen observation skills are necessary to capture key details. It is important to reassure adults that their patient records are available only with their consent and may be useful someday if needed for legal action. Nurses should document subjective data in quotes as much as possible (eg, "pt states…"). When documenting objective data, it is important to be detailed, descriptive, and note findings without bias.

4. Nurses and other health care professionals are "mandated reporters" when child, elder, or vulnerable-adult abuse or neglect is disclosed, assessed, or suspected. Mandated reporters must call the protective services hotline when they suspect abuse or neglect. Provided the report is done in good faith and without malice, the nurse and other professionals mandated by the state to report are protected by the state.

5. Cultural differences between patients and caregivers may lead to an erroneous suspicion of abuse. For example, a nurse might observe a patient and caregiver having an aggressive conversation that includes shouting. Some cultures consider such behavior acceptable, whereas others consider it verbal abuse. Views on financial or personal autonomy of patients, their right to make decisions independently, or the amount of respect they deserve may also differ among cultural or socioeconomic groups.

6. Safety planning is key to intervention. If a patient is in an unsafe or potentially unsafe situation, nurses must suggest and encourage a safety plan. The first step is to ask the patient what he or she has done in the past to be safe and then build on this. Basic components of safety plans usually include the following: Charged cell phone with pre-programmed emergency phone numbers (or these numbers readily available but not necessarily identifiable to the perpetrator) for police, support people, and safe housing; Copies of important or difficult-to-replace documents such as birth certificate or insurance papers stored in a safe place (possibly with support person); Change of clothes for self (and children) packed and hidden; Extra set of house and car keys; Transportation plan; Extra money hidden in a safe location; Escape plan from potential house or apartment exits; Escape locations/safe places. Each patient will have individualized safety needs. It is very important for the nurse to explain to the patient that research shows that danger of violence is particularly high when victims leave or have left a relationship with a perpetrator. This fact makes patient teaching and safety planning even more essential aspects of nursing interventions.

7. Poly-victimization is highest in children who report rape and dating violence. About 25% of children experience four or more different kinds of victimization. Trauma symptoms such as anxiety, depression, anger, and aggression are "red flags" of poly-victimization.

8. Female U.S. immigrants and refugees, particularly those who do not speak English or have U.S. legal documents, are especially vulnerable to IPV. Rates of IPV may be higher in female immigrants than in female U.S. citizens for several reasons. Some cultures more visibly accept violence against women than does the U.S. culture. In addition, U.S. immigrants who attempt to escape IPV face significant barriers. For example, they may not have access to bilingual safety shelters, financial assistance, food, or other support services. It is also unlikely that they have assistance from certified interpreters during court proceedings, when reporting complaints to police, or even when acquiring information about their rights and the legal system. Lastly, perpetrators of IPV may use their partners' immigration status as a tool of control and force women to remain in the relationship, making it difficult for victims to escape the violence.

Activity D

1. C
2. D
3. D
4. A
5. B
6. C
7. A

CHAPTER 13: SKIN, HAIR, AND NAILS ASSESSMENT

Activity A

1. A. keratinocytes; melanocytes; B. protein; C. eumelanin; pheomelanin; D. lifespan; genders; E. infecting microorganisms, chemical irritants, and moisture loss.
2. A. Arrector pili; B. curlier; C. epidermal layer; D. highly vascular; pink color

Activity B

1. 1 = C; 2 = F; 3 = G; 4 = A; 5 = B; 6 = E; 7 = D
2. 1 = B; 2 = D; 3 = C; 4 = A

Activity C

1. A. Acne with comedones; B. Papular and pustular acne; C. Dysplastic nevus; D. Pyogenic granuloma; E. Erythema nodosum; F. Pruritic urticarial papules and plaques of pregnancy

Activity D

1. The Braden scale scores patients from 1 to 4 in six subscales: sensory perception, moisture, activity, mobility, nutrition, and friction.
2. Common nursing diagnoses associated with skin problems include **Risk for infection**, **Pain**, **Impaired tissue integrity**, and **Impaired skin integrity.**
3. If performing a complete skin assessment, inspect all body areas, beginning at the crown of the head, parting the hair to visualize the scalp, and progressing caudally to the feet. Make sure to assess the underside of the foot and to separate the toes. Note general skin color. The normal finding is that skin pigmentation is consistent throughout the body. Patients with darker skin may normally have hypopigmented skin on the palms of their hands and soles of their feet. Abnormal findings include changes in skin pigmentation in any areas, vitiligo, flushing, erythema, cyanosis, pallor, rubor, brawniness, jaundice, or uremic frost.
4. *Primary lesions* arise from previously normal skin and include maculae, papules, nodules, tumors, polyps, wheals, blisters, cysts, pustules, and abscesses. *Secondary lesions* are changes that appear following a primary lesion (eg, formation of scar tissue, crusts from dried burn vesicles). Primary lesions may be further described as nonelevated, elevated-solid, or fluid-filled.
5. The dyes used in tattooing may cause an allergic reaction and result in swelling, redness, and tenderness at the tattoo site. Tattoo dyes are not FDA-approved for injection into the skin and may contain pigments suitable for automobile paints and other chemicals. Tattoos applied without known sterile equipment or single use dyes increase the risk for blood-borne diseases such as *Hepatitis B* and *HIV*.

6. During subjective data collection, nurses have the opportunity to integrate health teaching with history taking. For the integumentary system, a major focus of such teaching relates to the prevention of skin cancers, including melanoma.

7. Emergency skin findings are those that indicate acute dehydration, cyanosis, or impaired skin integrity (acute lacerations). They require prompt evaluation and interventions of fluids, oxygen, skin repair, or a combination.

Activity E

1. C
2. D
3. B
4. A
5. C
6. A
7. D

CHAPTER 14: HEAD AND NECK WITH LYMPHATICS ASSESSMENT

Activity A

1. A. quickly; accurately; B. immobilized; cleared; C. complete history; history; physical; essential; D. myocardial infarction
2. (In any order) Hypermetabolism; Tachycardia; Diarrhea; Anxiety; Fever; Weakness; Psychosis; Coma and death.

Activity B

1. 1 = H; 2 = F; 3 = G; 4 = E; 5 = B; 6 = C; 7 = A; 8 = D
2. 1 = B; 2 = C; 3 = D; 4 = A

Activity C

1. If test results are negative, the nurse should assess for complete range of motion of the neck, looking for any muscle tension, loss of mobility, or pain. The nurse should recall that cardiac disease may present with referred pain to the neck or jaw, making it important to assess for signs of cardiovascular disease.

2. Contributing factors include a more subtle onset, chronic diseases, and the idea that typical signs and symptoms (fatigue, cold intolerance, constipation, or depression) may be attributed to the process of aging. Additionally the older adult is more prone to hyperthyroidism.

3. Detection of maternal (and fetal) hypothyroidism is of major importance because of potential damage to fetal neural development, an increased incidence of miscarriage, and preterm birth.

4. Facial asymmetry may indicate damage to CN VII or a serious condition such as a *stroke*.

5. Signs and symptoms of hypothyroidism include fatigue; anorexia; cold intolerance; dry skin; brittle,

coarse hair; menstrual irregularities; weight gain or difficulty losing weight; and decreased libido.

6. Diagnosis of a cervical spine injury is challenging; many cases go undiagnosed, especially in those lacking adequate health insurance. Patients at risk include those following a fall or collision, and patients with osteoporosis, advanced arthritis, cancer, or degenerative bone disease.

7. Newborns have two *fontanels*, areas of the skull with a soft and non-ossified matrix. Fontanels enable the head and underlying structures to grow as the child develops. Assessing the size of the anterior and posterior fontanels at each evaluation of the infant is important to determine if ossification is happening at the appropriate time. The posterior fontanel closes by 3 months of age, while the anterior fontanel closes by 18 months of age.

Activity D

1. C
2. A
3. D
4. B
5. C
6. C
7. A

CHAPTER 15: EYES ASSESSMENT

Activity A

1. A. Eyelids; B. palpebral fissure; C. limbus; D. lacrimal apparatus
2. A. superior rectus; B. inferior rectus; C. superior oblique; D. medial rectus; E. inferior oblique; F. lateral rectus

Activity B

1. 1 = C; 2 = D; 3 = E; 4 = A; 5 = G; 6 = B; 7 = F.
2. 1 = B; 2 = C; 3 = A
3. 1 = E; 2 = D; 3 = A; 4 = C; 5 = F; 6 = B

Activity C

1. Gradual vision loss, while significant, does not usually require an emergent referral. Further, ascertaining the source of the trauma/injury helps determine whether the problem is emergent (immediate medical attention), urgent (medical attention within few hours), or non-urgent (appointment as soon as possible). Rapid assessment of the eye involves assessing for foreign bodies, lacerations, or hyphema (blood in the eye), testing extra-ocular movements, and examining the optic disc. Trauma that involves a penetrating injury or suspected fracture of the orbital bone requires an *emergent referral*. If a patient describes loss of vision, it is critical to ascertain a timeline of vision loss. Sudden loss of vision requires an emergent referral.

2. Older adults have changes both in eye structures and vision. Eyelids may droop and become wrinkled from loss of skin elasticity. The eyes sit deeper in the orbits from loss of subcutaneous fat. Eyebrows become thinner, and the outer thirds of the brows may be absent. Conjunctivae are thinner and may appear yellowish from decreased perfusion. The iris may have an irregular pigmentation. Tearing decreases as a result of loss of fatty tissue in the lacrimal apparatus. Vision may decline. Because the pupil is smaller, there is loss of accommodation, decreased night vision, and decreased depth perception. The lens enlarges and transparency decreases, making vision less acute.

3.
- Superior rectus muscle: Inserts anterior, superior surface; action is elevation and adduction.
- Inferior rectus muscle: Inserts anterior, inferior surface; action is depression and abduction.

4. Eye color differs among people of various genetic backgrounds, with lighter eyes more prevalent in more Northern countries. Genetic background also influences the diameters of eyelids and eyebrows.

5. Assessment of the patient's diet helps to identify any vitamin deficiencies that could affect the eyes.

6. Diabetes mellitus increases risks for eye problems, including diabetic retinopathy, cataracts, and glaucoma. Sunlight exposure also increases risks, so use of sunglasses is important, especially if the patient lives in a sunny climate. Poor diet has been linked to eye problems. Foods that promote eye health include deep-water fish, fruits, and vegetables (eg, carrots, spinach). Because the lens has no blood supply, staying well hydrated keeps the lens supple and moist.

7. High-velocity injuries are typically penetrating. Blunt-force trauma often results in fracture of the orbit. Trauma that involves a penetrating injury or suspected fracture of the orbital bone requires an emergent referral.

Activity D
1. B
2. D
3. A
4. C
5. A
6. A
7. C

CHAPTER 16: EARS ASSESSMENT

Activity A
1. A. cranial nerve (CN) VIII; B. vestibular function; C. bony labyrinth; D. cochlea; E, semicircular canals; vestibule
2. (In any order) Tympanic membrane; Cochlear window; Oval window; Eustachian tube

Activity B
1. 1 = E; 2 = D; 3 = G; 4 = F; 5 = B; 6 = C; 7 = A
2. 1 = B; 2 = C; 3 = A

Activity C
1.

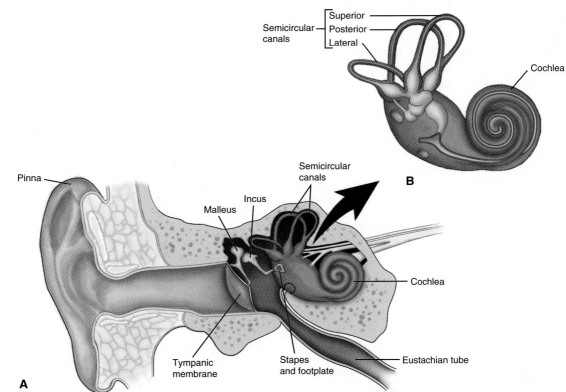

Activity D

1. The eustachian tube connects the middle ear to the nasopharynx and allows for pressure regulation of the middle ear. The ability to equalize pressure keeps the tympanic membrane intact with atmospheric variances. The eustachian tube opens briefly with swallowing and yawning; otherwise, this conduit remains closed.

2. Hearing is a complex experience. The external ear channels sound waves into the external auditory canal through the tympanic membrane, to ossicles in the inner ear via the oval window, then to the cochlea. The basal membrane in the cochlea vibrates the receptor hair cells of the organ of Corti, which transfer the signal into electrical impulses for the auditory nerve. The auditory nerve then delivers those impulses to the auditory cortex in the temporal lobe of the brain, which interprets them as and assigns meaning to the sound. The brainstem detects origination of the sound and can distinguish from which ear the electrical impulses originated, even though there may be only a slight delay of sound from one ear to the other. The cochlea interprets two components of sound: amplitude (volume) and frequency (pitch). *Amplitude* is the change in atmospheric pressure against the tympanic membrane and is directly related to the intensity of a sound. Decibels (dB) are the measurement units of amplitude. *Frequency,* the number of cycles per second the sound waves make, is measured in units of hertz (Hz). Normal conversation occurs between 10 to 60 dB and 200 to 5,000 Hz. A jet engine is approximately 140 dB; a whisper is approximately 30 dB.

3. The most common cause of conductive hearing loss in adults is auditory trauma related to excessive noise exposure, particularly at work. This problem is increasing among younger people as well.

4. Otosclerosis is a form of conductive hearing loss common in older adults. It results from the slow fusion of any combination of the ossicles in the middle ear. The fusion leads to obstruction of the transmission of sound waves from the tympanic membrane to the oval window and inner ear.

5. The cartilage and skin around the external ear may be less pliable in older adults. The stiff hairs in the canal may require a smaller otoscope tip to separate them and increase visualization of the tympanic membrane. The membrane itself may seem more opaque and less mobile.

6. The superior portion of the pinna should be congruent with the outer canthus of the eye. There should be no more than a 10-degree deviation from the medial fold of the lobe to attachment of the superior portion of the helix. More than 10-degree deviation requires further investigation–it can signify a genetic defect in the renal system. It can also indicate neurodevelopmental challenges.

Activity E

1. C
2. B
3. B
4. D
5. B
6. A
7. D
8. D

CHAPTER 17: NOSE, SINUSES, MOUTH, AND THROAT ASSESSMENT

Activity A

1. A. Milia; B. Choanal atresia; C. Ankyloglossia; D. Allergen; E. Vestibule; F. Kiesselbach's plexus; G. Sinus ostia; H. Rosenmiller's fossa; I. Adenoids; J. Stensen's duct

Activity B

1. 1 = D; 2 = E; 3 = A; 4 = C; 5 = B
2. 1 = C; 2 = D; 3 = B; 4 = A
3. 1 = C; 2 = E; 3 = D; 4 = A; 5 = F; 6 = G; 7 = B

Activity C

1. Loss of subcutaneous fat may cause the nose to appear more prominent in older adults. Edentulous (without any teeth) older adults may develop a pursed-lip appearance as mouth and cheeks fold inward. Overclosure of the mouth may lead to maceration of the skin at the corners of the mouth; this condition is called angular cheilitis. Teeth may appear yellow as worn enamel reveals the dentin layer. They also may appear larger as the gums recede. Teeth may loosen with bone resorption and move with palpation.

   The tongue and buccal mucosa may appear smoother and shiny from papillary atrophy and thinning of the buccal mucosa. This condition is called smooth, glossy tongue and may result from deficiencies of riboflavin, folic acid, and vitamin B12. Fissures may appear in the tongue with increasing age. This condition, called scrotal tongue, can become inflamed with the accumulation of food or debris in the fissures.

2. Diagnostic testing for allergic sensitivity is helpful in managing persistent upper-respiratory inflammation. Allergy testing may be performed via skin or blood. Various approaches to allergy skin testing include percutaneous or prick testing and intradermal testing. A blending of both types of skin testing is performed typically when evaluating upper-respiratory conditions. Radioallergosorbent testing (RAST) is a blood test that measures allergen specific IgE antibody, which is elevated in reaction to allergens to which the patient is sensitive.

3. Some outcomes commonly related to nose, mouth, sinus, and throat problems include the following:

- The patient's oral mucous membranes are pink and intact.
- The patient swallows with no evidence of aspiration.
- The patient states breathing is more comfortable and less congested.

4. People with allergies should damp dust and vacuum at home weekly, change or clean furnace filter monthly, avoid feather pillows and down comforters, wash sheets and blankets weekly in hot water, avoid "dust catchers" (eg, stuffed animals), consider using high efficiency particulate air (HEPA) filters in the bedroom and vacuum cleaner, and use hardwood floors in the bedroom. They can discourage and eliminate mold growth by repairing leaks, using dehumidifiers in damp basements, cleaning shower grouting weekly, decreasing houseplants, cleaning refrigerator drip pans, meticulously cleaning or avoiding portable humidifiers, adjusting whole house humidity to 40% or less, avoiding wool fabrics, avoiding foods that contain mold, and eliminating completely foods suspected of producing acute life-threatening symptoms. To decrease pet dander, patients should have only outdoor pets, remove pets from the bedroom, groom or bathe pets regularly (not by the allergic person), and wash hands after touching pets. Finally, patients can decrease exposure to pollens by keeping windows closed, grooming pets, and avoiding attic fans.

5.

Technique	Screening or RN Assessment	Focused or APRN Assessment
Inspect the nose.	X	
Inspect the nose with otoscope and nasal speculum.		X
Palpate the nose.		X
Inspect the sinuses.		X
Palpate/percuss the sinuses.		X
Inspect the mouth.	X	
Palpate the mouth.		X
Inspect the throat.	X	
Inspect/evaluate swallowing.		X

6. The *throat (oropharynx)* is the common channel for the respiratory and digestive systems. It begins at the inferior border of the soft palate and uvula. The throat includes the base of the tongue, pharyngoepiglottic and glossoepiglottic folds, anterior and posterior pillars, and palatine tonsils. The *tonsils* are in the back of the throat between the anterior and posterior pillars. The tissue appears more granular and less smooth than the surrounding mucous membranes. Lymphatic tissue of the tonsils and adenoids provide immunologic defense.

7. The upper respiratory system and mouth function as the entry point for air and food into the body. These organs serve as a common channel until air reaches the lungs and food reaches the esophagus. The upper respiratory tract warms, filters, humidifies, and transports air to the lower respiratory tract. The nose is the sensory organ for smell, while the mouth is the sensory organ for taste.

Activity D

1. D
2. A
3. B
4. D
5. C
6. C
7. C

CHAPTER 18: THORAX AND LUNGS ASSESSMENT

Activity A

1. A. vesicular breath sounds; B. stridor; C. whispered pectoriloquy; D. bronchovesicular breath sounds; E. crackles; F. egophony; G. adventitious breath sounds; H. bronchial breath sounds; I. wheezes; J. bronchophony

Activity B

1.

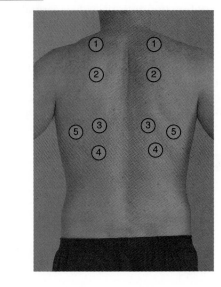

2.

A. Tachypnea
B. Bradypnea
C. Eupnea
D. Hyperventilation
E. Hypoventilation
F. Cheyne-Stokes respirations
G. Biot's respirations

Activity C

1. Some areas for health promotion and patient teaching during respiratory assessment include smoking cessation, prevention of occupational exposure, prevention of asthma, and immunizations.
2. Five factors that place a client at risk for respiratory problems are smoking, family history, past medical history, lifestyle, and occupational exposure.
3. Characteristics of a cough and sputum to note include where the cough comes from (sinuses, throat, or lungs); what it feels or sounds like; how bad it is; how often it happens; when it is worse; when it started; how long it has lasted; what makes it better; any other accompanying symptoms; what the patient thinks has caused the problem; if the amount of sputum has increased or decreased; the color and consistency of the sputum; any odor; and any changes in sputum amount, consistency, or color.
4. Ronchal fremitus is a coarse vibration produced by passage of air through or around thick exudates in the airways, such as in pneumonia.
5. Respiratory patterns in infants vary based on feeding, sleep state, and body temperature. Because of this irregularity, respirations in infants should be counted for 1 minute.
6. Retractions would be noted in the supraclavicular or intercostals muscles, between the ribs, and in the area just above the sternal notch.
7. Pulmonary function tests provide information about the patient's ability to move air into and out of the lungs. Total vital capacity, inspiratory volume, and expiratory reserve are measured for patients at risk for disease or dyspneic symptoms
8. Older adults are at increased risk for pulmonary. complications during stress. Attention must be paid to maintaining effective ventilation, keeping lung volumes high, clearing secretions, and positioning to prevent aspiration.

Activity D

1. D
2. B
3. A
4. D
5. B
6. C
7. A

CHAPTER 19: HEART AND NECK VESSELS ASSESSMENT

Activity A

1. A. gallop; B. murmur; C. split; D. click; E. bruit; F. Rub; G. Snap

Activity B

1. 1 = F; 2 = A; 3 = D; 4 = E; 5 = H; 6 = C; 7 = B; 8 = G
2. 1 = F; 2 = A; 3 = B; 4 = C; 5 = E; 6 = D

Activity C

1. The sequence is 7, 5, 1, 4, 2, 3, 6.

Activity D

1. Increased age, male gender, and African-American, Mexican-American, American Indian, native Hawaiian, or Asian-American heritages are risk factors for cardiovascular disease.
2. Cardiac emergencies that necessitate rapid assessment and intervention include acute coronary syndrome, acute severe heart failure, hypertensive crisis, cardiac tamponade, unstable cardiac arrhythmias, cardiogenic shock, systemic or pulmonary embolism, and aortic dissection.
3. Palpate the carotid arteries one at a time. Palpating them together poses a risk for obstructing both arteries, reducing blood flow to the brain and potentially causing dizziness or loss of consciousness. Palpate the carotid artery medial to the sternomastoid muscle in the neck between the jaw the clavicle. Avoid compressing over the carotid sinus. Stimulation of the sinus also causes parasympathetic stimulation, which may lead to reduced pulse rate and bradycardia. Older adults and patients sensitive to this stimulation may develop periods of life-threatening asystole. Palpate the strength of the pulse and grade it as with peripheral pulses.
4. S3 is quiet, low pitched, often difficult to hear, and usually audible in patients with heart failure. S4, usually an abnormal sound, results from a noncompliant ventricle as a consequence of hypertension, hypertrophy, or fibrosis. The pericardial friction rub is the most important physical sign of *acute pericarditis*. It may have up to three components during the cardiac cycle and is high-pitched, scratching, and grating.
5. Murmurs in adults usually indicate disease. If the heart valve fails to totally close, during systole the blood leaks back through the valve and causes a whooshing sound (similar to Korotkoff sounds heard during assessment of blood pressure). Similarly, a valve may fail to totally open, causing turbulence during diastole as the blood rushes against a partially closed valve to fill the heart. Therefore, these murmurs may occur during either systole or diastole. Murmurs also may result from vibration of

tissue or excessive flow as in pregnancy. Additionally they may occur in any of the four valves.

Systolic murmurs occur during contraction between S1 and S2 when the mitral and tricuspid valves are closed and the aortic and pulmonic valves are open. Diastolic murmurs occur during filling from the end of S2 to the beginning of the next S1, when the mitral and tricuspid valves are open and the aortic and pulmonic valves are closed.

6. Common nursing diagnoses include impaired cardiac tissue perfusion, decreased cardiac output related to impaired electrical conduction, activity intolerance, anxiety/fear related to fear of death, and decreased self-esteem.

Activity E

1. C
2. B
3. C
4. C
5. A
6. B
7. B

CHAPTER 20: PERIPHERAL VASCULAR AND LYMPHATIC ASSESSMENT

Activity A

1. A. arterioles; B. endothelial; C. low-pressure; D. pressure gradient; E. bicuspid valves; F. thoracic ducts
2. A. African Americans; B. Genetics; C. 50 years; obesity; D. Hypertension.

Activity B

1. 1 = D; 2 = A; 3 = B; 4 = E; 5 = C.
2. 1 = C; 2 = D; 3 = B; 4 = A.
3. 1 = C; 2 = A; 3 = F; 4 = B; 5 = E; 6 = D.
4. Location = B; Borders = A; Ulcer base = A; Drainage = B; Gangrene = B; Pain = A; Skin = B; Pulses = A.

Activity C

1. The lymphatic system consists of the lymph nodes and lymphatic vessels, as well as the spleen, tonsils, and thymus. It maintains fluid and protein balance and functions with the immune system to fight infection. The lymphatic vessels carry lymph in the tissues back to the bloodstream. The pathways of these vessels often run parallel to the arteries and veins. The thoracic ducts at the junctions of the subclavian and internal jugular veins return the lymph fluid to the circulation. The lymphatic vessels contain valves to maintain unidirectional flow. Skeletal muscle contraction, passive movement, and increases in heart rate all support lymph flow. Only the superficial lymph nodes are accessible for palpation. Lymphatic flow in the arms drains into the epitrochlear, axillary, and infraclavicular nodes. In the lower extremities, the lymph drains primarily into the inguinal nodes.

2. Calcification of the arteries, or *arteriosclerosis*, causes them to become more rigid in older adults. Less arterial compliance results in increased systolic blood pressure, which often is compounded by the coexistence of atherosclerotic disease in the arteries supplying the brain, heart, and other vital organs. Incidence of peripheral arterial disease (PAD) increases dramatically in the seventh and eighth decades of life.

3. If a patient is experiencing symptoms of complete arterial occlusion such as pain, numbness, coolness, or color change of an extremity, stop the assessment and get help. This is a limb-threatening situation. If the patient is experiencing symptoms of deep vein thrombosis (DVT) such as pain, edema, and warmth of an extremity, stop the assessment and get help. Immediate intervention to start anticoagulants is necessary. A pulmonary embolism may result from a DVT. Be alert for any signs of a pulmonary embolism including acute dyspnea, chest pain, tachycardia, diaphoresis, and anxiety. This life-threatening emergency requires immediate intervention.

4. The health history includes key information for the development of health-promotion measures including the educational needs of the patient. Identifying cardiovascular risk factors and evaluating the patient's understanding of them provides a basis for the development of a plan to eliminate modifiable risk factors and to control as much as possible the severity of those that cannot be changed. This approach may prevent disease through early intervention or lessen progression and complications. The subjective portion of the assessment lends itself well to incorporating patient education into the discussion. The setting of a private one-on-one meeting with the patient focusing on risk factors and symptoms provides the ideal opportunity to initiate the patient education process, which is an integral component of nursing care. *Healthy People* goals are not specific for peripheral vascular disease, but instead focus on areas of risks for such disease, such as smoking, overweight, and lack of regular exercise.

5. Questions to ask relative to family history of peripheral vascular disease include the following:
   • Do you have a family history of cardiovascular problems?
      • Who had the illness?
      • Was the illness arterial, venous, or lymphatic?
      • How was it treated?
      • What was the outcome?
   • Do you have a family or personal history of diabetes?
      • Who had/has the illness?
      • How is it treated?
      • How well is it controlled?
      • Have there been any complications related to diabetes?

- Do you have a family or personal history of hypertension?
  - Who had/has the illness?
  - How is it treated?
  - How well is it controlled?
  - Have there been any complications related to hypertension?
- Do you or does anyone in your family have an elevated cholesterol level?
  - Who had/has the elevated cholesterol level?
  - How is it treated?
  - How well controlled is it?

6. The most modifiable risk factors are smoking, high-fat diet, and limited activity level. Cessation of smoking can significantly delay the progression of atherosclerosis. Nurses ask patients about their readiness to quit smoking. They offer various resources to assist patients with smoking cessation, including individual and group counseling, support groups, medical treatment, and nicotine-replacement therapy. Diet modification includes weight management and decreasing the consumption of foods high in saturated fats. Monitoring of cholesterol and triglyceride levels is important; these patients need a thorough understanding of the relationship that diet, activity, and genetic factors have to cholesterol levels and the development of atherosclerosis. Nurses also discuss with patients the preventative role of exercising four to five times a week as recommended by the American Heart Association.

7. To achieve desired outcomes, evidence-based interventions are applied. Examples include monitoring peripheral pulses every 4 hours, assessing and documenting degree of edema using scale every 4 hours, evaluating pain on a 10-point scale, providing patient education on risk factors, keeping limbs warm and having the patient wear skid-free slippers, and performing meticulous foot care once a day.

Activity D

1. A
2. D
3. C
4. C
5. A
6. C
7. C

CHAPTER 21: BREASTS AND AXILLAE ASSESSMENT

Activity A: Fill in the Blank

1. A. sternal; mid-axillary; axilla; B. four quadrants; horizontal; vertical; C. Montgomery's glands; D. Cooper's ligaments; fibrous bands.

2. A. lateral axillary (brachial) nodes; B. central axillary (midaxillary); C. posterior axillary (subscapular); D. anterior axillary (pectoral).

Activity B

1. A = Y; B = Y; C = N; D = Y; E = Y; F = N; G = N

Activity C

1. The most common breast concerns that cause women to seek medical evaluation are a newly discovered lump, pain, and nipple discharge. In any of these situations, it is important for the health care provider to perform a focused health history and examination. The greatest fear a woman has related to these symptoms is that she has breast cancer, although often the cause is benign. Specific questions to ask depend on presenting symptoms.

2. Before beginning, the nurse provides as much privacy as possible and answers any questions that patients may have. This is an opportune time to ask female patients if they perform monthly SBE. If not, instructing patients in it and watching return demonstrations can provide an opportunity to verify technique and provide helpful correction as indicated. The breast examination involves inspection and palpation. It is important to expose both breasts fully initially during inspection to assess for symmetry, but then to cover or drape one breast while palpating the other.

3. The breasts often symbolize the development of sexuality and reproductive capacity. The adolescent girl often will compare her growth to that of others. Early-maturing girls may experience more dissatisfaction with their physical appearance, because most of their peers have the slim body shape that cultural norms perpetuate. Late-maturing girls may worry that they will be "flat." Timing of breast development in girls has a social stigma; girls who mature either too early or too late may be concerned.

4. As women age, glandular, alveolar, and lobular tissues in the breasts decrease. After menopause, fat deposits replace glandular tissue that continues to atrophy as a result of decreased ovarian hormone, estrogen, and progesterone secretion. The inframammary ridge thickens, making this area easier to palpate. The suspensory ligaments relax, causing breasts to sag and droop. Breasts also decrease in size and lose elasticity. Nipples become smaller, flatter, and less erectile. Axillary hair may stop growing at this time. These changes are more apparent in the eighth and ninth decades of life.

5. Mammography consists of two x-rays (digital or conventional film). If a palpable mass has been detected or if the woman has nipple discharge, magnification and additional views are necessary. A woman between 30 to 40 years may benefit from a mammogram if a mass is suspected, depending on breast density. Ultrasound is used with women younger than 40 years, who tend

to have denser breast tissue, those with silicone breast implants, pregnant women, and as a guide when performing a core needle biopsy (CNB). This non-invasive test produces a picture through high-frequency sound waves of the internal breast structures to help practitioners differentiate between a solid and cystic mass. Fine-needle aspiration (FNA) and CNB are biopsies in which a needle is inserted into the abnormal site to collect a sample of cells for analysis to determine if cancer exists. An excisional biopsy is similar to a lumpectomy, in which the lump or suspicious area and a portion of the surrounding tissue are removed and examined. Magnetic resonance imaging (MRI) is a supplemental tool to mammography. This non-invasive, painless test uses a magnetic field (not x-ray), radio waves, and a computer to detect and stage breast cancer and other breast abnormalities.

6. During midpuberty, one or both male breasts commonly and temporarily enlarge as a result of changing hormone levels, a condition referred to as *gynecomastia*. Pubescent males also may develop breast buds or tenderness, which also is usually temporary. The breasts may also enlarge in adolescent males from adipose tissue related to obesity. It is important to investigate feelings related to body image and sexual identity in adolescent males with enlarged breasts. Gynecomastia is physically benign but can cause emotional distress. Reassurance that this is temporary and normal may help alleviate the distress.

7. Nurses are aware of variations in breast development related to ethnicity. For example, African-American females mature earlier than Caucasians. Variations in the color of the skin and nipple relate to ethnic background. Differences exist in the incidence and outcomes of breast cancer. Hispanic, Asian, and American Indian women have a lower risk for developing breast cancer. African-American women experience a lower incidence but higher mortality rate from breast cancer than Caucasian women do. African-American women 35 to 44 years have a breast cancer death rate more than twice that of Caucasian women in the same age group. This may be from breast cancer being diagnosed at a more advanced stage in the African-American population, possibly from them having less access to breast health care. Breast cancer is the leading cause of death among Filipino women.

Activity D
1. C
2. D
3. C
4. A
5. B
6. D
7. D

CHAPTER 22: ABDOMINAL ASSESSMENT

Activity A
1. A. xiphoid process; superior margin; B. liver, pancreas, gall bladder; C. waste products; 48 hours; D. bowel activity; E. dentition; chew

Activity B
1.

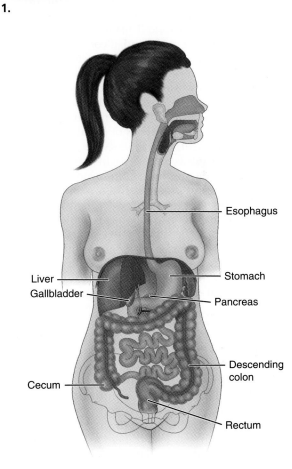

Activity C
1. 1 = C; 2 = E; 3 = B; 4 = F; 5 = D; 6 = G; 7 = A
2. 1 = B; 2 = C; 3 = D; 4 = A; 5 = F; 6 = E
3. 1 = C; 2 = A; 3 = B.

Activity D
1. The abdomen is a large cavity extending from the xiphoid process of the sternum down to the superior margin of the pubic bone. It is bordered in the back by the vertebral column and paravertebral muscles, and at the sides and front by the lower rib cage and abdominal muscles. Four layers of large, flat muscles form the ventral abdominal wall and are joined at the midline by a tendinous seam, the linea alba.

2. Genitourinary organs within the abdominal cavity include the kidneys, ureters, and bladder; the spermatic cord in males; and the uterus and ovaries in females. Disease processes in these organs can produce abdominal symptoms. The kidneys control blood pressure through the production of renin, stimulate red blood cell production by secreting erythropoietin, and remove waste products filtered by the kidneys from the body. The ureters and bladder aid with removal of waste products in the form of urine. The spermatic cord protects the vas deferens, blood vessels, lymphatics, and nerves that run from scrotum to penis. The ovaries produce ova and secrete estrogen and progesterone. The uterus allows fertilization of the ova with sperm and, if conception occurs, provides an environment for fetal development.

3. The digestive process consists of mechanical and chemical digestion. *Mechanical digestion* means the breakdown of food through chewing, peristalsis, and churning. *Chemical digestion* means the breakdown of food through a series of metabolic reactions with hydrochloric acid, enzymes, and hormones. The digestive process begins in the mouth where food is ingested and mastication (chewing) begins. During this process saliva mixes with the food and a bolus of food forms. The bolus passes into the oropharynx and esophagus, which propels the bolus via slow peristaltic movements into the stomach. In the stomach the bolus is churned into a liquid, mixed with digestive juices and hydrochloric acid produced there. The liquid form is called *chyme*.

4. The abdominal muscles relax, allowing the uterus to protrude into the abdominal cavity to accommodate the growing fetus. The medially located rectis abdominis muscles become separated. As the fetus grows and takes up more room in the abdominal cavity, the stomach rises and may impinge on the diaphragm. Uterine compression of the bowels results in diminished bowel sounds and decreased bowel activity, which partly contributes to constipation. Venous pressure in the lower abdomen increases, which may lead to hemorrhoids and further problems with elimination. During pregnancy the appendix is displaced upward and laterally to the right, which can complicate the diagnosis of appendicitis in pregnant women. A darkly pigmented line, the linea nigra, appears in the midline of the anterior abdomen from pubis to umbilicus in many pregnant women. Near the end of pregnancy, the umbilicus may become everted and striae (stretch marks) may develop on the skin of the abdomen.

5. In older adults, production of saliva and stomach acid is reduced, and gastric motility and peristalsis slow. All these changes can lead to problems with swallowing, absorption, and digestion. Elderly people also have changes in dentition. Chewing difficulties, accompanied by limited financial resources, can dramatically alter dietary choices and may result in painful mastication. All these factors along with generally reduced muscle mass and tone may contribute to constipation.

6. Food-borne illnesses affect the very young, elderly, and immunocompromised patients most seriously. Risk of food-borne illness has increased from emerging pathogenic organisms, improper food storage or preparation, an increasing global supply of foods, and inadequate training of food handlers. The *Healthy People* goal for this risk factor is to reduce infections by food-borne pathogens. Education about food handling in retail areas and at home, food labeling, and proper food preparation are the methods identified to achieve these goals.

7. Hepatitis A and B immunizations are recommended for all infants; people whose work may expose them to blood, body fluids, or unsanitary conditions (ie, health care, food services, sex workers); and those traveling to parts of the world where these illnesses are prevalent.

Activity E

1. B
2. C
3. C
4. D
5. A
6. B
7. C

CHAPTER 23: MUSCULOSKELETAL ASSESSMENT

Activity A

1. A. compact bone; cancellous bone; B. glenohumeral; glenoid fossa; C. tibiotalar joint; D. subluxation; partial dislocation.
2. A. structural; functional; B. symmetry; C. scoliometer; D. palpation; abnormal protrusions.

Activity B

1. A. Consume the daily recommended amount of calcium and vitamin D. Limit caffeine, which increases excretion of calcium.
   B. Perform at least 30 minutes of weight-bearing exercise three times per week.
   C. Avoid smoking and excess alcohol consumption.
   D. Discuss your risk for osteoporosis with your health care provider.
   E. Have a bone density test and take medication when appropriate.

Activity C

1. 1 = D, 2 = C, 3 = A, 4 = B
2. 1 = E, 2 = D, 3 = F, 4 = B, 5 = A, 6 = C

Activity D

1. Scoliosis is the lateral curvature of the spine, usually affecting both the thoracic and lumbar parts, with a deviation in one direction in the thoracic and in the other direction in the lumbar spine. Scoliosis

may be structural, caused by a defect in the spine, or functional, caused by habits (eg, consistently carrying a heavy backpack on one shoulder).

To screen for scoliosis, inspect the patient's back. While the patient stands, look for symmetry of the hips, scapulae, shoulders, and any skin folds or creases. The patient then needs to bend forward with the arms hanging toward the floor. Look for any lateral curves or protrusions on one side. Then, the patient should slowly stand up while inspection of the spine continues. A scoliometer may be used to obtain a measurement of the number of degrees that the spine is deviated. A deviation in the thoracic area usually has a corresponding deviation on the other side in the lumbar area. During palpation of the spine, feel for any abnormal protrusions or deformities.

2. Knowledge of previous surgeries provides additional information, allows the nurse to anticipate findings during the physical assessment, and enables the nurse to alter assessment procedures as needed to protect the patient.

3. Assess both extremities at the same time to evaluate for symmetry. Bilateral assessment for muscle tone and strength is necessary for comparison. Note the size and shape of extremities and muscles, as well as alignment and any deformity or asymmetry.

4. Joints are palpated for contour and size; muscles are palpated for tone. Feel for any bumps, nodules, or deformity. Ask if there is any tenderness during touch.

5. Stand in front of the patient and palpate both shoulders, noting any muscular spasm, atrophy, swelling, heat, or tenderness. Start at the clavicle and methodically explore the acromioclavicular joint, scapula, greater tubercle of the humerus, area of the subacromial bursa, biceps groove, and anterior aspect of the glenohumeral joint.

6. Painful joints in the fingers are common in *osteoarthritis*. A firm mass over the dorsum of the wrist may be a *ganglion*. *Rheumatoid arthritis* may cause edema, redness, and tenderness of the finger and wrist joints.

7. While standing, assess the iliac crest, size and symmetry of the buttocks, and number of gluteal folds. Assist the patient to the supine position with legs straight. Look for any swelling, lacerations, lesions, deformity, size of the muscle, and symmetry. Look at the hips from the anterior and posterior views. While the patient is supine, palpate the hip joints, iliac crests, and muscle tone. Feel for any bumps, nodules, and deformity. Ask if there is any tenderness with touch. Feel for crepitus when moving the joint.

Activity E
1. A
2. C
3. B
4. D
5. B
6. A
7. C
8. D

CHAPTER 24: NEUROLOGICAL ASSESSMENT

Activity A
1. A. muscles and skin; deliberate motor actions; B. interconnecting neurons; C. outside of the brain; directed toward the center of the brain; D. synapses
2. A. precentral gyrus; B. postcentral gyrus; C. cerebral cortex; D. frontal lobe; E. parietal lobe; F. occipital lobe; G. temporal lobe

Activity B
1. 1 = C, 2 = E. 3 = A, 4 = B, 5 = D
2. 1 = C, 2 = D, 3 = A, 4 = B, 5 = F, 6 = E
3. 1 = E, 2 = F, 3 = D, 4 = A, 5 = B, 6 = C

Activity C
1. Because of the crossing of the fibers in the medulla, right-sided sensations are perceived on the left side of the brain, and left-sided sensations are perceived on the right side of the brain. Additionally, specialized ascending tracts for pain and temperature (spinothalamic) and coordination of movement (spinocerebellar) enter the dorsal ganglia, synapse with another neuron, and cross the spinal column here (instead of in the medulla as with the dorsal columns). The information is carried to the sensory cortex on the opposite site of the brain. Thus, all sensory information is perceived on one side of the brain for the opposite side of the body.

2. Although the dermatomes provide a general idea of the innervation by each nerve, some overlap exists; C1 to C3 controls movement in and above the neck; C4 to C6 is at the level of the shoulder and diaphragm for breathing independently; C7 to C8 is at the level of the fingers and hand grasp to perform self care and transfers with arms; T1 to T6 provides trunk stability for balance when sitting; T6 to T12 is for the thoracic muscles and upper back for respiratory and transfer strength; L1 to L2 is at the level of legs and pelvis; L3 to L4 is hamstrings and ankles.

3. Reflexes are involuntary responses to stimuli. They maintain balance and tone, such as the sucking reflex of a baby when the cheek is stroked. Reflexes also provide quick responses in potentially harmful situations, such as withdrawing of the foot when stepping on a sharp object. The simplest type of reflex arc involves a receptor-sensing organ, afferent sensory neuron, efferent motor neuron, and effector motor organ.

4. The abbreviated acute assessment includes rapid assessment of level of consciousness (LOC) using the Glasgow Coma Scale (GCS); if the patient can respond verbally, basic orientation; basic speech/language assessment; pupillary reaction; gross assessment of extremity strength; and gross assessment of sensation. If consciousness is impaired,

assessing selected cranial nerves may help differentiate neurological from metabolic causes. Also, vital signs are part of this acute assessment, because they may be either a cause or result of the acute change. As soon as is practical, obtaining health history information helps identify potential sources of the problem.

5. A *head injury* is suspected if there is a witnessed loss of consciousness of longer than 5 minutes; history of amnesia of longer than 5 minutes; abnormal drowsiness; more than three episodes of vomiting; suspicion of non-accidental injury; or seizure in a patient with no history of epilepsy.

6. Risk factors for stroke are similar to those for cardiovascular disease; thus, prevention also involves modification of unhealthy lifestyle choices. Patients should control blood pressure through weight reduction, healthy diet, and use of antihypertensive medications as prescribed. At every visit, nurses should ask patients about smoking and, for those with a positive response, about the desire for cessation. Nurses should provide all patients with information about a diet low in saturated fat and high in fruits and vegetables. They should ask overweight and obese patients about their willingness to reduce calories. Additionally, nurses should advise all patients to exercise aerobically 3 to 7 times a week for 20 to 60 minutes per session.

7. The history of the present illness or problem should elucidate a detailed account of each symptom, its nature (location, quality, and severity), date of onset, precipitating factors, and duration (constant, intermittent, or worse at any particular time of day). Nurses also should note what, if anything, makes the symptom worse or better, and what has been the general pattern of progression (rapid, static, progressively worse, remitting, exacerbating).

During assessment of the neurological system, nurses should inquire about common symptoms in all patients to screen for the early presence of disease. If a patient is concerned about specific neurological problems, nurses assess these focused areas with follow-up questions. A thorough history of symptoms assists with identifying the current problem or diagnosis. Nurses should direct questioning toward a history of problems with headaches, weakness or paralysis, loss of sensation, and involuntary movements or sensations.

Activity D

1. C
2. A
3. B
4. C
5. D
6. B
7. C
8. D

CHAPTER 25: MALE GENITALIA AND RECTAL ASSESSMENT

Activity A

1. A. bulbourethral glands; B. anorectal junction; saw-tooth-like; C. rectal columns; internal hemorrhoidal plexus; D. somatic sensory nerves

Activity B

1. 1 = C; 2 = E; 3 = A; 4 = B; 5 = D; 6 = G; 7 = F
2. 1 = E; 2 = D; 3 = F; 4 = C; 5 = B; 6 = A

Activity C

1.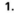

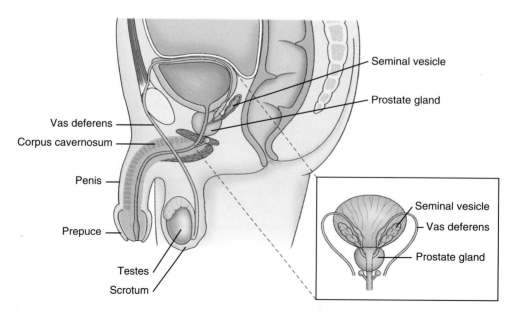

Activity D

1. Testicular growth begins and the scrotal skin thins and becomes pendulous. The testes become active and begin to secrete testosterone, which promotes bone maturation and epiphyseal closure. Genital hair begins to appear at the base of the penis. As physical development continues, genital hair darkens and extends over the entire pubic area; it is at this time that the prostate gland enlarges. When maturation is complete, genital hair is curly, dense, and coarse, with a diamond-shape from umbilicus to anus. Growth and development of the scrotum and testes are complete and the length and width of the penis is increased.

2. Older men may experience distention of the rectum from degeneration of afferent neurons in the rectal wall, which interferes with relaxation of the internal sphincter. The distention can cause an elevated pressure threshold for the feeling of rectal distention, causing retention of stool. At the same time the autonomically controlled internal sphincter loses tone, the external sphincter cannot, by itself, control the bowels; this may result in incontinence. Pubic hair becomes finer, grey, and less plentiful. Pubic alopecia may also occur. Testosterone levels decline with aging, which may affect both libido and sexual function. Erection becomes more dependent on tactile stimulation and less responsive to erotic cues. The penis may decrease in size and testes drop lower in the scrotum. The fibromuscular structures of the prostate gland atrophy. Ironically benign hyperplasia of the glandular tissue often obscures the atrophy of aging.

3. Six conditions can result in an *acute scrotum*: ischemia, trauma, infectious conditions, inflammatory conditions, hernia, and acute situations accompanying a chronic condition (eg, testicular tumor with rupture). Although differential diagnosis is broad, an accurate physical assessment and history can often accurately define the condition. Imaging studies can correlate with the clinical assessment and expedite therapeutic decisions.
Signs and symptoms of the acutely ill genitourinary patient can range from subtle to obvious. An example of subtle signs is a patient complaining of fatigue or shortness of breath upon exertion. More obvious behaviors are a patient who complains of sudden and severe testicle pain (eg, possible testicle torsion). Patients presenting with an acute problem are anxious and tense; staying calm will help the patient relax and promote clear thinking.

4. Surgery is used to treat enlarged prostate, testicular cancer, hydrocele, variocele, and undescended testicle. Some men choose permanent sterilization through vasectomy. Rectal or anal conditions requiring surgery include hemorrhoids, anorectal fissures, and carcinoma of the rectum and anus.

5. Nurses may hesitate to initiate conversation about sexual history. Nevertheless, this information is important to help identify high-risk sexual practices, establish patient norms, and provide education. Sexual dysfunction can present as anxiety, anger, or depression. In addition, physical problems can lead to sexual problems. The nurse must be careful not to impose personal standards on the patient.

6. Steps for testicular self-examination (TSE) are as follows: 1. TSE is best performed after a warm shower or bath. Heat relaxes the scrotum, which makes the TSE easier; 2. Examine each testicle one at a time with both hands. Place the index and middle fingers under the testicle with the thumbs placed on top. Roll the testicle gently from side to side. You should not feel pain. Remember that one testicle may be larger; this finding is normal; 3. Cancerous lumps usually are on the sides of the testicle, but can show up on the front. Become familiar with the location of the epididymis; this soft, tubelike structure behind the testes collects and carries sperm. If you become familiar with this structure you won't mistake it for a lump; 4. Make an appointment with a physician, preferably a urologist, as soon as possible if you find a lump or any of the following warning signs: enlargement of the testes, pain or discomfort, heaviness in the scrotum, a dull ache in the groin, significant loss of size of one testicle, or a sudden collection of fluid in the scrotum.

Activity E

1. C
2. D
3. B
4. A
5. D
6. A
7. C

CHAPTER 26: FEMALE GENITALIA AND RECTAL ASSESSMENT

Activity A

1. A. mons pubis; B. clitoris; C. vaginal introitus; D. frenulum
2. A. vesicovaginal septum; urethra; bladder. B. peritoneum; myometrium; endometrium. C. isthmus; ampulla; fimbriae.

Activity B

1. 1 = E; 2 = D; 3 = A; 4 = C; 5 = B
2. 1 = C; 2 = F; 3 = A; 4 = B; 5 = D; 6 = E

Activity C

1.

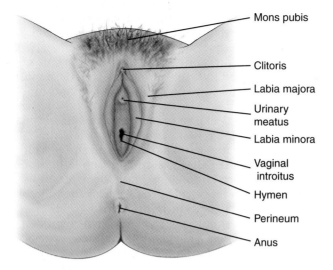

- Mons pubis
- Clitoris
- Labia majora
- Urinary meatus
- Labia minora
- Vaginal introitus
- Hymen
- Perineum
- Anus

Activity D

1. The vagina is a tube of muscular tissue that extends from vaginal introitus to uterus. The three-layer vaginal muscle wall is extremely expandable especially during childbirth. It is lined by glandular mucous membrane, within which are folds called ruggae. These ruggae become less prominent in advanced years. The vagina is approximately parallel to the lower portion of the sacrum. This position is the reason the anterior wall of the vagina measures 7 cm while the posterior wall is about 9 cm. The vesicovaginal septum separates the anterior wall of the vagina from the urethra and bladder. The rectovaginal septum separates the posterior wall of the vagina from the rectum.

2. Age of onset of puberty in girls has continued to decline. The U.S. median age at menarche is 12.4 years. African-American girls may begin puberty before 8 years. Onset of menses correlates with estrogen release by the hypothalamic-pituitary-ovarian (HPO) axis. Budding of the breast occurs first, followed by development of pubic hair. Onset of menses follows breast budding by approximately 2 to 3 years. Tanner's stages of maturation are used in the assessment of preadolescent and adolescent females.

3. Menopause is defined as 12 consecutive months without menses. As estrogen levels decrease the uterus becomes smaller, the ovaries shrink, the normal vaginal ruggae flatten, and the epithelium atrophies. These normal changes may lead to problems such as vaginal infections, urinary tract infections, dyspareunia, and lowered libido. Older women are at increased risk for endometrial cancers and need education regarding abnormal signs and symptoms.

4. Nurses should educate the patient about problems that can arise from douching, such as vaginal infections, imbalance of normal vaginal flora (pH), and the possibility of transferring a vaginal infection into the uterus. The consequence can be pelvic inflammatory disease.

5. Dysuria (burning with urination) or frequent UTIs may be related to bladder trauma from intercourse. Educate the patient to empty her bladder before and after intercourse to reduce trauma and introduction of bacteria into the urethra.

6. Screening, treating, and counseling of and about chlamydia and gonorrhea are currently recommended for all sexually active adolescents. *Chlamydia trachomatis* is currently the most common and frequently reported bacterial sexually transmitted infection (STI) in the United States. Approximately 2.8 million cases are reported annually. Of those, occurrence is highest in patients 15 to 24 years. Because of the asymptomatic nature of this infection, risk for it is high. Long-term infection can cause pelvic inflammatory disease (PID) and subsequent potential infertility.

7. Osteoporosis is a bone disorder characterized by decreased bone mass, which leads to fragility and potential fracture especially in females. Bone mineral density (BMD) screening is a simple and cost efficient test recommended for all women 65 years or older. Those at risk for osteoporosis (Caucasian or Asian women with a family history of osteoporosis, thin frame, tobacco use, glucocorticoid use, or any fracture after age 45 years) should be screened as well.

Activity D

1. D
2. C
3. B
4. A
5. C
6. D
7. A
8. C

CHAPTER 27: PREGNANT WOMEN

Activity A

1. A. sex (gender); B. placement; functional grade; C. covers; cesarean; D. "flutters"

2. conducting intake interviews, dating the pregnancy, taking a detailed history, obtaining consents for prenatal testing, arranging for referrals if needed, educating the patient about the practice, triage, gather preliminary data, conducting and interpreting non-stress tests, education.

Activity B
1. 1 = E; 2 = D; 3 = A; 4 = C; 5 = B
2. 1 = C; 2 = D; 3 = A; 4 = B

Activity C
1. Pregnant women are advised to sleep on their sides during the third trimester. Unfortunately, many women find this position uncomfortable and feel like they wake up more tired than when they went to sleep. Help alleviate discomfort of by teaching about strategic placement of pillows. In addition to the pillow under her head, the woman can put a thick pillow between the legs, which places the upper leg parallel with the mattress and relieves strain on the abdominal muscles and ligaments. Wedging another pillow behind the woman's back allows her to lie at a 45-degree angle with her back supported, without impeding venous return. A pillow under the abdomen further supports the suspensory ligaments. When the nurse uses pillows to show the woman how this feels, most women can relax and are less anxious about getting a good night's sleep.
2. Ectopic pregnancy occurs when the fertilized egg never leaves the fallopian tube. Signs of this potentially life-threatening condition include lower abdominal pain on one side and spotting of blood. Confirmation of ectopic pregnancy is considered an obstetric emergency requiring hospitalization and termination of the pregnancy to save the mother's life.
3. The embryo travels from the fallopian tube and implants in the uterine lining, often with a resulting small bleed. Typically, the process from ovulation to implantation takes approximately 2 weeks, so implantation bleeding can occur at the same time the woman expects her period. From weeks 2 to 8 after conception, all major fetal organs form. Therefore, it is very important for women to avoid teratogens during this period (which can be difficult because many are not even aware that they are pregnant this early). At 10 weeks, the placenta weighs only on average 20 g, yet this may be sufficient for it to produce enough progesterone to maintain a pregnancy. By 12 weeks' gestation, the placenta has grown sufficiently to take over production of progesterone, and the corpus luteum is reabsorbed. Most women who have had morning sickness start feeling better once the placenta takes over progesterone production.
4. The fetus begins the second trimester 3 inches long and weighing less than 1 oz (0.8 g). By the end of the second trimester, the fetus is about 15 inches long and weighs more than 2 lbs (1,000 g). Major organs develop to the point that the fetus may survive (with help) outside the womb. At about 20 weeks, the woman's uterus reaches the umbilicus, and she begins to "show." She also clearly feels fetal movements ("quickening"). Unless a cesarean is required, it makes no difference where the placenta implants as long as it does not cover the cervical opening (os).
5. The fetus gains weight rapidly, but more slowly than in the second trimester. It begins the trimester weighing about 2 lbs, and at birth averages about 7½ lbs. Fetal organs grow and mature, muscles increase in size and strength, and a protective fat layer forms to assist with temperature control after birth. Skin thickens and forms a more protective barrier. During the last 4 weeks of pregnancy, the mother transfers IgG antibodies to the fetus to assist in the formation of the immune system. Integration of nervous and muscular functions proceeds rapidly. A key task of the third trimester is maturation of the fetal lungs. With normal amniotic fluid volume, functionality of the lungs depends on their ability to form surfactant.
6. Many providers perform a fetal survey by ultrasound at 20 weeks' gestation. By this time, the fetus is large and developed enough so that all major organs are visible, including the sex organs that indicate gender. In some cases, functionality of organs can also be assessed. If ultrasound identifies certain abnormalities, preparations can be made to improve fetal chances for survival at birth. The fetal survey also indicates placement, functional grade, and size of the placenta.
7. Naegele's Rule says to subtract 3 months from the first day of the LMP and add 7 days to the result to arrive at a due date for pregnancy.
8. Conditions in pregnancy that require immediate attention include ectopic pregnancy, pyelonephritis, hemorrhage, and regular and painful contractions before 37 weeks.

Activity D
1. A
2. B
3. D
4. C
5. A
6. B

CHAPTER 28: NEWBORNS AND INFANTS

Activity A
1. A. first year; accelerated; B. cephalocaudally; central to distal; gross to fine; C. listening; watching; interacting; D. Denver Developmental II.
2.
   - Is the newborn term gestation (37 weeks or greater)?
   - Is the amniotic fluid clear?
   - Is the newborn breathing or crying?
   - Does the newborn have good muscle tone?

Activity B
1. 1 = C; 2 = E; 3 = A; 4 = B; 5 = D
2. 1 = E; 2 = D; 3 = A; 4 = B; 5 = C
3. 1 = D; 2 = E; 3 = A; 4 = C; 5 = B

Activity C

1. It is important to determine whether these areas are progressing steadily. Milestones serve as guidelines so that developmental delays can be identified early and appropriate interventions instituted.
2. Normal weight range for a full-term newborn is 5 lb 8 oz to 8 lb 13 oz (2,500 to 4,000 g). Average length is 19 to 21 inches (48 to 53 cm). Most infants gain approximately 1 to 2 lbs per month, double their birth rate by 6 months, and triple their birth rate by 1 year. By the end of the 12th month, most infants have increased their length by approximately 50%.
3. Respiratory distress in the newborn and infant often progresses rapidly to severe distress requiring bag and mask or mechanical ventilation. Nurses must intervene early at the first sign of distress to avert an emergency resuscitation, if possible.
4. Infants should have regular examinations with a pediatrician or another health care professional with specialized pediatric training, such as a Pediatric Advanced Practice Registered Nurse. Ideally, parents schedule an initial visit before the baby is born. At this visit, the primary care provider obtains the family and prenatal history, gives anticipatory guidance, inquires about the chosen feeding method, and encourages breastfeeding.
5. Safe sleep habits for infants help prevent SIDS. Infants should always be placed on their backs to sleep. The mattress should be firm. Pillows, soft toys, excessive blankets, and bedding should not be in the crib when the infant is asleep. The infant should not sleep in the same bed with a sleeping adult. It is too easy for the tiny face to be covered inadvertently and for the infant to be smothered.
6. Parents should be informed that it is important for their infant to receive vaccines at the ages and times recommended to ensure the highest level of protection against vaccine-preventable diseases. If the infant misses an immunization or gets behind schedule, there is a catch-up schedule available on the AAP Web site. Because immunizations are normally administered in conjunction with routine checkups, determine if the parents are keeping regularly scheduled appointments. Next, check the immunization record. The initial record is typically provided to the parents before the newborn is discharged home when the first immunization is given. If the record is not up-to-date, ask if the parents are familiar with the immunization schedule. Provide a schedule, if needed, and help the parents determine where they can go to have the infant immunized.

Activity D

1. C
2. A
3. C
4. A
5. A
6. D
7. B
8. B

CHAPTER 29: CHILDREN AND ADOLESCENTS

Activity A

1. A. predictable times; B. 2 years: C. articulation.
2. A. respiratory; heart; B. tertiary care center. C. nasal flaring; retractions.

Activity B

1. 1 = D; 2 = C; 3 = A; 4 = B
2. 1 = C; 2 = E; 3 = A; 4 = B; 5 = D

Activity C

1. Transfer to a tertiary care center is indicated for children in respiratory distress; once they cannot compensate for oxygen requirements, they may soon require mechanical ventilation.
2. Legal consent for health care treatment is 18 years of age. Most states, however, permit contraception and treatment for sexually transmitted infections (STIs) at 13 years.
3. Premature and small-for-gestational-age babies may have long-term sequelae if their transition to extrauterine life was difficult.
4. Questions to ask are as follows: Is the child infected with HIV? Is the child in close contact with people known or suspected to have TB? Is the child in close contact with people known to be alcohol dependent or intravenous drug users or to reside in a long-term care facility, correctional or mental institution, nursing home/facility, or other long-term residential facility? Is the child foreign-born and from a country with high TB prevalence? Is the child from a medically underserved low-income population, including a high-risk racial or ethnic minority population (eg, African American, Hispanic, Native American)? Is the child/adolescent alcoholic dependent, an intravenous drug user, or a resident of a long-term-care facility, correctional or mental institution, nursing home/facility, or other long-term residential facility?
5. Adolescents are more likely than adults to have multiple sexual partners and short-term relationships, to engage in unprotected intercourse, and to have partners at high risk for STIs.
6. For children who have not received the full roster of recommended vaccines, the nurse should encourage catch-up doses. He or she should document administration and dates of the vaccines and provide this information to caregivers/parents for their own records in addition to maintaining the health record at the place of regular health care.
7. The infant seat should be in the back facing backward for the first year minimally. Depending upon the car seat, it may be in the back seat facing backward until the child is 30 to 35 lbs. A child may be turned facing forward after 1 year of age if in the correct car seat. At 4 years of age or 40 lbs, the child

may graduate from a car seat to booster seat. He or she should be seated and restrained with a seat belt in such a seat, which is designed for use until children are at least 4'9".

Activity D

1. B
2. A
3. B
4. D
5. D
6. C
7. B
8. C

CHAPTER 30: OLDER ADULTS

Activity A

1. A. 30 days; 20 days; B. mitotic activity; C. sweat; capillary fragility; D. photoaging
2. A. dry eyes; B. lens; opaque; C. accommodating; glare. D. lipid; iris.

Activity B

1. 1 = C; 2 = D; 3 = B; 4 = A
2. 1 = N; 2 = Y; 3 = Y; 4 = Y; 5 = N

Activity C

1. The size and function of the kidney decrease with age. Nephrons in the cortex are fewer, while abnormal glomeruli increase. The body responds to the sclerotic changes in the glomeruli by increasing the size of the remaining healthy glomeruli.
2. Older adults often lose height. Gradual compression of the spinal column is related to narrowing of intervertebral discs. Beginning at around 30 years, bone absorption starts to exceed bone formation. In women, this bone loss accelerates in the decade immediately following menopause. Decreased lean body mass also occurs with aging. There is a loss of type II muscle (fast-twitch) fibers as compared with type I muscle (slow-twitch, fatigue-resistant) fibers, which leads to muscle wasting. Regeneration of muscle tissues slows with age, but studies show that exercise can increase lean muscle mass even in frail older adults.
3. With aging, the number of neurons and glial cells gradually decline, and these cells show structural changes. Nevertheless, current studies do not support the notion of extensive brain atrophy in normal aging. Atrophy is common in people with degenerative neurological diseases. The overall number of neuronal synapses decreases, while lipofuscin granules in the nerve cells accumulate.

There is increased production and accumulation of oxyradicals in all body systems.

4. The pituitary gland decreases in size, weight, and vascularity. Secretion of growth hormone and circulating levels of insulin-like growth factor (IGF) decreases. Plasma levels of the adrenal steroids (DHEA and DHEA-S) show a significant decline with aging. Prevalence of glucose intolerance and type 2 diabetes increases.
5. Falls, especially if accompanied by fracture, are the most common reason for admission of older adults to emergency departments. Chronic conditions also may be exacerbated; for example, worsening of COPD or congestive heart failure can be an acute condition. Infection, chest pain, abdominal pain, and delirium should be assessed and treated rapidly. Because older adults may not mount an immune response, infection may be present even in the absence of fever.
6. Although some acute situations do not allow for finding a quiet space, an environment that is calm and quiet is essential for conducting an interview with an older person. It is essential to reduce or eliminate background noise as much as possible when carrying on conversations. This includes turning off the television or radio in the patient's room and closing the door to reduce sounds of telephones, beepers, alarms, or pagers. Cold or drafty environments are uncomfortable and can distract the older adult from tasks at hand. The older adult needs to be warm and comfortable during the interview.
7. When older adults are hospitalized or more seriously ill, the nurse should gather as much information as possible from previous records so that he or she can review and clarify findings with the older adult, rather than trying to gain all the information from the patient's memory. This helps the older person to conserve energy. If the older adult is acutely ill and fatigues easily, the nurse may need to return and complete the interview later.
8. In many cultures, an older person would never be called by his or her first name at a first meeting and especially would not be addressed as "Sam" or "Nancy" by a young stranger. The nurse should set a tone of respect for the older person at the beginning of the interview by introducing himself or herself and then calling the patient by his or her formal name. The nurse can then clarify how the patient would like to be addressed in the interview.

Activity D

1. D
2. B
3. A
4. B
5. C
6. B

CHAPTER 31: HEAD-TO-TOE ASSESSMENT OF THE ADULT

Activity A

1. A. cyanotic; pale; B. difficult (labored); C. strained; D. anxious; E. distress

Activity B

1. 1 = D; 2 = B; 3 = A; 4 = C

Activity C

1. 1 = D; 2 = A; 3 = C; 4 = B
2. 1 = Y; 2 = N; 3 = Y; 4 = N; 5 = Y

Activity D

1. Screening and resulting teaching are primary prevention services that nurses offer as part of their professional responsibilities.
2. The nurse assesses past health history to provide context for how the current problem might be related. He or she assesses findings considering the information previously reviewed in the chart. For example, the nurse might say, "I'm going to ask you some questions about your health history. I noticed that your chart says that you have an allergy to Zofran. Tell me about that." This is a way of verifying information and obtaining further details.
3. The most important focus areas for health-related patient teaching involve adequate nutrition, increasing physical activity, maintaining weight, and reducing stress. Avoidance of behaviors that contribute to disease (eg, smoking, overuse of alcohol) is important as well. Another focal point for teaching is prevention of disease through immunizations including childhood immunizations and pneumococcal and influenza vaccines. Prevention of accidental injury involves interventions such as recommending bicycle helmets, avoiding drinking and driving, and using seatbelts. Primary prevention of disease and promotion of health are priorities for increased quality and quantity of life. An additional specialized focus area is promotion of health during pregnancy and breastfeeding. Maintaining health during pregnancy is vital for both mother and baby. Teaching regarding importance of prenatal appointments and screenings and promotion of breastfeeding are key topics.
4. The nurse focuses questions on issues and symptoms specific to the patient. In this way, the patient is viewed as a person who has multiple things that are affected by the health status. These questions are related to the primary problems and concerns for the patient.
5. It is important to be honest when there are difficulties, such as, "Your blood pressure is a little high. We can talk more about that after we're finished." Instead of giving false reassurances, the nurse instead provides objective data. Nevertheless, the nurse avoids sharing conclusions before collecting all data, because the initial problem list may change during the interaction. The nurse evaluates the response of the individual and family to actual or potential health problems and also performs assessments related to the direct care role.
6. Because acuity of the hospitalized patient is often increased, the nurse prioritizes which data to collect related to the presenting problems and performs a basic screening of other body systems. He or she uses clinical judgment about which items to include and to omit. Techniques are adapted based on the individual patient situation. The admitting assessment is usually documented in a separate area of the patient chart, and may include input from other health care professionals.
7. Because of the complications of immobility and being in a hospital environment, the nurse performs a short screening assessment at the beginning each shift. He or she does so for all patients. This assessment typically takes 5 to 10 minutes to provide a basis for comparison in the event of a sudden change in condition. This screening enables the nurse to identify patient acuity; need for immediate treatment, teaching, or discharge planning; and care priorities. The nurse completes and documents this assessment on an assessment form.

Activity D

1. B
2. D
3. B
4. A
5. C
6. D
7. A
8. D

Laboratory Manual for

Nursing Health Assessment: A Best Practice Approach

SHARON JENSEN, MN, RN
Instructor
School of Nursing
Seattle University
Seattle, Washington

Wolters Kluwer | Lippincott Williams & Wilkins
Health
Philadelphia • Baltimore • New York • London
Buenos Aires • Hong Kong • Sydney • Tokyo

Executive Editor: Elizabeth Nieginski
Product Director: Renee A. Gagliardi
Design Coordinator: Joan Wendt
Illustration Coordinator: Brett Macnaughton
Manufacturing Coordinator: Karin Duffield
Prepress Vendor: SPi Technologies

Printed in China

ISBN-13: 978-0-7817-8060-5
ISBN-10: 0-7817-8060-8

Care has been taken to confirm the accuracy of the information presented and to describe generally accepted practices. However, the author, editors, and publisher are not responsible for errors or omissions or for any consequences from application of the information in this book and make no warranty, expressed or implied, with respect to the currency, completeness, or accuracy of the contents of the publication. Application of this information in a particular situation remains the professional responsibility of the practitioner; the clinical treatments described and recommended may not be considered absolute and universal recommendations.

The author, editors, and publisher have exerted every effort to ensure that drug selection and dosage set forth in this text are in accordance with the current recommendations and practice at the time of publication. However, in view of ongoing research, changes in government regulations, and the constant flow of information relating to drug therapy and drug reactions, the reader is urged to check the package insert for each drug for any change in indications and dosage and for added warnings and precautions. This is particularly important when the recommended agent is a new or infrequently employed drug.

Some drugs and medical devices presented in this publication have Food and Drug Administration (FDA) clearance for limited use in restricted research settings. It is the responsibility of the health care provider to ascertain the FDA status of each drug or device planned for use in his or her clinical practice.

LWW.com

9 8 7 6 5 4 3 2 1